ANATOMICAL BASIS OF CARDIAC INTERVENTIONS, VOLUME 1

Kalyanam Shivkumar, MD, PhD, Series Editor

Atlas of
CARDIAC ANATOMY

Shumpei Mori, MD, PhD

Kalyanam Shivkumar, MD, PhD

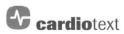

Cardiotext Publishing, LLC
750 2nd St. NE, Suite 102
Hopkins, Minnesota 55343
USA

https://www.cardiotextpublishing.com

Any updates to this book may be found at: https://cardiotextpublishing.com/electrophysiology-heart-rhythm-mgmt
/atlas-of-cardiac-anatomy

Comments, inquiries, and requests for bulk sales can be directed to the publisher at: info@cardiotextpublishing.com.

Library of Congress Control Number: 2022935373

ISBN: 978-1-942909-57-6

eISBN: 978-1-942909-58-3

Printed in the United States of America

5 6 7   28 27 26 25 24

DEDICATION

*Dr. Mori dedicates this work to his parents, Toshihiko and Ruriko Mori,
his wife, Hwaryung, and their children, Toshitada and Toshiteru.*

*Dr. Shivkumar dedicates this work to the memory of his parents,
Ramanathan Kalyanam Iyer (1932–1992) and Saraswathi Venkataraman (1934–2020),
his wife, Preethi, and their son, Tejas.*

ONLINE ACCESS

The first edition of this title is available gratis in a digital edition under Creative Commons license **Attribution-NonCommercial-NoDerivatives 4.0 International**.

Please visit cardiotextpublishing.com/electrophysiology-heart-rhythm-mgmt/atlas-of-cardiac-anatomy for access and license information.

TABLE OF CONTENTS

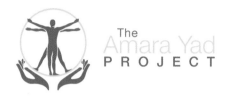

Amara Yad (The Immortal Hand) is a physician-led initiative with a single goal: To honor the victims of medical exploitation through corrective action. As its first act, Amara Yad will publish a new generation of open-access digital anatomic atlases of the highest quality. These digital atlases will be made available gratis to all users to support the life-saving mission of the profession, made possible with the generous backing of the Amara Yad Project initiated by the UCLA Cardiac Arrhythmia Center in 2022.

THE HISTORY

Between 1938 and the end of World War II, University of Vienna anatomist Eduard Pernkopf published a series of anatomical atlases. He used the bodies of over 1,300 murdered victims of Nazi terror as subjects for his work.

The Nazi history of the Pernkopf atlas series was concealed in the 1950s. Swastikas and SS insignia proudly displayed in the illustrators' signatures of those atlases were erased (partially) from prints in subsequent editions of the atlas. For decades, physicians used Pernkopf's atlases without the knowledge that bodies depicted in those works belonged to the victims of Nazi atrocities. The atlases were regarded as preeminent anatomical resources, a clinical necessity, and remained in use even after their depraved origins had been exposed. Importantly, no effort was made to surpass this work and provide a definitive resource for the world.

TODAY

Anatomic atlases are an indispensable resource for medical professionals. At UCLA, the production of clear and accurate atlases that support the lifesaving mission of the profession is made possible by the University's Willed Body Donor Program, U.S. federal research support for science, financial gifts from donors, and volunteer efforts of students and faculty.

We dedicate this inaugural volume of the Amara Yad Project to the noble humans who have so generously willed their bodies for science and education. We also specifically honor the victims of medical exploitation in Pernkopf's atlases. We shift the focus away from the images of their bodies and toward their enduring human dignity.

www.uclahealth.org/heart/arrhythmia/amara-yad

ACKNOWLEDGMENTS

At the outset, we would like to thank the family of Dr. Wallace A. McAlpine—his daughters Ms. Laurel Flowers, Ms. Kim Renteria Clark, and Ms. Leigh McAlpine Whitten, and his son Mr. Fraser McAlpine—for helping us locate Dr. McAlpine's works. In 2013, Dr. Bruce Lytle at the Cleveland Clinic helped locate the physical collection and subsequently the collection was officially transferred to UCLA for the multi-year digitization project. We gratefully acknowledge the Cleveland Clinic Foundation for this gesture. We would also like to acknowledge the Leonetti O'Connell Foundation and Dr. Craig Gordon and family for their unrestricted gifts that made this expensive project a reality.

This project also made it obvious to us that it is a true privilege to be part of a team at UCLA, with inspiring colleagues. Our electrophysiology mentor, Professor Noel G. Boyle, deserves special mention for encouraging us to pursue this project in the first place. We thank all the faculty, staff, and trainees at the UCLA Cardiac Arrhythmia Center, UCLA Cardiac Interventional Programs, and the UCLA Departments of Surgery and Radiology for our useful interactions. The interactions and feedback from our exceptional trainees over the years at UCLA are much appreciated.

We would like to express our deep gratitude to the selfless individuals who have donated their bodies and tissues for the advancement of education and research. Special thanks to One Legacy Foundation and the NIH SPARC Program, which formed the basis for obtaining donor hearts for research and for funding this effort. Special thanks to the Surgical Sciences Laboratory at UCLA (Professor Warwick J. Peacock and Dr. Grace Chang). We are grateful to Professor Michael C. Fishbein at Department of Pathology and Laboratory Medicine at UCLA for his valuable guidance, and all the staff members of the UCLA Donated Body Program, Translational Research Imaging Center (Department of Radiology) at UCLA, and Translational Pathology Core Laboratory at UCLA. We thank Ms. Michelle Betwarda at the UCLA Cardiac Arrhythmia Center for her administrative acumen and tenacity, which ensured the acquisition and digitization of the McAlpine Collection. We thank Mr. Michael Papalucas, who expertly digitized the original slides made by Dr. McAlpine, as well as Ms. Delilah Cohn, who enhanced a subset of those digital images. We are grateful to Dr. Hatsue Ishibashi-Ueda at the Department of Diagnostic Pathology at Hokusetsu General Hospital, Professor Taka-aki Matsuyama at the Department of Legal Medicine at Showa University School of Medicine, and Ms. Diane E. Spicer at the Heart Institute at Johns Hopkins All Children's Hospital and at the Department of Pediatric Cardiology at Heart Center at University of Florida for their guidance on pressure perfusion–fixation. We appreciate the patience, dedication, and expertise provided by Cardiotext Publishing and the team led by Mr. Mike Crouchet for the output that is "bespoke" for this volume. Special thanks to Professors Francis E. Marchlinski and William G. Stevenson for their encouragement and for graciously writing the Foreword for this book.

Shumpei Mori, MD, PhD
Kalyanam Shivkumar, MD, PhD

ABOUT THE AUTHORS

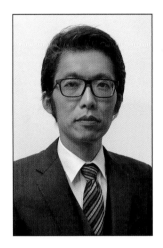

Shumpei Mori, MD, PhD

Associate Professor
Director, Specialized Program for Anatomy & Imaging
UCLA Cardiac Arrhythmia Center
Los Angeles, California

Dr. Mori is a physician scientist who is serving as the Director of the Specialized Program for Anatomy & Imaging at UCLA Cardiac Arrythmia Center. His field of specialization is cardiac anatomy and advanced clinical imaging. He has a long track record of publications and has published several books. He currently serves as an editor of *Clinical Anatomy* and Section Editor at the *Journal of the American College of Cardiology: Clinical Electrophysiology.*

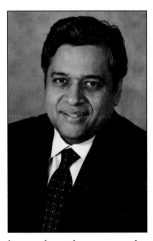

Kalyanam Shivkumar, MD, PhD

Professor of Medicine (Cardiology), Radiology & Bioengineering
Director, UCLA Cardiac Arrhythmia Center & EP Programs
Director & Chief, UCLA Cardiovascular & Interventional Programs
Los Angeles, California

Dr. Shivkumar is a physician scientist serving as the inaugural director of the UCLA Cardiac Arrhythmia Center & EP Programs (since its establishment in 2002) and as the Director and Chief of UCLA's Cardiovascular and Interventional Programs. He leads a team that provides state-of-the-art clinical care and has developed several innovative therapies for the non-pharmacological management of cardiac arrhythmias and other cardiac diseases. He has a long track record of research publications and books. He has been elected as a member of the American Society of Clinical Investigation (ASCI), the Association of American Physicians (AAP), the Association of University Cardiologists (AUC), and is as an honorary fellow of the Royal College of Physicians, London (FRCP). He currently serves as the Editor-in-Chief of the *Journal of the American College of Cardiology: Clinical Electrophysiology.*

FOREWORD

An understanding of cardiac anatomy is fundamental to the practice of cardiology. Detailed and nuanced knowledge is required for effective diagnosis, interpretation of cardiac imaging, and treatment with interventional and surgical approaches. Since Andreas Versalius referred to the heart as the "center of life" in his 1543 atlas of anatomy, *De humani corporis fabrica libri septem*, anatomy was taught from drawings, descriptions, and dissection. Photographs and elegantly detailed drawings were important parts of the medical curriculum.

In 1975, Wallace McAlpine published a major contribution to the field, *Heart and Coronary Arteries: An Anatomic Atlas for Clinical Diagnosis, Radiological Investigation, and Surgical Treatment*, with beautifully detailed photographic images of cardiac anatomy made possible by "perfusion–fixation" of the heart, adapting a technique that he had observed applied to lung specimens. He developed a systematic approach to photographic examination of the explanted heart that included reference to anatomic position as well as views to clarify individual aspects of anatomy. We owe a debt of gratitude to Dr. Shivkumar and his colleagues for "rediscovering" these images more than three decades later and making the collection available through the UCLA Cardiac Arrhythmia Center. Inspired by Dr. McAlpine's opus, Drs. Shivkumar and Mori have now gone further to provide new images obtained by applying Dr. McAlpine's technique to extend and display detailed investigation of anatomic regions that have assumed even greater importance as cardiac imaging, intervention, and surgery have advanced.

The electrophysiology community, for example, focused on detailed electrical recordings and came to appreciate the importance of anatomic relationships through their efforts to define the locations and mechanisms of complex arrhythmias during catheter manipulation. This experience was coupled with efforts to explore the optimum location for pacing and defibrillator lead placement to restore electrical synchrony, improve cardiac function, and effectively terminate arrhythmias. No anatomic aspect of the heart has gone unexplored with electrode catheters, although admittedly, this exploration was frequently attempted with a limited understanding of the details of cardiac anatomy, morphology, and relationships. An awareness of surrounding anatomic structures came from manifestations of collateral injury observed after thermal energy ablation and was frequently not adequately anticipated based on an awareness of anatomic proximity. The need for an improved understanding of cardiac anatomy, morphology, and relationships became obvious in our field to optimize the success and minimize the risks of our interventional procedures. Similarly, interventional treatment of valvular heart disease, advances in surgical therapies, advances in complex imaging, and neurocardiology have brought to the fore the need for detailed knowledge of the heart's anatomy.

The presentation of the cardiac anatomy in this new atlas uses a crucial attitudinal approach that includes the fluoroscopically familiar right anterior oblique and left anterior oblique views and sequentially peels back anatomic structures with progression of the figures to allow the reader to create visual images of anatomic structures that are merely reflected by silhouettes on fluoroscopy. It is like having the lights turned on in a dark, yet familiar room. Structures and important anatomic relationships, only imagined based on catheter manipulation under fluoroscopy, are displayed and appropriately labeled. All chambers are beautifully shown. Further facilitating this understanding are the images of strategically placed electrode catheters that aid in the understanding of obstacles to effective catheter placement, stability, and contact required for a successful procedure. The authors also take the additional important step of identifying the anatomically typical relationship of the precordial ECG leads. This effort is critical to provide an understanding of how basic ECG P wave and QRS analysis can aid in the localization of arrhythmias within the heart's complex anatomic structures.

A few areas of special interest and emphasis in this atlas are also worth highlighting. Millions of people have benefited from coronary artery interventions to improve blood flow, but the coronary arteries and veins are also becoming important conduits for other interventional therapies. Effective implementation of optimal cardiac pacing and catheter-based ablation are facilitated by understanding of the anatomy of the coronary vasculature, which is beautifully delineated, along with the obstacles and challenges to its complete access. Options for management of the embolism risk by left atrial appendage occlusion techniques continue to evolve, based on recognition of the anatomic considerations and variability. This structure is highlighted in detail. For years, the pericardial space was largely the purview of cardiac surgeons. Percutaneous access to the pericardial space is now an important means of accessing parts of the heart for ablation and strategies using this access for other interventions are emerging. The detailed assessment of the pericardial space is another welcome addition.

Approaches to valvular heart disease are rapidly progressing and are also based on understanding of the anatomy and its relation to pathophysiology. Interventional cardiologists and surgeons will find a wealth of enlightening pictures clarifying the anatomy of the valves and their supporting apparatus, knowledge that forms the cornerstone of the evolving approaches to catheter-based interventional treatment. Finally, the cardiac nervous system is well recognized as playing a role in tachy- and bradyarrhythmias, electrical storms, and neurocardiogenic syncope. Approaches have emerged to therapeutically target the cardiac nervous system and a detailed delineation of the complexity on cardiac innervation is appreciated.

This atlas should be studied in detail and its images "burned into the brain" of everyone who performs interventional procedures, from trainees to the most experienced operators. The images should be referred to frequently and will create a valuable roadmap that must be followed. The appeal of the images will, of course, extend beyond the proceduralist to include all those with a serious interest in cardiac anatomy who want to take this clear and concise educational journey.

We congratulate Drs. Shivkumar and Mori on the wonderful achievement that is this atlas. It will help us better understand the anatomy crucial to diagnosing and treating our patients as well as advance cardiovascular science. We are excited that the first volume in the **Anatomical Basis of Cardiac Interventions** series, which details the anatomy of the normal adult heart, will be followed by future volumes that extend this important exploration.

Francis E. Marchlinski, MD
Richard T. and Angela Clark President's Distinguished Professor
University of Pennsylvania

William G. Stevenson, MD
Professor of Medicine
Vanderbilt University

PREFACE

This volume serves as a core foundation of anatomy that can stand alone or be studied in conjunction with future volumes in this series, the **Anatomical Basis of Cardiac Interventions**. Specific areas such as interventional electrophysiology, structural heart disease, interventional imaging, cardiac surgery, and cardiac neuroanatomy will be presented in greater detail.

Our sentiment about the field of anatomy is best summarized by the words of the anatomists McMinn and Hutchings who stated that "beauty of form is not limited to the exterior."* Every moment spent on this project has been joyful for us as learners who are mesmerized by the beauty of the heart. Among fundamental biological sciences, anatomy is perhaps "timeless" because it is not going to change. Our intention is that the first volume will not only serve as a foundational resource for new entrants to the field, but also for experienced operators who could obtain new insights. We hope that the reader will concur with the wise words of our beloved UCLA Coach John Wooden who said, "It's what you learn after you know it all that counts!"

Shumpei Mori, MD, PhD
Kalyanam Shivkumar, MD, PhD
University of California, Los Angeles
March 2022

*R.M.H. McMinn & R.T. Hutchings: *A Color Atlas of Human Anatomy*, Chicago: Year Book Medical Publishers ©1988.

A GUIDE FOR READERS

The inspiration for *Atlas of Cardiac Anatomy*, the first volume in the **Anatomical Basis of Cardiac Interventions** series, can be traced to the iconic anatomical atlas created by Dr. Wallace A. McAlpine in his 1975 book, *Heart and Coronary Arteries: An Anatomical Atlas for Clinical Diagnosis, Radiological Investigation, and Surgical Treatment.*

Atlas of Cardiac Anatomy includes many previously unpublished images from more than 2,900 remarkable images of the heart from the Wallace A. McAlpine Collection at UCLA Cardiac Arrhythmia Center.

Dr. McAlpine used a pressure perfusion–fixation method to maintain the physiological morphology of the hearts. He photographed them at a dedicated photo studio that he established in the basement of his home.

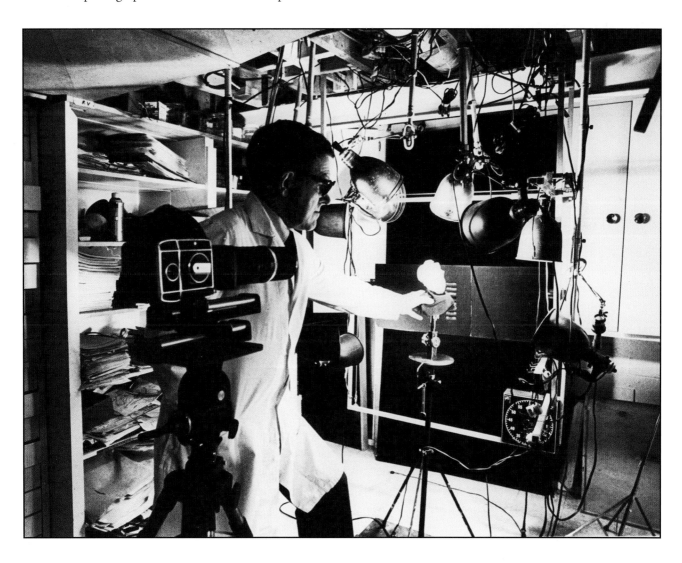

The hearts were placed on a special tripod with a rotational mount that allowed him to record serial photographs of the hearts viewed at slightly different angles and also show the progressive dissection viewed from the same direction.

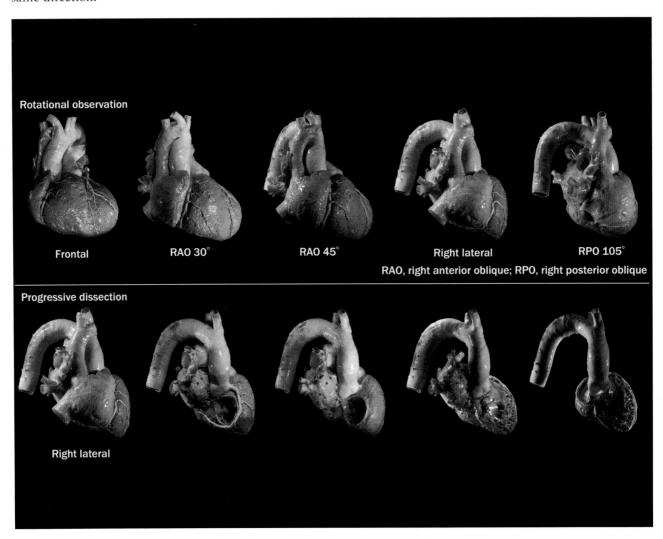

Rotational observation

Frontal   RAO 30°   RAO 45°   Right lateral   RPO 105°

RAO, right anterior oblique; RPO, right posterior oblique

Progressive dissection

Right lateral

In 2020, to honor his timeless contribution and inspired by his artistic masterpieces, UCLA Cardiac Arrhythmia Center replicated an anatomical laboratory, including a set-up for pressure perfusion–fixation of the hearts. In addition to the restored images from the original Wallace A. McAlpine Collection, the current series of atlases includes new photographs. Approximately 50 years after his iconic work, these new photographs are based on the technique pioneered by Dr. McAlpine to complement the cardiac anatomy approach.

An appreciation of cardiac anatomy using an attitudinal approach, a central theme of Dr. McAlpine's work, is the cornerstone of all the books in this series. Images of the heart are viewed from the anterior, right anterior oblique, and left anterior oblique directions. They show the relationship with the heart and precordial electrocardiographic leads. The structural anatomy of the heart is described sequentially following the direction of blood flow, starting from the sinus venarum and eventually ending at the aortic valve. We then focus on coronary arteries, coronary veins, pericardial space, and cardiac innervation thereby setting the foundation for the subsequent volumes in this series. Images and captions are prepared not only from the standpoint of cardiologists focused on cardiac anatomy and imaging but also from the viewpoint of cardiologists from various interventional fields, including clinical cardiac electrophysiologists, who especially need to have extensive foundational knowledge, as their work involves mapping almost all regions of the human heart (endocardial and epicardial).

The Orientation of the Heart Within the Chest

We would like to specify the location of the heart in the thorax as a prelude for this book and provide an orientation for the directions featured in the first 3 sections. In contrast to the rest of the images in this atlas, these images are reconstructed from a cardiac computed tomography dataset, showing the real-life anatomy of the living, blood-filled heart without losing its structural relationship with surrounding structures, including the thoracic cage, lungs, and esophagus.

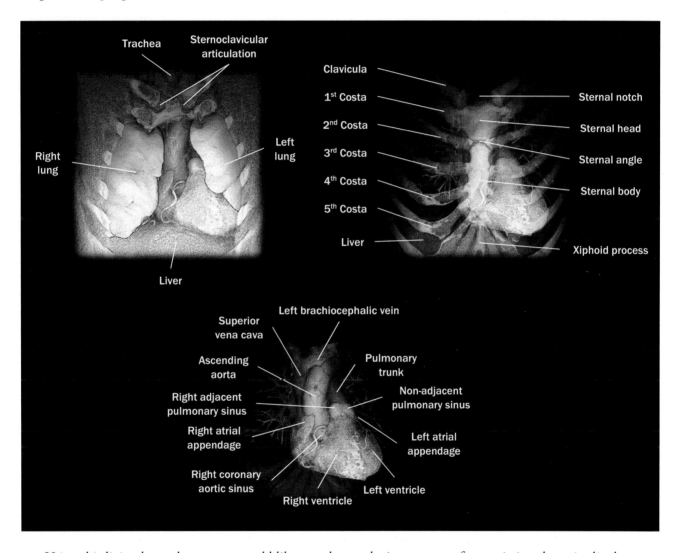

Using this living heart dataset, we would like to enhance the importance of appreciating the attitudinal aspects of the heart viewed from representative directions.

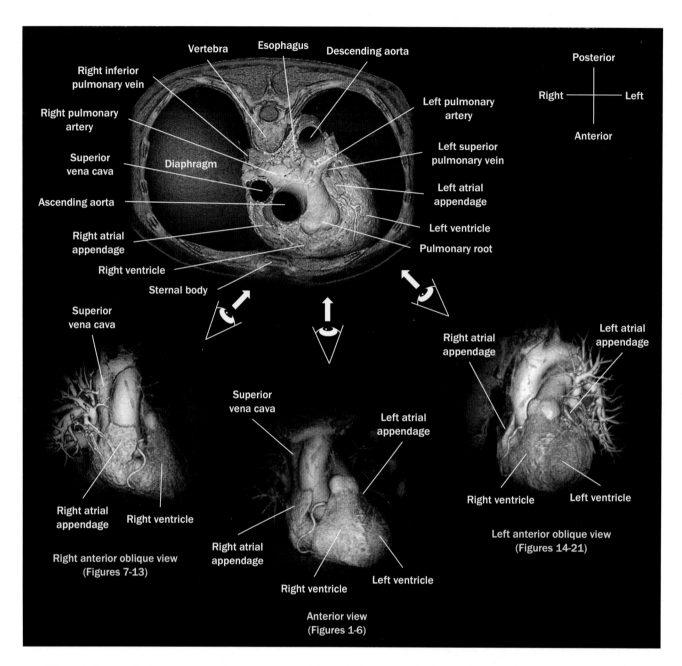

Thus, it is equally important to have anatomical knowledge not only focused on cardiac structure, but also the adjacent cardiac/noncardiac structures. In this regard, it is remarkable that Dr. McAlpine, in his original work, had imaged a heart with surrounding structures as demonstrated in this book.

Anaglyphs (Stereoscopic Images)

A component of *Atlas of Cardiac Anatomy* is a set of 25 anaglyphs (stereoscopic images) that correspond with specific photographs marked with the icon in the caption.

Anaglyphs provide a 3D effect when viewed with 3D glasses (a red lens and a cyan lens). This publication does not include 3D glasses, but a variety of 3D glasses are available at various online retailers.

The reader can view anaglyphs at https://cardiotextpublishing.com/atlas-of-cardiac-anatomy-anaglyphs.

We hope this book is useful not only for cardiac electrophysiologists and interventional practitioners, but also for anyone taking care of patients with cardiac disease.

1

Anterior View of the Heart

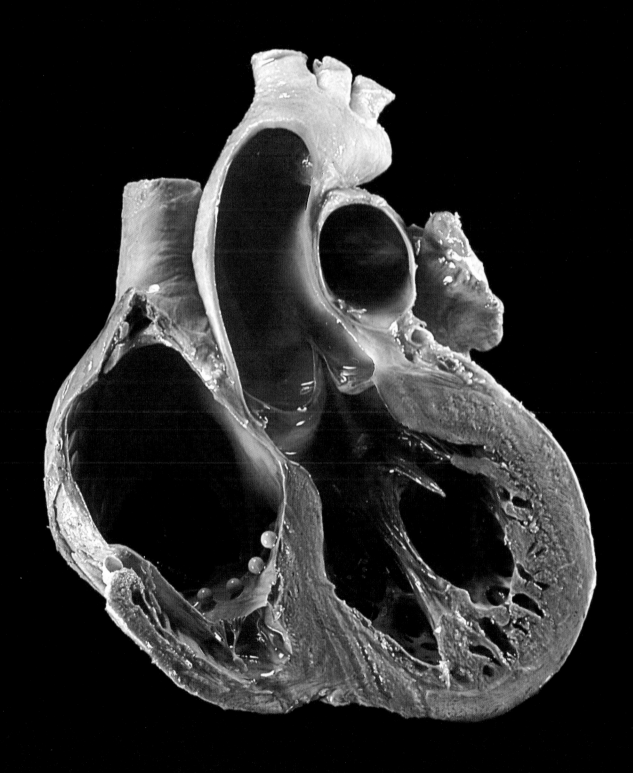

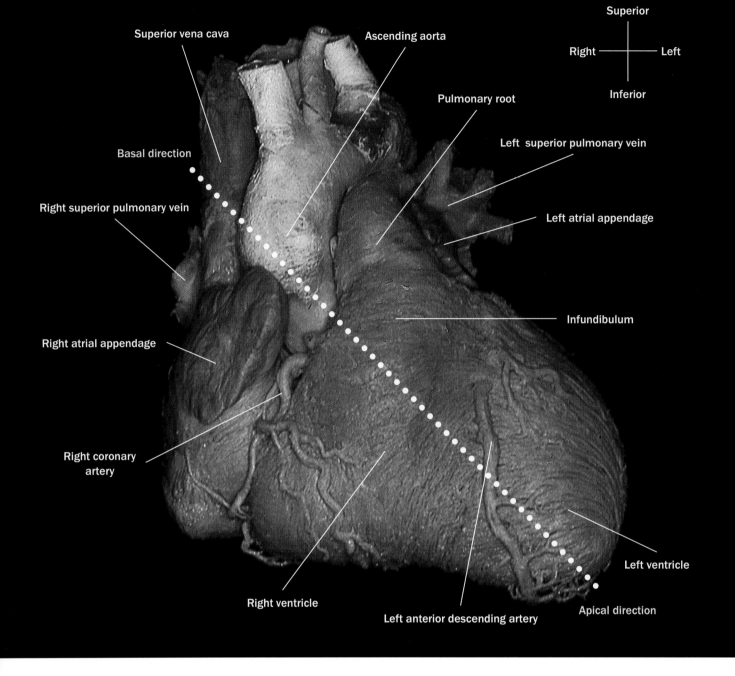

Superior

Right ——|—— Left

Inferior

Figure 1 Appropriate directional terminology to describe three-dimensional cardiac anatomy.[1]

The left and right images show the heart viewed from the anterior and superior directions, respectively. The direction indicators show the appropriate standard terminology to describe the direction related to the heart. According to the general rule to describe the human body, anterior, posterior, superior, inferior, right, and left are used to indicate the direction toward ventral, dorsal, cranial, caudal, right, and left, respectively. The cardiac axis, the line connecting the aortic root and cardiac

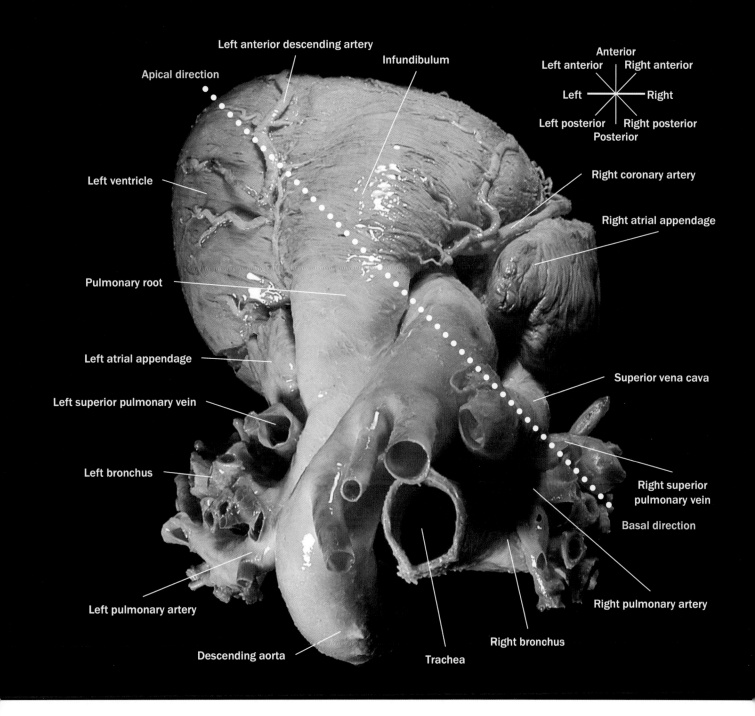

Apical direction

Left anterior descending artery

Infundibulum

Anterior
Left anterior   Right anterior

Left ————————— Right

Left posterior   Right posterior
Posterior

Left ventricle

Right coronary artery

Right atrial appendage

Pulmonary root

Left atrial appendage

Superior vena cava

Left superior pulmonary vein

Left bronchus

Right superior
pulmonary vein

Basal direction

Left pulmonary artery

Right pulmonary artery

Descending aorta

Trachea

Right bronchus

apex (white dotted lines), directs toward left antero-inferior direction.[2] This left antero-inferior direction is also described as the apical direction, with opposite direction being described as the basal direction. The atrial and ventricular septa are aligned along this cardiac axis. Thus, the right anterior and left posterior directions are also described as lateral, relative to the septal or medial structures close to the atrial and ventricular septa.

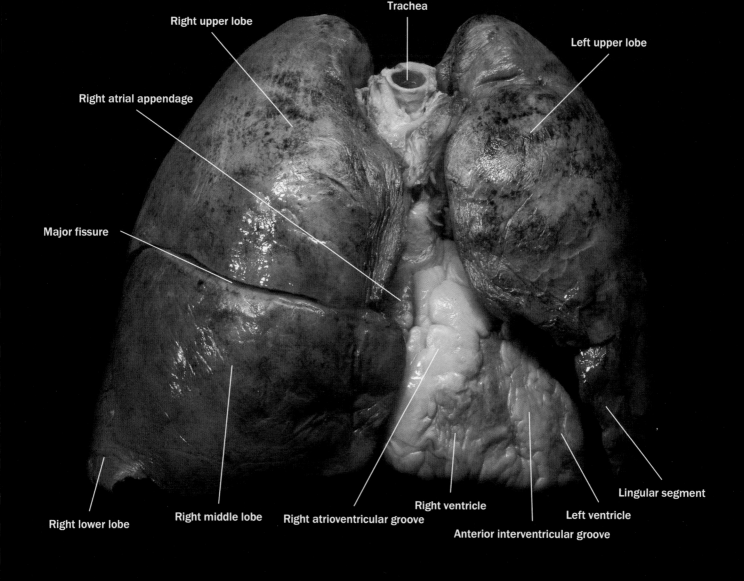

Trachea

Right upper lobe

Left upper lobe

Right atrial appendage

Major fissure

Lingular segment

Right ventricle

Left ventricle

Right lower lobe Right middle lobe Right atrioventricular groove

Anterior interventricular groove

Figure 2 En-bloc resection of the thoracic organs viewed from the anterior direction.[1]

The heart is located in the center of the thorax, covered bilaterally by the lung lobes except the anterior wall of the right ventricle and mid-apical anterior wall of the left ventricle. The anterior part of the pericardium and pleura are removed. The right atrioventricular groove extends between the right middle lobe and left upper lobe. Thus, the right atrioventricular groove and basal anterior wall of the right ventricle are located just posterior to the sternum. The apical anterior left ventricle is adjacent to the lingular segment of the left lung. The cardiac apex points to the left antero-inferior direction. This regional anatomy makes it feasible to observe the heart from the left parasternal and apical echocardiographic windows.[3]

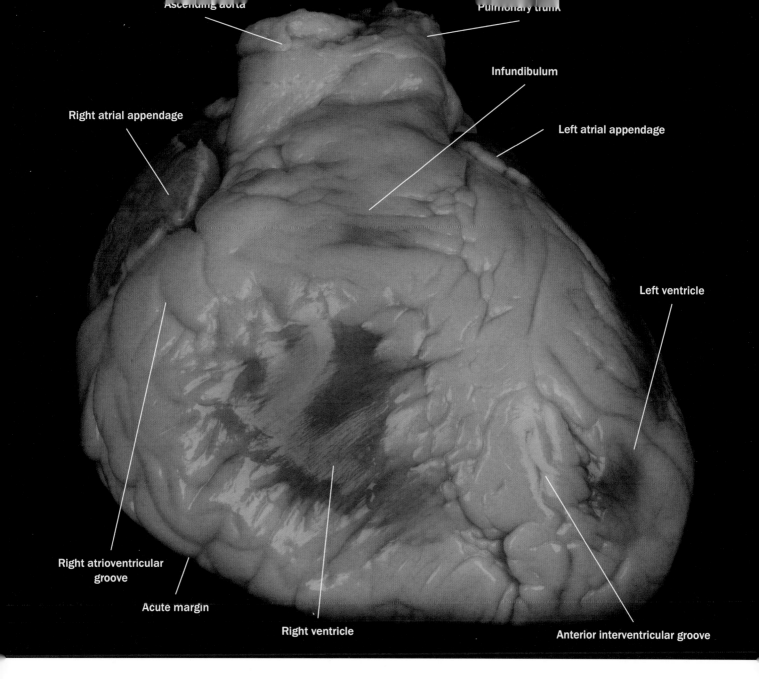

Ascending aorta

Pulmonary trunk

Infundibulum

Right atrial appendage

Left atrial appendage

Left ventricle

Right atrioventricular
groove

Acute margin

Right ventricle

Anterior interventricular groove

Figure 3 Anterior view of the heart with epicardial adipose tissue.

The apex of the right atrial appendage is located adjacent to the ascending aorta. The apex of the left atrial appendage is adjacent to the pulmonary root. Rich epicardial adipose tissue is distributed along the coronary vessels, including the right atrioventricular groove, anterior interventricular groove, and acute margin. Localized regions in the right ventricular anterior free wall, left ventricular apical anterior wall, and left ventricular supero-lateral free wall at the mid-ventricular level also lack the epicardial adipose tissue.

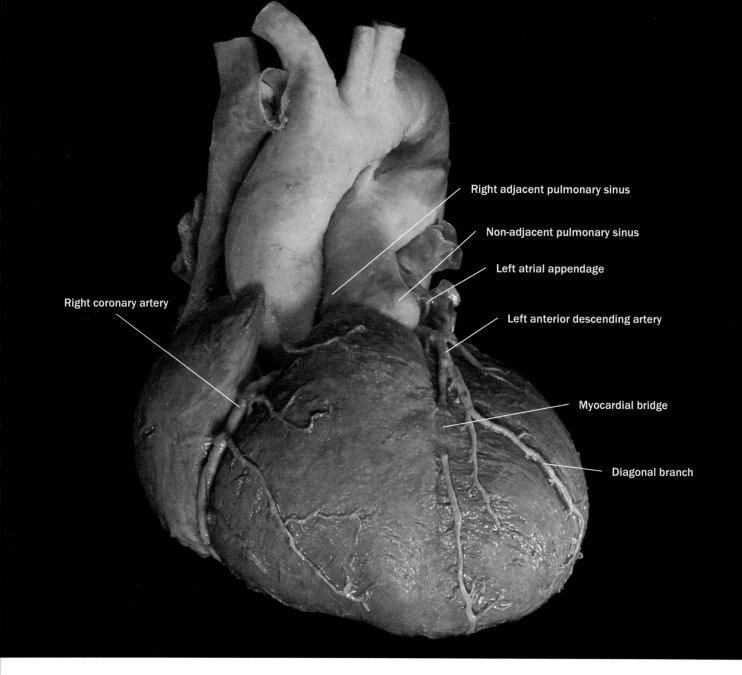

Right adjacent pulmonary sinus

Non-adjacent pulmonary sinus

Left atrial appendage

Left anterior descending artery

Right coronary artery

Myocardial bridge

Diagonal branch

Figure 4 The heart viewed from the anterior direction.[1]

The directional indicator shows the appropriate standard terminology to describe the direction related to the heart. The right ventricle is located most anterior, and the left atrium is located most posterior. Both chambers are midline structures located between the sternum and vertebral column, rather than being described as right- and left-side structures. The anterior view is the best *en face* view of the posterior wall of the left atrium. This view can separate both the left and right pulmonary veins. The bottom of the left atrium is located superior to that of the right atrium. The right border of the cardiac contour is composed of the superior vena cava and the right atrial appendage. The left border of the cardiac contour is composed of the aortic arch, left pulmonary artery overriding the left main bronchus, left atrial appendage, and left ventricle.[4] The apices of the right and left atrial appendages are adjacent to the ascending aorta and pulmonary root, respectively. The aortic root is wedged centrally between the right and left atrioventricular junctions.[5] The aortic root is located posterior to the right ventricular outflow tract, also referred to as the infundibulum, and right postero-inferior to the pulmonary root.[6] The left pulmonary artery is located superior relative to the right pulmonary artery, as it needs to override

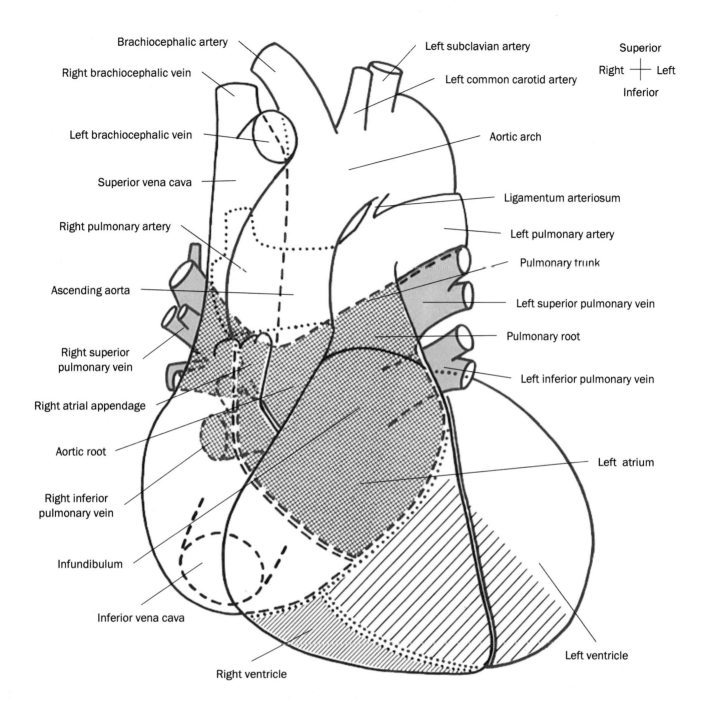

Brachiocephalic artery

Right brachiocephalic vein

Left brachiocephalic vein

Superior vena cava

Right pulmonary artery

Ascending aorta

Right superior pulmonary vein

Right atrial appendage

Aortic root

Right inferior pulmonary vein

Infundibulum

Inferior vena cava

Right ventricle

Left subclavian artery

Left common carotid artery

Superior

Right ─┼─ Left

Inferior

Aortic arch

Ligamentum arteriosum

Left pulmonary artery

Pulmonary trunk

Left superior pulmonary vein

Pulmonary root

Left inferior pulmonary vein

Left atrium

Left ventricle

the left main bronchus.[7] The pulmonary bifurcation and right pulmonary artery lie superior to the left atrial roof. The right pulmonary artery passes inferior to the aortic arch toward the right direction. The proximal part of the left coronary artery is located postero-inferior to the pulmonary root and trunk. The mid- to distal part of the left anterior descending artery literally descends anterior, after emerging at the left border of pulmonary root after skirting the left and non-adjacent pulmonary sinuses.[8] The orifice of the right coronary artery is posterior to the right ventricular outflow tract. The proximal right coronary artery is directed toward the right anterior direction to run along the right atrioventricular groove. In case of deep aortic wedging, the proximal right coronary artery directs toward right antero-superior direction, showing the shepherd's crook appearance.[5] In such case, the left atrial roof and fossa ovalis are located superior relative to the aortic root.[5]

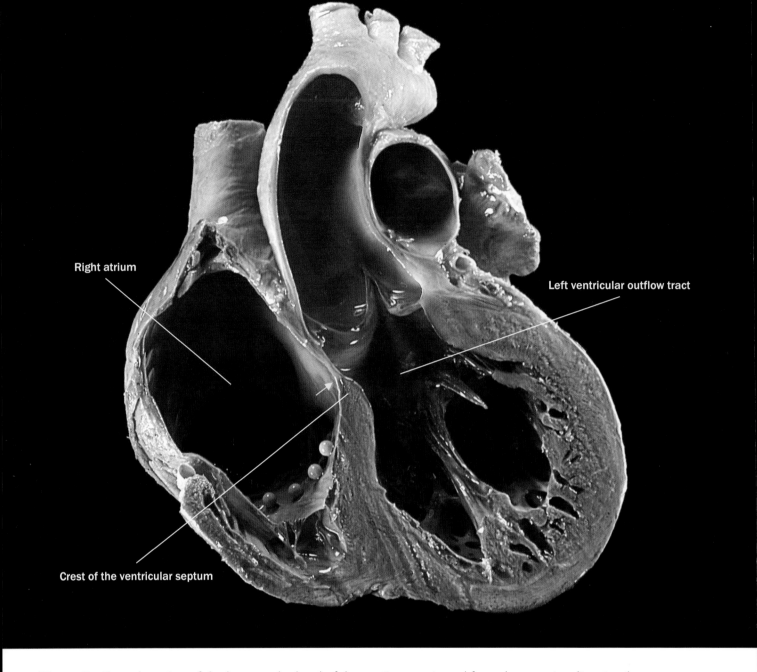

Right atrium

Left ventricular outflow tract

Crest of the ventricular septum

Figure 5 Frontal section of the heart at the level of the aortic root viewed from the anterior direction.[1]

The atrioventricular portion of the membranous septum is observed inferior to the right coronary aortic sinus. It separates the right atrium from the left ventricular outflow tract.[9] The crest of the ventricular septum inferior to the membranous septum is the general location of the atrioventricular conduction axis. Thus, the angle created between the membranous septum and the crest of the ventricular septum (yellow arrow) is where the His-bundle catheter is fixed.[10] The non-coronary aortic sinus is located most infero-posterior compared to other two coronary aortic sinuses.[11] The fossa ovalis is located to the right and posterior to the non-coronary aortic sinus. The primary septum at the floor of the fossa ovalis tilts toward the right antero-inferior direction. The left coronary aortic sinus is supported by the left ventricular free wall. This muscular support has less than half the thickness of the other part of the left ventricular free wall.[12] This region, when complicated with annular calcification, is vulnerable to free wall rupture during transcatheter aortic valve implantation.[13] The epicardial part of this basal superior left ventricular free wall related to the left coronary aortic sinus is

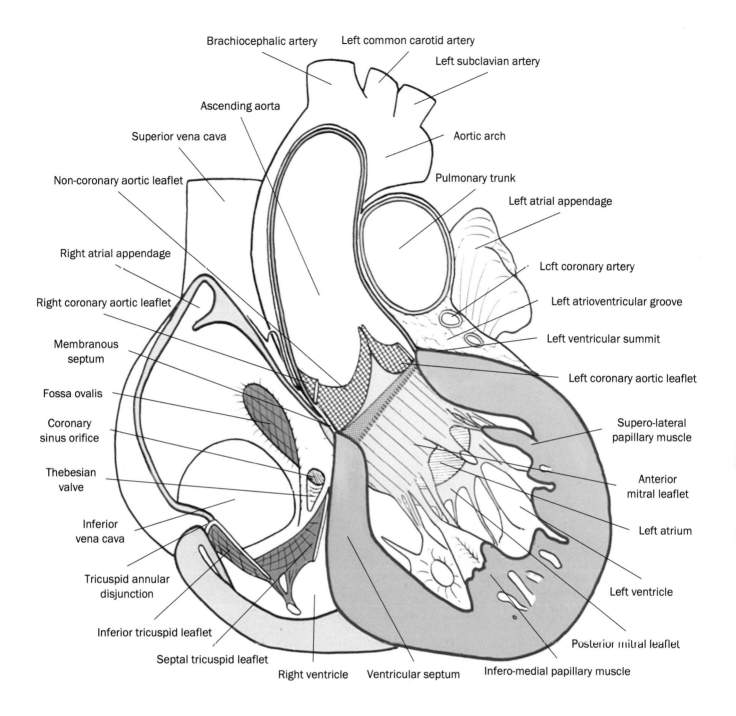

Brachiocephalic artery

Left common carotid artery

Left subclavian artery

Ascending aorta

Superior vena cava

Aortic arch

Pulmonary trunk

Non-coronary aortic leaflet

Left atrial appendage

Right atrial appendage

Left coronary artery

Left atrioventricular groove

Right coronary aortic leaflet

Left ventricular summit

Membranous septum

Left coronary aortic leaflet

Fossa ovalis

Supero-lateral papillary muscle

Coronary sinus orifice

Anterior mitral leaflet

Thebesian valve

Left atrium

Inferior vena cava

Left ventricle

Tricuspid annular disjunction

Inferior tricuspid leaflet

Posterior mitral leaflet

Septal tricuspid leaflet

Right ventricle   Ventricular septum   Infero-medial papillary muscle

referred to as the left ventricular summit.[1,14] The proximal left coronary artery and coronary venous tributaries are located superior to the left ventricular summit within the thick epicardial adipose tissue of the left atrioventricular groove. Thus, the proximal left coronary artery and coronary venous tributaries running this region are surrounded in the compartment created by the left coronary aortic sinus, left ventricular summit, pulmonary root and trunk, and left atrial appendage.[15] Based on this structural anatomy, radiofrequency catheter ablation of the left ventricular summit is feasible via the coronary venous system. Also, dilatation of the pulmonary root and pulmonary trunk can compress the proximal left coronary artery.[16] The anterior mitral leaflet is in continuity with the interleaflet triangle between the left and non-coronary aortic sinuses. Papillary muscles of the left ventricle are related to the left ventricular free wall, not to the ventricular septum. Tricuspid annular disjunction is also noted.[17]

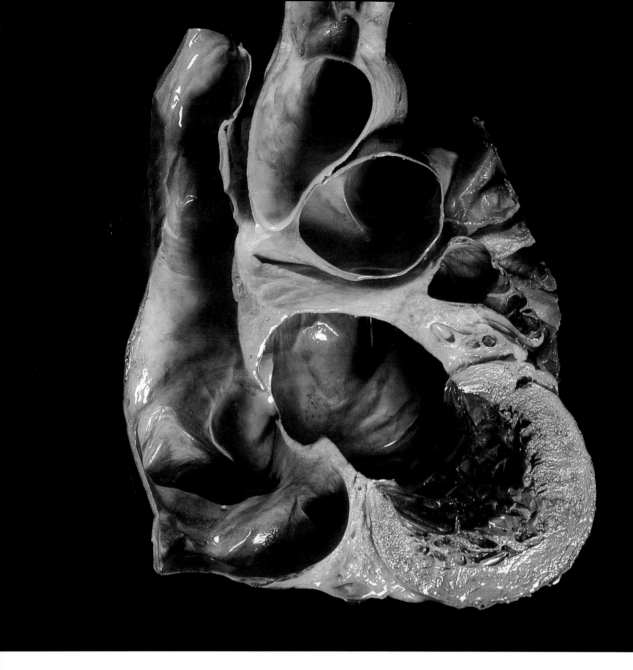

Figure 6 Frontal section of the heart at the level of the inferior pyramidal space viewed from the anterior direction.[1]

The inferior pyramidal space is the epicardial adipose tissue wedging toward the central fibrous body, also referred to as the right fibrous trigone,[1,18,19] from the diaphragmatic surface of the heart. The inferior pyramidal space arises from the crux created between the inferior regions of both atrioventricular grooves, inferior interatrial groove, and inferior interventricular groove. Inferior pyramidal space intervenes between the right atrium and basal left ventricle. Therefore, this region is not the atrioventricular septum, but the atrioventricular sandwich[10] according to the anatomical definition of the septum, which is the partition between the cardiac chamber that can be penetrated without exiting to the extracardiac space. The middle cardiac vein and atrioventricular nodal artery are observed within this space. The primary septum at the floor of the fossa ovalis and antero-inferior muscular buttress (anterior limbus of the fossa ovalis) is the membranous and muscular

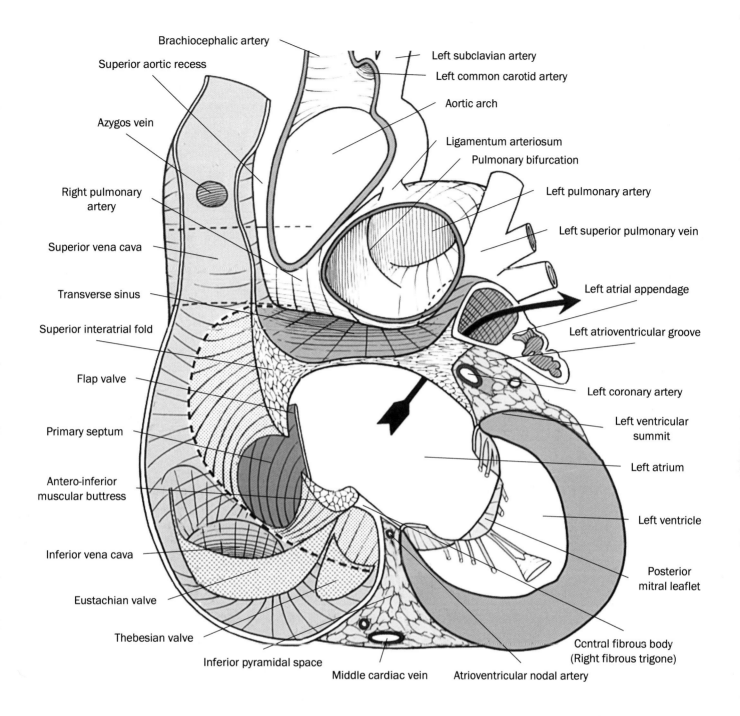

Brachiocephalic artery
Superior aortic recess
Azygos vein
Right pulmonary artery
Superior vena cava
Transverse sinus
Superior interatrial fold
Flap valve
Primary septum
Antero-inferior muscular buttress
Inferior vena cava
Eustachian valve
Thebesian valve
Inferior pyramidal space
Middle cardiac vein

Left subclavian artery
Left common carotid artery
Aortic arch
Ligamentum arteriosum
Pulmonary bifurcation
Left pulmonary artery
Left superior pulmonary vein
Left atrial appendage
Left atrioventricular groove
Left coronary artery
Left ventricular summit
Left atrium
Left ventricle
Posterior mitral leaflet
Central fibrous body (Right fibrous trigone)
Atrioventricular nodal artery

components of the true atrial septum.[20] The secondary septum superior to the fossa ovalis is not the true septum, but the superior interatrial fold located right atrial side relative to the flap valve of the primary septum. The circumflex artery and coronary venous tributary are observed within the left atrioventricular groove sandwiched between the left atrial appendage and the left ventricular summit. The distal pulmonary trunk, pulmonary bifurcation, and right pulmonary artery are located at the roof of the left atrium, with the intervening transverse sinus. Superior extension of the transverse sinus between the ascending aorta and superior vena cava is the superior aortic recess, also referred to as the aorto-caval recess.[21] The Eustachian and Thebesian valves guard the orifice of the inferior vena cava and coronary sinus,[22] respectively.

References

1. McAlpine WA. Digitized collection of all the images created by Dr. McAlpine at UCLA. Copyright UCLA Cardiac Arrhythmia Center. Part of this collection appeared in *Heart and Coronary Arteries: An Anatomical Atlas for Clinical Diagnosis, Radiological Investigation, and Surgical Treatment.* New York: Springer-Verlag; 1975.

2. Mori S, Anderson RH, Tahara N, et al. Diversity and determinants of the three-dimensional anatomical axis of the heart as revealed using multidetector-row computed tomography. *Anat Rec* (Hoboken). 2017;300:1083–1092.

3. Mori S, Tretter JT, Spicer DE, et al. What is the real cardiac anatomy? *Clin Anat.* 2019;32:288–309.

4. Mori S, Spicer DE, Anderson RH. Revisiting the anatomy of the living heart. *Circ J.* 2016;80:24–33.

5. Mori S, Anderson RH, Takaya T, et al. The association between wedging of the aorta and cardiac structural anatomy as revealed using multidetector-row computed tomography. *J Anat.* 2017;231:110–120.

6. Anderson RH, Mohan TJ, Sánchez-Quintana D, et al. The anatomic substrates for outflow tract arrhythmias. *Heart Rhythm.* 2019;16:290–297.

7. Mori S, Anderson RH, Nishii T, et al. Isomerism in the setting of the so-called "heterotaxia": The usefulness of computed tomographic analysis. *Ann Pediatric Cardiol.* 2017;10:175–186.

8. Dong X, Tang M, Sun Q, et al. Anatomical relevance of ablation to the pulmonary artery root: Clinical implications for characterizing the pulmonary sinus of Valsalva and coronary artery. *J Cardiovasc Electrophysiol.* 2018;29:1230–1237.

9. Mori S, Nishii T, Takaya T, et al. Clinical structural anatomy of the inferior pyramidal space reconstructed from the living heart: Three-dimensional visualization using multidetector-row computed tomography. *Clin Anat.* 2015;28:878–887.

10. Mori S, Fukuzawa K, Takaya T, et al. Clinical structural anatomy of the Inferior pyramidal space reconstructed within the cardiac contour using multidetector-row computed tomography. *J Cardiovasc Electrophysiol.* 2015;26:705–712.

11. Mori S, Fukuzawa K, Takaya T, et al. Clinical cardiac structural anatomy reconstructed within the cardiac contour using multi-detector-row computed tomography: Atrial septum and ventricular septum. *Clin Anat.* 2016;29:342–352.

12. Toh H, Mori S, Tretter JT, et al. Living anatomy of the ventricular myocardial crescents supporting the coronary aortic sinuses. *Semin Thorac Cardiovasc Surg.* 2020;32:230–241.

13. Hayashi K, Bouvier E, Lefevre T, et al. Potential mechanism of annulus rupture during transcatheter aortic valve implantation. *Catheter Cardiovasc Intern.* 2013;82:E742–E746.

14. Yamada T, McElderry HT, Dipalladium H, et al. Idiopathic ventricular arrhythmias originating from the left ventricular summit: Anatomic concepts relevant to ablation. *Circ Arrhythm Electrophysiol.* 2010;3:616–623.

15. Mori S, Fukuzawa K, Takaya T, et al. Clinical cardiac structural anatomy reconstructed within the cardiac contour using multi-detector-row computed tomography: Left ventricular outflow tract. *Clin Anat.* 2016;29:353–363.

16. Kroni W, Sigurdsson G, Horwitz PA. Left main coronary artery compression by an enlarged pulmonary artery. *JACC Cardiovasc Intern.* 2013;6:e3–e4.

17. Anabel EW, Childless M, Daugaard LA, et al. Tricuspid annulus disjunction: novel findings by cardiac magnetic resonance in patients with mitral annulus disjunction. *JACC Cardiovasc Imaging.* 2021;14:1535–1543.

18. Zimmerman J, Bailey CP. The surgical significance of the fibrous skeleton of the heart. *J Thorac Cardiovasc Surg.* 1962;44:701–712.

19. Racker DK. The AV junction region of the heart: A comprehensive study correlating gross anatomy and direct three-dimensional analysis. Part I. Architecture and topography. *Anat Rec.* 1999;256:49–63.

20. Mori S, Nishii T, Tretter JT, et al. Demonstration of living anatomy clarifies the morphology of interatrial communications. *Heart.* 2018;104:2003–2009.

21. Mori S, Hanna P, Dacey MJ, et al. Comprehensive anatomy of the pericardial space and the cardiac hilum: Anatomical dissections with intact pericardium. *JACC Cardiovasc Imaging.* 2021. DOI: 10.1016/j.jcmg.2021.04.016. Online ahead of print.

22. Anderson RH, Webb S, Brown NA. Clinical anatomy of the atrial septum with reference to its developmental components. *Clin Anat.* 1999;12:362–374.

2

Right Anterior Oblique View of the Heart

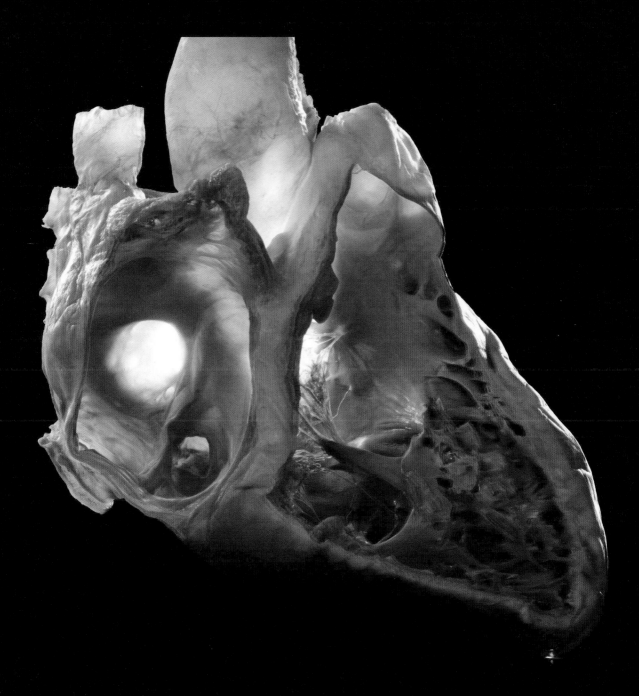

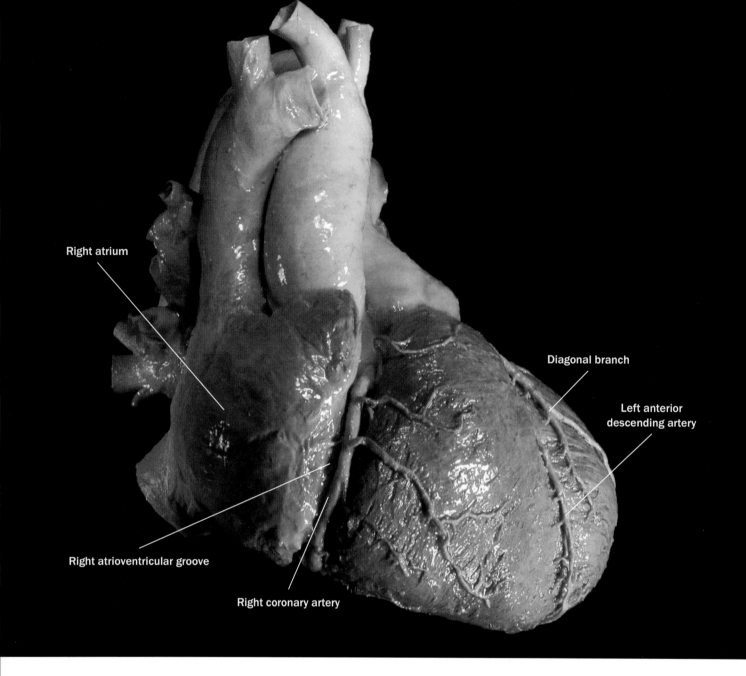

Right atrium

Diagonal branch

Left anterior
descending artery

Right atrioventricular groove

Right coronary artery

Figure 7 The heart viewed from the right anterior oblique direction.[1]

The directional indicator shows the appropriate standard terminology to describe the direction related to the heart. The right anterior oblique direction is optimal angulation to separate the atria from the ventricles, or to obtain an *en face* view of the atrial and ventricular septa. The atrioventricular groove intervenes between the atrium and ventricle. During fluoroscopic procedure, the atrioventricular groove can be appreciated as the radiolucent band.[2] Although the right and non-coronary aortic sinuses are separated, this view cannot separate the left coronary aortic sinus from the right and non-coronary aortic sinuses.[3] The bottom of the left heart is located superior to the bottom of the right heart. In contrast to the vertically aligned superior vena cava, the orifice of the inferior vena cava is located posterior relative to the orifice of the superior vena cava, and its axis directs toward the apex of the right atrial appendage. In this right anterior oblique image, corresponding roughly to the right anterior oblique 30-degree view, the right-hand border of the cardiac contour is not composed of the right ventricle. The mid-apical superior and supero-lateral wall of the left ventricle composes this part of the contour.[3] Thus, the right-hand part of the cardiac silhouette relative to the left anterior descending artery is the region of the left ventricle, where is perfused by the diagonal branches. The left-hand part of the cardiac silhouette relative to the

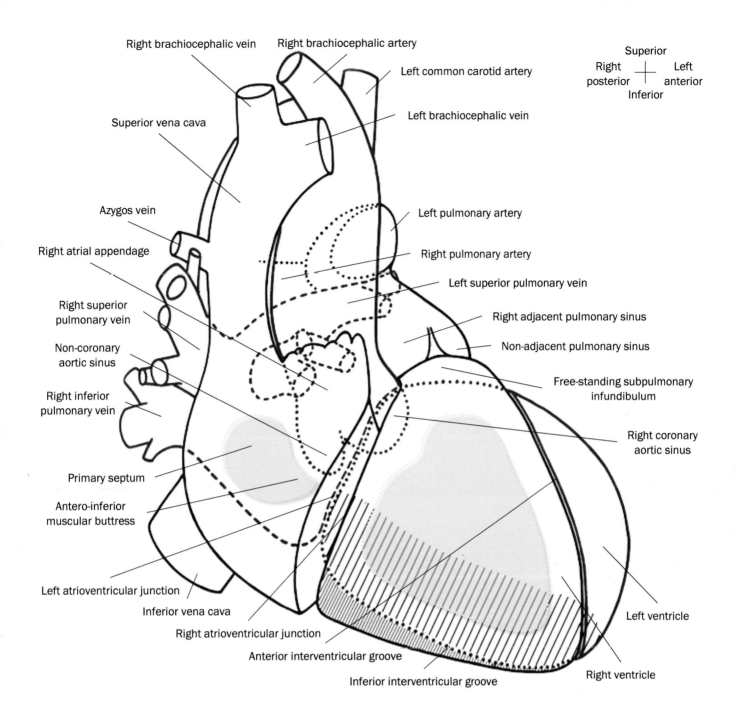

Right brachiocephalic vein

Right brachiocephalic artery

Left common carotid artery

Superior
Right posterior | Left anterior
Inferior

Left brachiocephalic vein

Superior vena cava

Azygos vein

Left pulmonary artery

Right pulmonary artery

Right atrial appendage

Left superior pulmonary vein

Right superior
pulmonary vein

Right adjacent pulmonary sinus

Non-adjacent pulmonary sinus

Non-coronary
aortic sinus

Free-standing subpulmonary
infundibulum

Right inferior
pulmonary vein

Right coronary
aortic sinus

Primary septum

Antero-inferior
muscular buttress

Left ventricle

Left atrioventricular junction

Inferior vena cava

Right atrioventricular junction

Anterior interventricular groove

Right ventricle

Inferior interventricular groove

left anterior descending artery is the right ventricle. This knowledge is important to avoid inadvertent damage of the right ventricular anterior free wall during the procedure targeting the right side of the ventricular septum, including ablation, pacing, and biopsy. Relative to the basal superior left ventricle, the pulmonary valve is lifted up by the encircling free-standing subpulmonary infundibulum. Thus, at the level just beneath the pulmonary valve, even facing direction away to the observer is not the septum, but a medial and posterior free wall of the right ventricular outflow tract. The yellow regions roughly demarcate the safe region that is true atrial and ventricular septa.[2] The right atrioventricular junction is shifted apical to the left atrioventricular junction, rendering the basal medial part of the left ventricular myocardium being adjacent to the floor of the triangle of Koch, intervened by the inferior pyramidal space.[4] The right coronary aortic sinus is located antero-superior relative to the non-coronary aortic sinus, which is located most postero-inferior. The pulmonary valve is located most superior among the all-cardiac valves.[5] The right superior pulmonary vein is located posterior to the superior vena cava just superior of its junction with the right atrium.

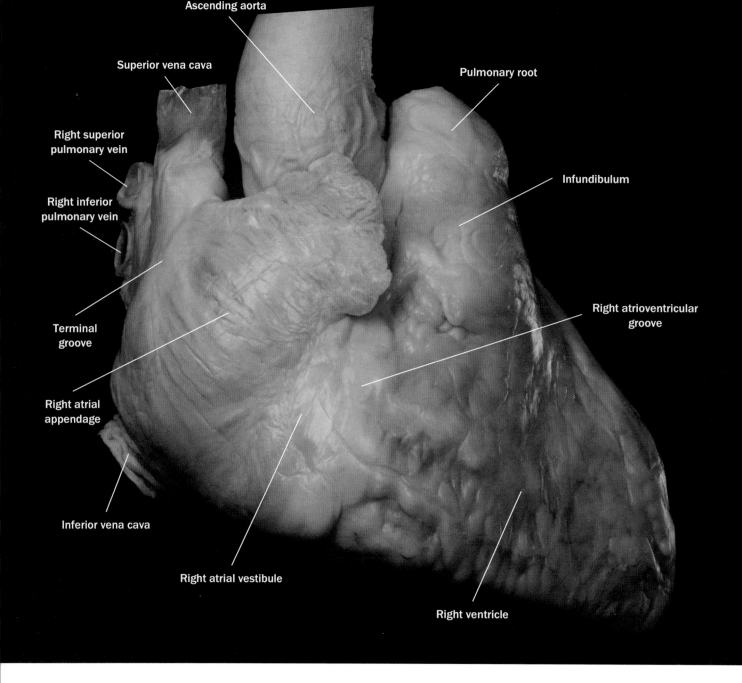

Ascending aorta

Superior vena cava

Pulmonary root

Right superior pulmonary vein

Infundibulum

Right inferior pulmonary vein

Right atrioventricular groove

Terminal groove

Right atrial appendage

Inferior vena cava

Right atrial vestibule

Right ventricle

Figure 8 Progressive dissection images of the heart viewed from the right anterior oblique direction: Outer aspect of the right heart. 🔲🔳 Anaglyph 1.

In this right anterior oblique image, corresponding to 45-degree to 50-degree views, shows an *en face* view of the right heart. In contrast to the vertical axis of the superior vena cava, the axis of the inferior vena cava tilts toward the apex of the right atrial appendage. The apex of the right atrial appendage covers the right side of the ascending aorta and superior part of the right atrioventricular groove, involving the proximal right coronary artery. Transillumination (right) clarifies

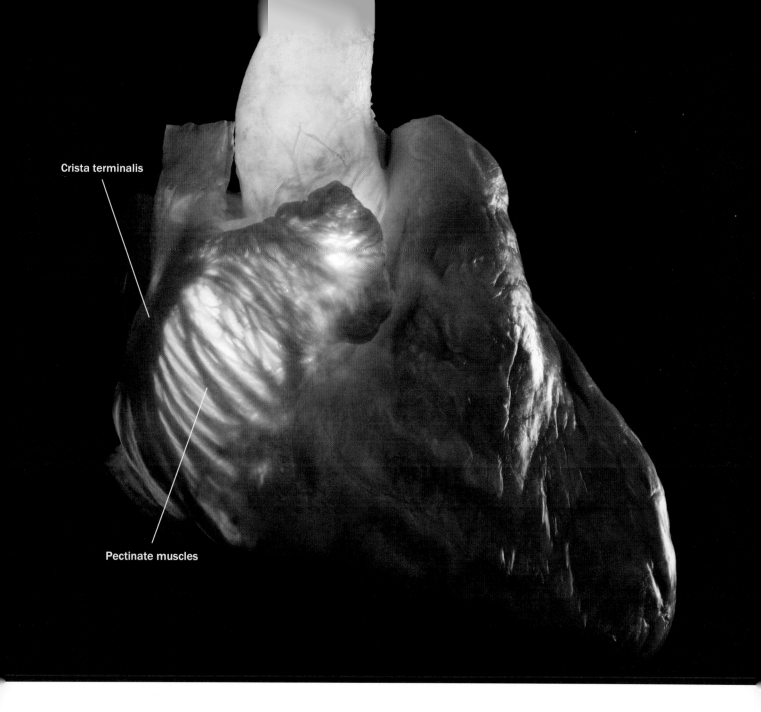

Crista terminalis

Pectinate muscles

the location of the crista terminalis that demarcates posterior margin of the right atrial appendage. The crista terminalis gives rise to multiple pectinate muscles traversing the free wall of the right atrial appendage directing toward the right atrial vestibule, the encircling smooth right atrial wall continuing to the attachment of the tricuspid valve.

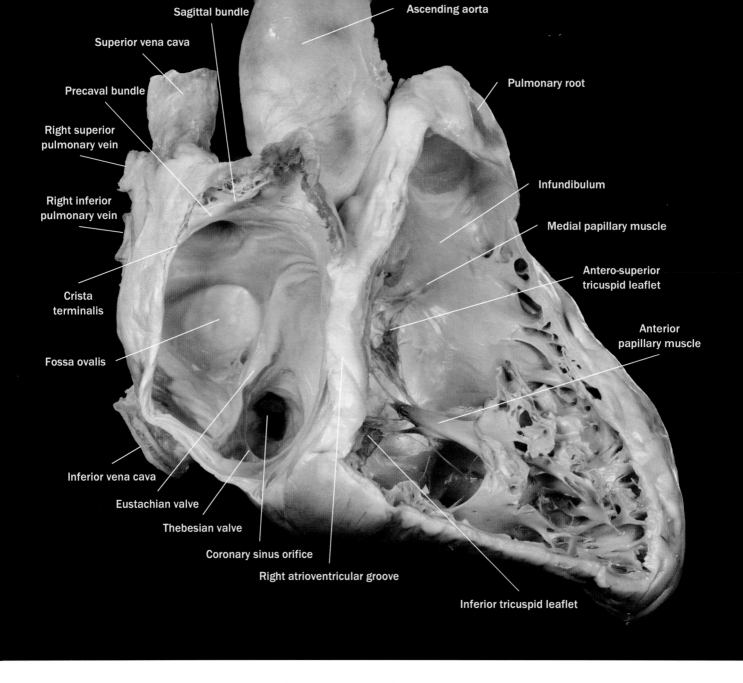

Figure 9 Progressive dissection images of the heart viewed from the right anterior oblique direction: Removal of the right heart free wall. [🔵◼️] Anaglyph 2.

Right atrial and ventricular free wall are removed except the right atrioventricular groove. These images show the medial aspect of the right atrium as well as trabeculations of the right ventricle. The anterior papillary muscle anchors the commissure between the antero-superior and inferior tricuspid leaflets. The medial part of the antero-superior leaflet is anchored by the medial papillary muscle located anterior to the right coronary aortic sinus. Transillumination (right) enhances the primary septum at the floor of the fossa ovalis, ascending aorta, aortic root, and membranous septum. The supero-medial aspect of the right atrial appendage, corresponding to the right aortic mound (torus aorticus), is also transilluminated through the aortic root. This indicates that this part of the right atrium is not the atrial septum, but

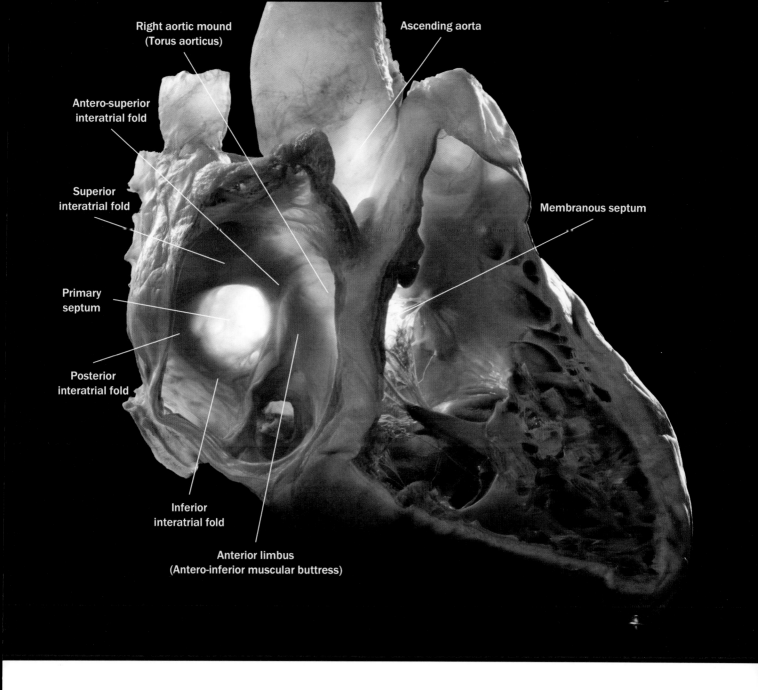

Right aortic mound
(Torus aorticus)

Ascending aorta

Antero-superior
interatrial fold

Superior
interatrial fold

Membranous septum

Primary
septum

Posterior
interatrial fold

Inferior
interatrial fold

Anterior limbus
(Antero-inferior muscular buttress)

the medial free wall of the right atrium facing to the aortic root, and specifically, the anterior half of the non-coronary aortic sinus. The ring-like negative transillumination surrounding the fossa ovalis corresponds to the secondary septum or interatrial fold/groove, except the anterior limbus of the fossa ovalis. The secondary septum is not the true septum, but the interatrial fold/groove, surrounding the fossa ovalis antero-superior, superior, posterior, and inferior. The anterior limbus corresponds to the antero-inferior muscular buttress, that connects to the central fibrous body at the bottom of the non-coronary aortic sinus. Only the primary septum at the floor of the fossa ovalis and the antero-inferior muscular buttress are the true anatomical atrial septum.[6]

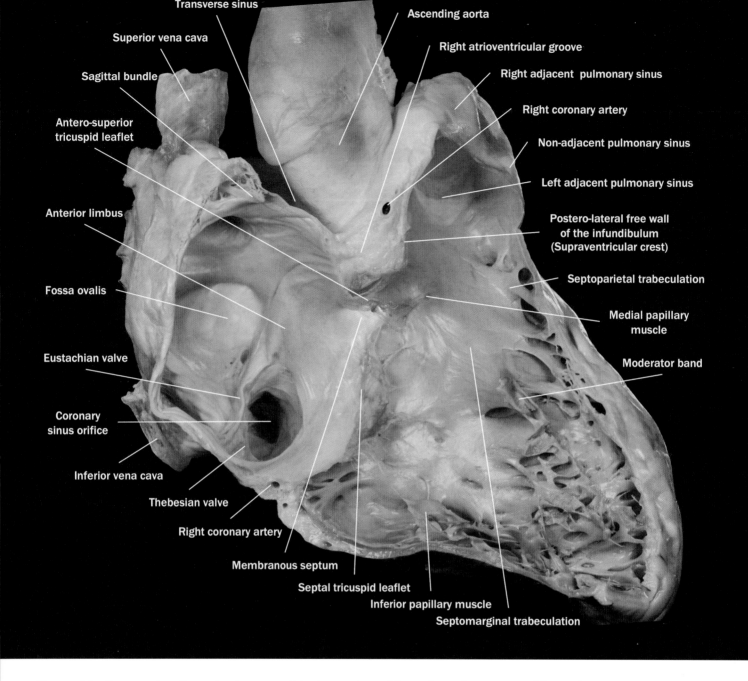

Transverse sinus

Ascending aorta

Superior vena cava

Right atrioventricular groove

Sagittal bundle

Right adjacent pulmonary sinus

Antero-superior tricuspid leaflet

Right coronary artery

Non-adjacent pulmonary sinus

Left adjacent pulmonary sinus

Anterior limbus

Postero-lateral free wall of the infundibulum (Supraventricular crest)

Fossa ovalis

Septoparietal trabeculation

Medial papillary muscle

Eustachian valve

Moderator band

Coronary sinus orifice

Inferior vena cava

Thebesian valve

Right coronary artery

Membranous septum

Septal tricuspid leaflet

Inferior papillary muscle

Septomarginal trabeculation

Figure 10   Progressive dissection images of the heart viewed from the right anterior oblique direction: Focus on the medial structures of the right heart. ▭▬ Anaglyph 3.

Further progressive dissection was performed by removing the lateral right atrioventricular groove, apex of the right atrial appendage, postero-lateral free wall of the right ventricular outflow tract (infundibulum), and anterior papillary muscle of the right ventricle. The membranous septum is located at the commissure between the antero-superior and septal tricuspid leaflets. The septal tricuspid leaflet is mainly anchored by multiple small septal papillary muscles or the chordae tendineae directly arising from the ventricular septum. The chordae tendineae from the inferior papillary muscle also anchor the septal leaflet. The sectional plane of the moderator band is observed. Transillumination (right) shows the relationship between the non-coronary aortic sinus (seen through the right atrium), right coronary aortic sinus (seen through the right atrioventricular groove and supraventricular crest), and the membranous septum. The non-coronary aortic sinus and right posterior part of the ascending aorta is adjacent to the supero-medial wall of the right atrial appendage with the intervening right-side transverse sinus. The right coronary aortic sinus is adjacent to the postero-

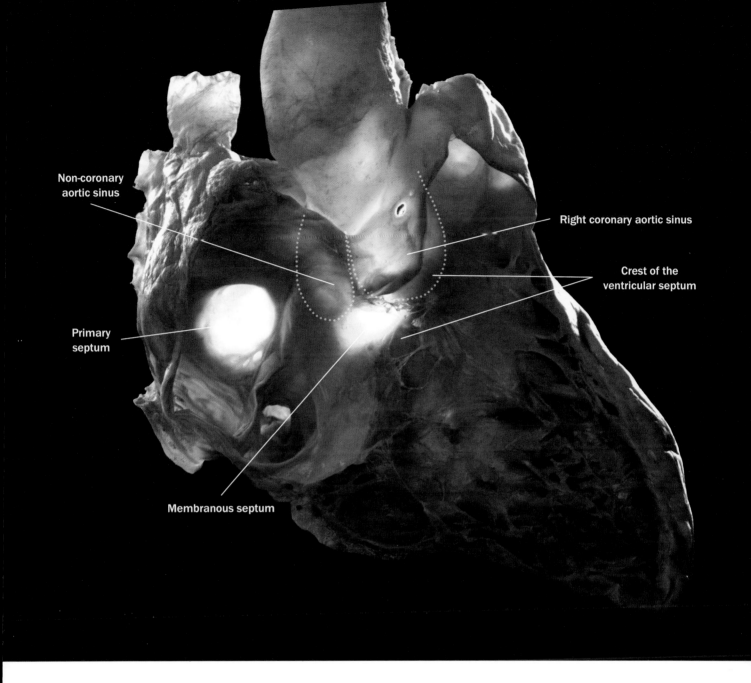

Non-coronary
aortic sinus

Right coronary aortic sinus

Crest of the
ventricular septum

Primary
septum

Membranous septum

lateral free wall of the right ventricular outflow tract, also referred to as the ventriculo-infundibular fold. The endocardial side of this region corresponds to the supraventricular crest covering the right coronary aortic sinus with its medial part.[7] The base of the right coronary aortic sinus is supported by the crest of the ventricular septum, corresponding to the septal part of the left ventricular ostium,[1] which is not transilluminated.[8] The medial papillary muscle is located at the base of the septomarginal trabeculation, anterior to the right coronary aortic sinus. The morphology of the septomarginal trabeculation varies among hearts, and it is not prominent in this particular heart. The medial papillary muscle is also referred to as the muscle of Lancisi, muscle of Luschka, and papillary muscle of the conus.[9] The medial papillary muscle commonly anchors the medial part of the antero-superior tricuspid leaflet with its prominent chordae tendinea.[10] The proximal right bundle branch runs close to the base of this medial papillary muscle before coursing within the septomarginal trabeculation and moderator band.[11]

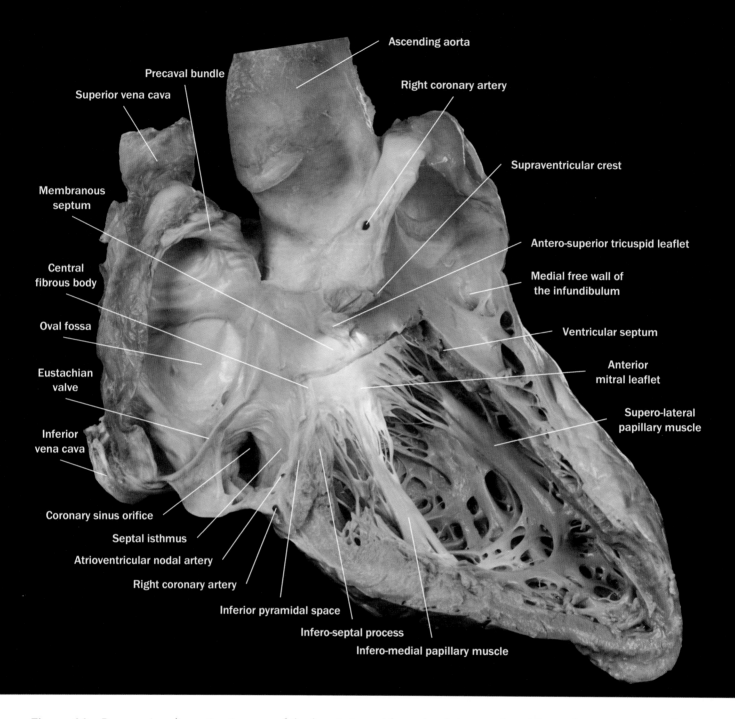

Ascending aorta

Precaval bundle

Superior vena cava

Right coronary artery

Supraventricular crest

Membranous septum

Antero-superior tricuspid leaflet

Medial free wall of the infundibulum

Central fibrous body

Ventricular septum

Oval fossa

Anterior mitral leaflet

Eustachian valve

Supero-lateral papillary muscle

Inferior vena cava

Coronary sinus orifice

Septal isthmus

Atrioventricular nodal artery

Right coronary artery

Inferior pyramidal space

Infero-septal process

Infero-medial papillary muscle

Figure 11   Progressive dissection images of the heart viewed from the right anterior oblique direction: Removal of the ventricular septum. 🔲🔲 Anaglyph 4.

The substantial part of the muscular ventricular septum is removed to show the left ventricle. The basal superior part of the section is made along the inferior margin of the membranous septum, where is the location of the atrioventricular conduction axis and proximal right bundle branch. The substantial part of the ventricular septum is observed in *en face* fashion from this direction. However, the ventricular septum located anterior to the right coronary aortic sinus lies superior relative to the left ventricular outflow tract as the right ventricular outflow tract overrides the left ventricular outflow tract. Therefore, *en face* view of the ventricular septum at this region cannot be obtained from this right anterior oblique direction. It is the right anterior oblique and cranial view that can show the *en face* view of this part of the ventricular septum. Therefore, so-called antero-septal region of the right ventricular outflow tract (infundibulum) facing the observer, is actually not the septum, defined as a structure that separates two chambers, but it is the medial free wall of the infundibulum. The ventricular surface of the anterior mitral leaflet is observed from this direction. Both the infero-medial and supero-lateral papillary muscles are also observed, indicating that they are related to the left ventricular free

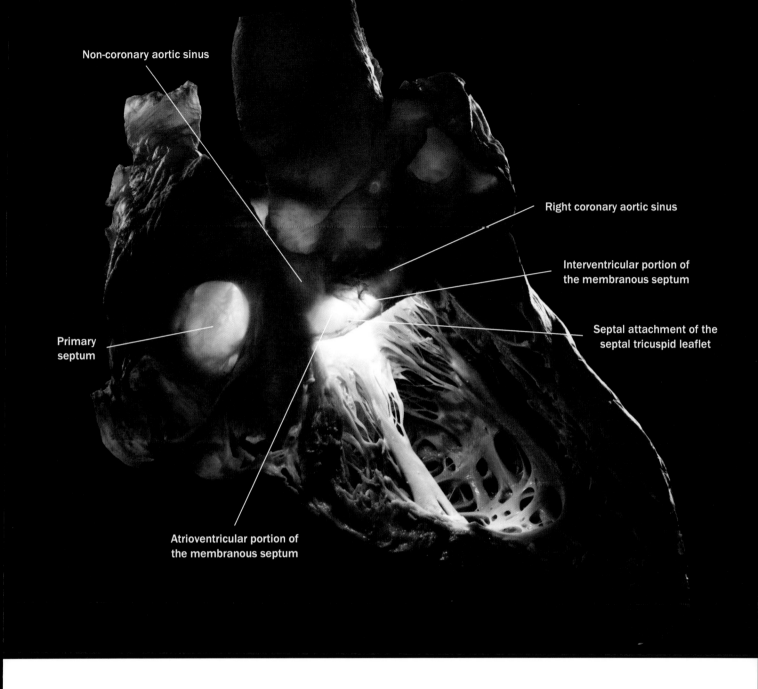

Non-coronary aortic sinus

Right coronary aortic sinus

Interventricular portion of the membranous septum

Primary septum

Septal attachment of the septal tricuspid leaflet

Atrioventricular portion of the membranous septum

wall,[5] aligned in a vertical fashion rather than horizontal fashion. The basal infero-medial left ventricular wall located anterior to the coronary sinus extends toward the central fibrous body at the base of the non-coronary aortic sinus. This basal infero-medial left ventricular muscle ascending toward the central fibrous body is referred to as the infero-septal process.[12] As this infero-septal process is adjacent to the septal isthmus, left ventricular arrhythmia originating from the epicardial side of this infero-septal process can be ablated from the septal isthmus.[13] Successful traversal of this region from the right atrium to the left ventricle has been reported.[14] However, it is important to appreciate that this region is the atrioventricular sandwich. The inferior pyramidal space, the wedging epicardial fibro-adipose tissue carrying the atrioventricular nodal artery, intervenes between the right atrium and the left ventricle.[15] The membranous septum is divided by the septal attachment of the septal tricuspid leaflet unequally into the atrioventricular and interventricular portions with various proportions of each portion.[16] Refer to Figure 67.

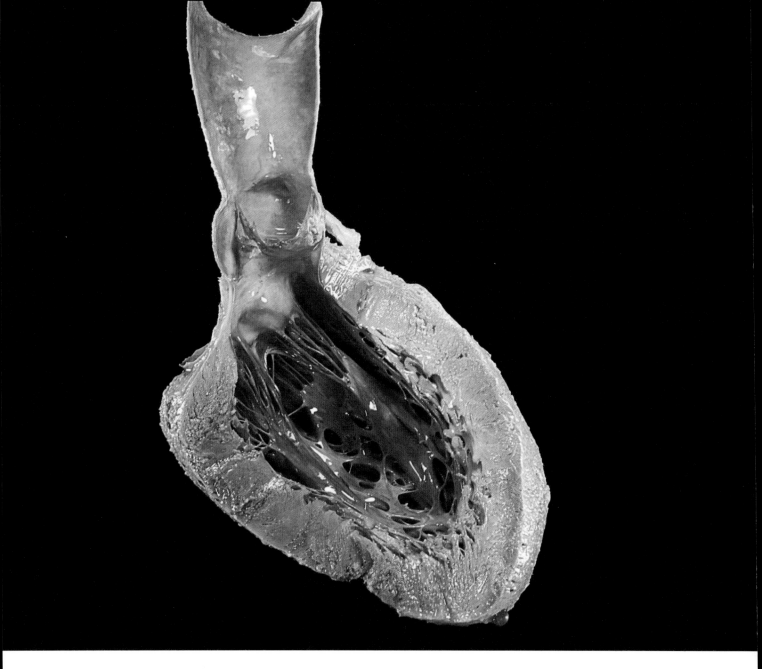

Figure 12 The left ventricle viewed from the right anterior oblique direction.[1]

In this section, the basal infero-medial left ventricle shows a peculiar shape. This is the region referred to as the infero-septal process.[12] It is in continuity with the right fibrous trigone, also referred to as the central fibrous body,[1,17] at the base of the non-coronary aortic sinus. The infero-medial and supero-lateral papillary muscles belong to the left ventricular free wall.[18] The interleaflet triangle between the right and left coronary aortic sinuses is supported by the basal left ventricular free

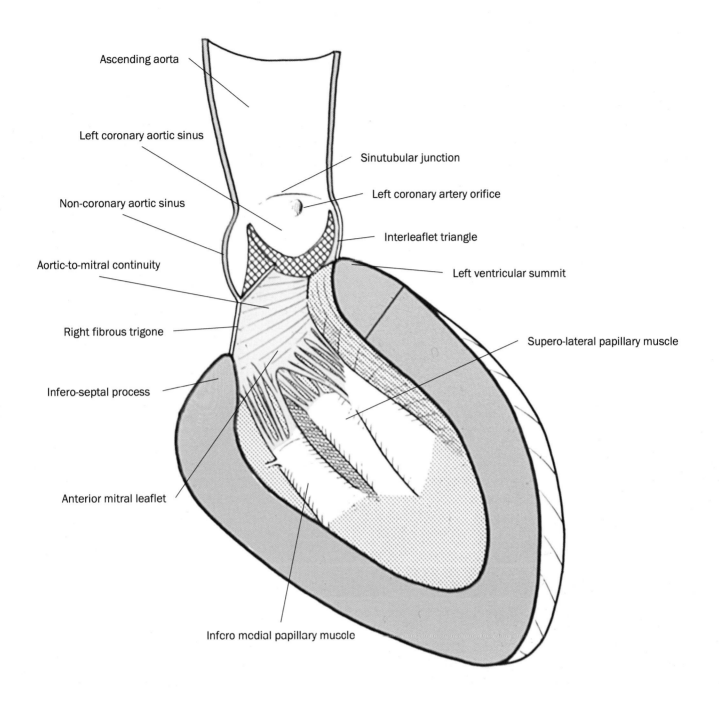

Ascending aorta

Left coronary aortic sinus

Non-coronary aortic sinus

Aortic-to-mitral continuity

Right fibrous trigone

Infero-septal process

Anterior mitral leaflet

Sinutubular junction

Left coronary artery orifice

Interleaflet triangle

Left ventricular summit

Supero-lateral papillary muscle

Infero-medial papillary muscle

wall.[7] This interleaflet triangle is close to the posterior attachment of the right ventricle, where the free-standing subpulmonary infundibulum separates from the left ventricle to lift up the pulmonary valve. Refer to Figure 81. The epicardial surface of this basal superior left ventricular free wall is referred to as the left ventricular summit.[1,19] The interleaflet tringle between the left and non-coronary aortic sinuses is in continuity with the anterior mitral leaflet. Refer to Figure 120.

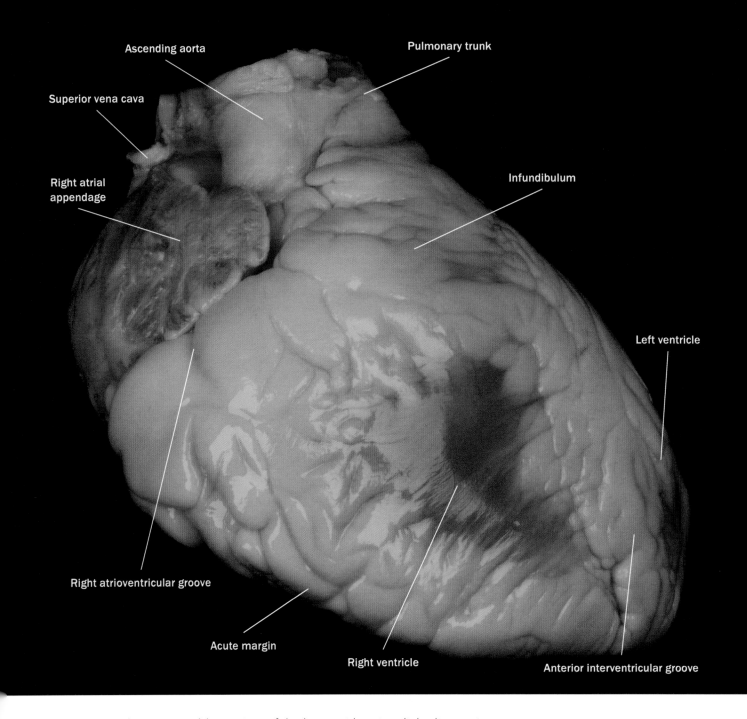

Superior vena cava

Right atrial
appendage

Ascending aorta

Pulmonary trunk

Infundibulum

Left ventricle

Right atrioventricular groove

Acute margin

Right ventricle

Anterior interventricular groove

Figure 13 Right anterior oblique view of the heart with epicardial adipose tissue.

The right atrial appendage is generally not covered with thick epicardial adipose tissue. Rich epicardial adipose tissue is distributed along the atrioventricular groove, anterior interventricular groove, and acute margin. Localized region in the right ventricular anterior free wall lacks epicardial adipose tissue.

References

1. McAlpine WA. Digitized collection of all the images created by Dr. McAlpine at UCLA. Copyright UCLA Cardiac Arrhythmia Center. Part of this collection appeared in *Heart and Coronary Arteries: An Anatomical Atlas for Clinical Diagnosis, Radiological Investigation, and Surgical Treatment.* New York: Springer-Verlag; 1975.

2. Mori S, Fukuzawa K, Takaya T, et al. Clinical cardiac structural anatomy reconstructed within the cardiac contour using multidetector-row computed tomography: Atrial septum and ventricular septum. *Clin Anat.* 2016;29:342–352.

3. Mori S, Fukuzawa K, Takaya T, et al. Optimal angulations for obtaining an *en face* view of each coronary aortic sinus and the interventricular septum: Correlative anatomy around the left ventricular outflow tract. *Clin Anat.* 2015;28:494–505.

4. Mori S, Nishii T, Takaya T, et al. Clinical structural anatomy of the inferior pyramidal space reconstructed from the living heart: Three-dimensional visualization using multidetector-row computed tomography. *Clin Anat.* 2015;28:878–887.

5. Mori S, Fukuzawa K, Takaya T, et al. Clinical cardiac structural anatomy reconstructed within the cardiac contour using multidetector-row computed tomography: The arrangement and location of the cardiac valves. *Clin Anat.* 2016;29:364–370.

6. Mori S, Nishii T, Tretter JT, et al. Demonstration of living anatomy clarifies the morphology of interatrial communications. *Heart.* 2018;104:2003–2009.

7. Mori S, Fukuzawa K, Takaya T, et al. Clinical cardiac structural anatomy reconstructed within the cardiac contour using multidetector-row computed tomography: Left ventricular outflow tract. *Clin Anat.* 2016;29:353–363.

8. Toh H, Mori S, Tretter JT, et al. Living anatomy of the ventricular myocardial crescents supporting the coronary aortic sinuses. *Semin Thorac Cardiovasc Surg.* 2020;32:230–241.

9. Wensink AC. The medial papillary complex. *Br Heart J.* 1977;39:1012–1018.

10. Tretter JT, Sarwar AE, Anderson RH, et al, Assessment of the anatomical variation to be found in the normal tricuspid valve. *Clin Anat.* 2016;29:399–407.

11. Shimizu S. [Topographical anatomy of the atrioventricular node of Tawara—findings by macro-microscopic dissection under dissecting microscope] (in Japanese). *Nihon Kyobu Geka Gakkai Zasshi.* 1989 Feb;37(2):227–233.

12. Li A, Zuberi Z, Bradfield JS, et al. Endocardial ablation of ventricular ectopic beats arising from the basal inferoseptal process of the left ventricle. *Heart Rhythm.* 2018;15:1356–1362.

13. Tavares L, Dave A, Valderrama M. Successful ablation of premature ventricular contractions originating from the inferoseptal process of the left ventricle using a coronary sinus approach. *Heart Rhythm Case Rep.* 2018;4:371–374.

14. Santangelo P, Hyman MC, Muser D, et al. Outcomes of percutaneous trans-right atrial access to the left ventricle for catheter ablation of ventricular tachycardia in patients with mechanical aortic and mitral valves. *JAMA Cardio.* 2020;6:1–6.

15. Mori S, Fukuzawa K, Takaya T, et al. Clinical structural anatomy of the inferior pyramidal space reconstructed within the cardiac contour using multidetector-row computed tomography. *J Cardiovasc Electrophysiol.* 2015;26:705–712.

16. Tretter JT, Mori S, Saremi F, et al. Variations in rotation of the aortic root and membranous septum with implications for transcatheter valve implantation. *Heart.* 2018;104:999–1005.

17. Zimmerman J, Bailey CP. The surgical significance of the fibrous skeleton of the heart. *J Thorac Cardiovasc Surg.* 1962;44:701–712.

18. Mori S, Spicer DE, Anderson RH. Revisiting the anatomy of the living heart. *Circ J.* 2016;80:24–33.

19. Bradfield JS. Redefining optimal targets for intramural ventricular arrhythmias: Planning for combat! *JACC Clin Electrophysiol.* 2020;6:1349–1352.

3

Left Anterior Oblique
View of the Heart

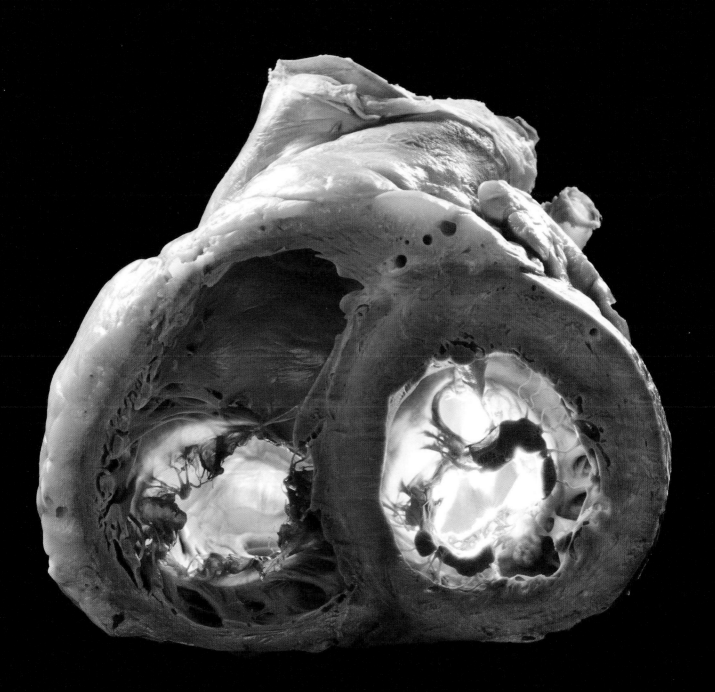

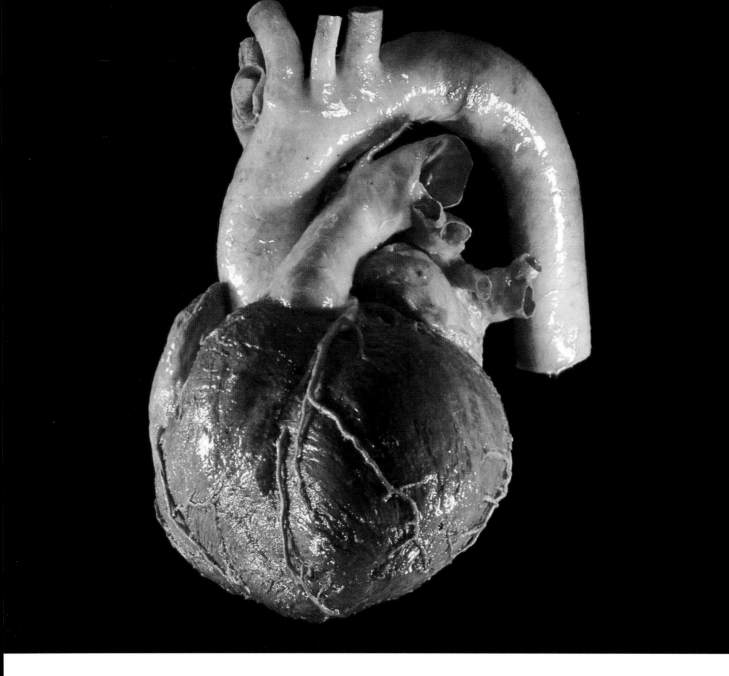

Figure 14 The heart viewed from the left anterior oblique direction.[1]

The view corresponds roughly to the left anterior oblique 60-degree view. As the atrial and ventricular septa directs toward the left antero-inferior direction, the left anterior oblique direction is optimal angulation to separate the right heart from the left heart. The directional indicator shows the appropriate standard terminology to describe the direction related to the heart (cross bar). In addition, the use of directional terms as lateral and medial or septal (dotted circle) is appropriate for atria and apical/inlet components of the ventricles.[2] This rule is not the case for the outlet component of the ventricles. As the right ventricular outflow tract crosses over the left ventricular outflow tract, the ventricular septum at this outflow component is not located vertically. Rather, it tilts toward the left posterior direction. Thus, during the procedure within the right ventricular outflow tract, the septum is located postero-inferior within the infundibulum (refer to Figure 11). Thus, left posterior direction relative to the right ventricular outflow tract should not be deemed as the septal direction, as it can be the medial free wall of the free-standing subpulmonary infundibulum. Even though this view is appropriate to obtain the *en face* view of the both atrioventricular valves, it is not appropriate to obtain the *en face* view of the left atrial posterior wall. The posterior wall of the left atrium is basically located parallel to the frontal plane with some anterior tilting at its roof. Therefore, to

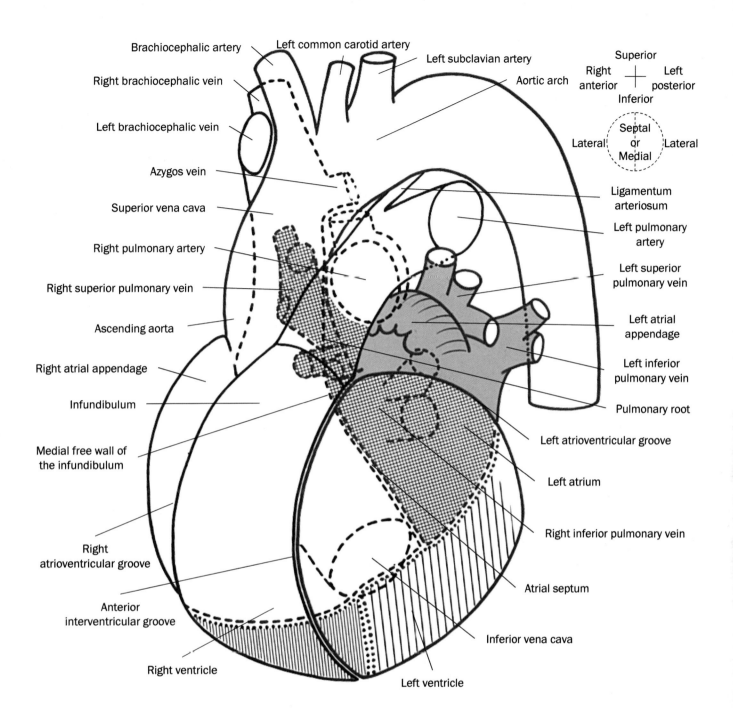

Brachiocephalic artery

Left common carotid artery

Left subclavian artery

Right brachiocephalic vein

Aortic arch

Superior

Right anterior — Left posterior

Inferior

Left brachiocephalic vein

Septal or Medial

Lateral — Lateral

Azygos vein

Ligamentum arteriosum

Superior vena cava

Left pulmonary artery

Right pulmonary artery

Left superior pulmonary vein

Right superior pulmonary vein

Ascending aorta

Left atrial appendage

Right atrial appendage

Left inferior pulmonary vein

Infundibulum

Pulmonary root

Medial free wall of the infundibulum

Left atrioventricular groove

Left atrium

Right inferior pulmonary vein

Right atrioventricular groove

Anterior interventricular groove

Atrial septum

Right ventricle

Inferior vena cava

Left ventricle

separate the right and left pulmonary veins, the more appropriate direction is the anterior view rather than this left anterior oblique view. The apices of the right and left atrial appendages are adjacent to the ascending aorta and pulmonary root, respectively. They guard the entrance/exit to the transverse sinus located posterior to the both arterial trunks. The physiological tilting of the atrial septum is illustrated along with the tilting of the proximal aorta to the right anterior direction. Therefore, the bottom of the left atrium is located superior to that of the right atrium, and the left atrium looks as if it rides on the right atrium. Due to this tilting, the orifice of the inferior vena cava is located medially compared to the orifice of the superior vena cava. Deep left anterior oblique direction is optimal direction to see the *en face* view of the aortic arch to separate the ascending aorta from the descending aorta. Beneath the arch, the right pulmonary artery runs away from the observer toward the right pulmonary hilum, running posterior to the right superior pulmonary vein and anterior to the right main bronchus. On the other hand, beneath the arch, the left main bronchus comes toward the observer to reach to left pulmonary hilum, running posterior to the left superior pulmonary vein. As the left pulmonary artery overrides the left main bronchus, it is eventually located posterior to the left main bronchus. Refer to Figure 93.

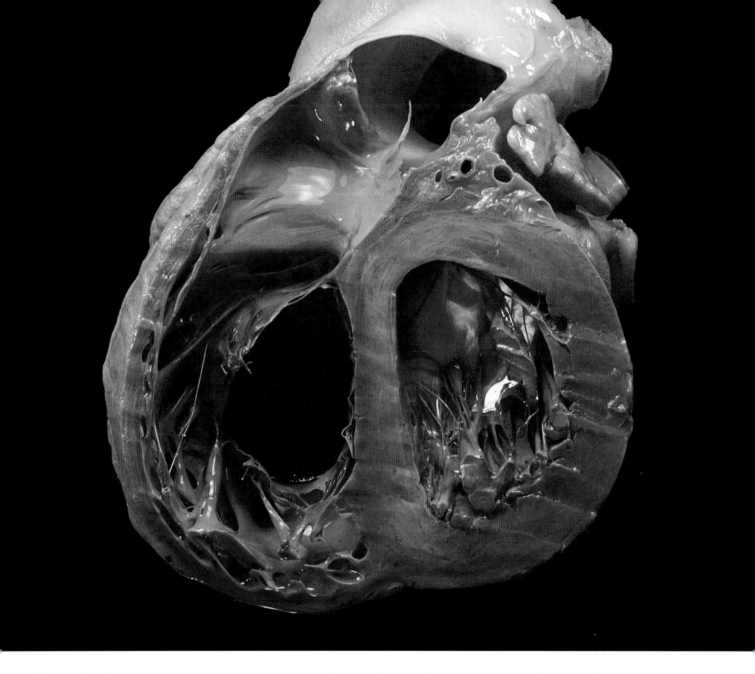

Figure 15 Plane section of the heart at the level of the medial papillary muscle viewed from the left anterior oblique direction.[1]

In the right ventricle, the medial part of the antero-superior tricuspid leaflet is anchored by the medial papillary muscle. The medial papillary muscle arises from the inferior limb of the septomarginal trabeculation located at the basal superior part of the ventricular septum. The inferior papillary muscle anchors the septal and inferior tricuspid leaflets. The commissure between the antero-superior and inferior tricuspid leaflets is anchored by the anterior papillary muscle.[3] The septal tricuspid leaflet attaches to the ventricular septum by its multiple small septal papillary muscles or the chordae tendineae originating from the ventricular septum. The supraventricular crest, corresponding to the ventriculo-infundibular fold or postero-lateral free wall of the infundibulum, separates the tricuspid valve from the pulmonary valve. The medial part of the supraventricular crest is located anterior to the right coronary aortic sinus. The superior part of the ventricular septum between the right and left ventricular outflow tract, corresponding to the location of the septomarginal trabeculation, tilts toward left posterior direction. Thus, superior to this basal supero-septum, medial side of the right ventricular outflow tract is not the septum,

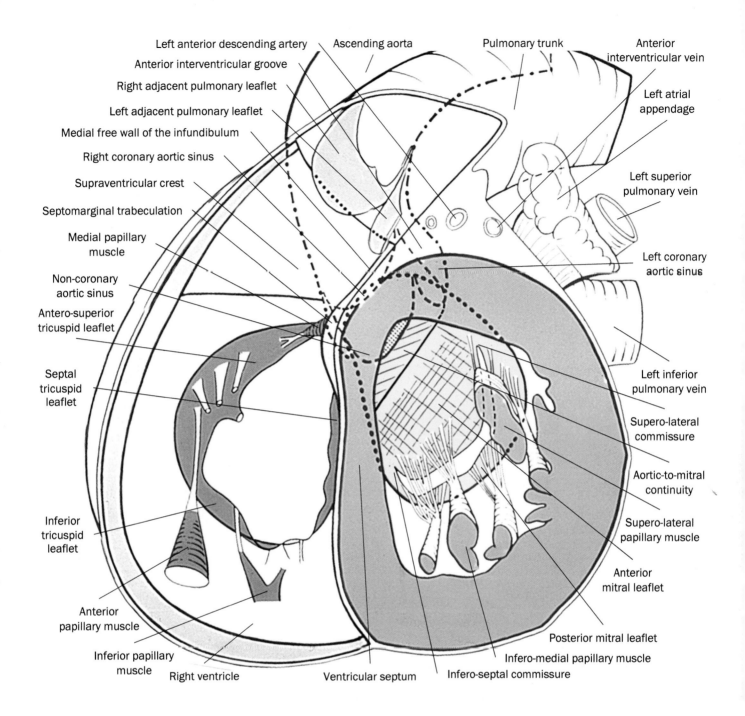

Left anterior descending artery
Anterior interventricular groove
Right adjacent pulmonary leaflet
Left adjacent pulmonary leaflet
Medial free wall of the infundibulum
Right coronary aortic sinus
Supraventricular crest
Septomarginal trabeculation
Medial papillary muscle
Non-coronary aortic sinus
Antero-superior tricuspid leaflet
Septal tricuspid leaflet
Inferior tricuspid leaflet
Anterior papillary muscle
Inferior papillary muscle
Right ventricle

Ascending aorta
Pulmonary trunk

Anterior interventricular vein
Left atrial appendage
Left superior pulmonary vein
Left coronary aortic sinus
Left inferior pulmonary vein
Supero-lateral commissure
Aortic-to-mitral continuity
Supero-lateral papillary muscle
Anterior mitral leaflet
Posterior mitral leaflet
Infero-medial papillary muscle
Infero-septal commissure

Ventricular septum

but the thin medial free wall adjacent to the anterior interventricular groove, including the left anterior descending artery and anterior interventricular vein.[4] In the left ventricle, multiple heads of the infero-medial and supero-lateral papillary muscles are observed. Each infero-medial and supero-lateral papillary muscle gives chordae tendineae to infero-medial and supero-lateral half of the mitral valves, respectively. The coaptation line of the anterior and posterior mitral leaflet is located nearly parallel to the alignment of both papillary muscles. The anterior and posterior mitral leaflets are also referred to as the aortic and mural leaflets of the mitral valve, respectively. This coaptation line is not horizontal as observed during transthoracic echocardiography; rather, it significantly tilts toward the vertical direction.[5] Therefore, the anterior mitral leaflet is located medial and superior relative to the posterior mitral leaflet, which is located lateral and inferior. The apex of the left atrial appendage is a free-floating structure within the pericardial space covering the superior to supero-lateral basal left ventricle.[6] It is independent of the epicardial adipose tissue of the left atrioventricular and anterior interventricular grooves.

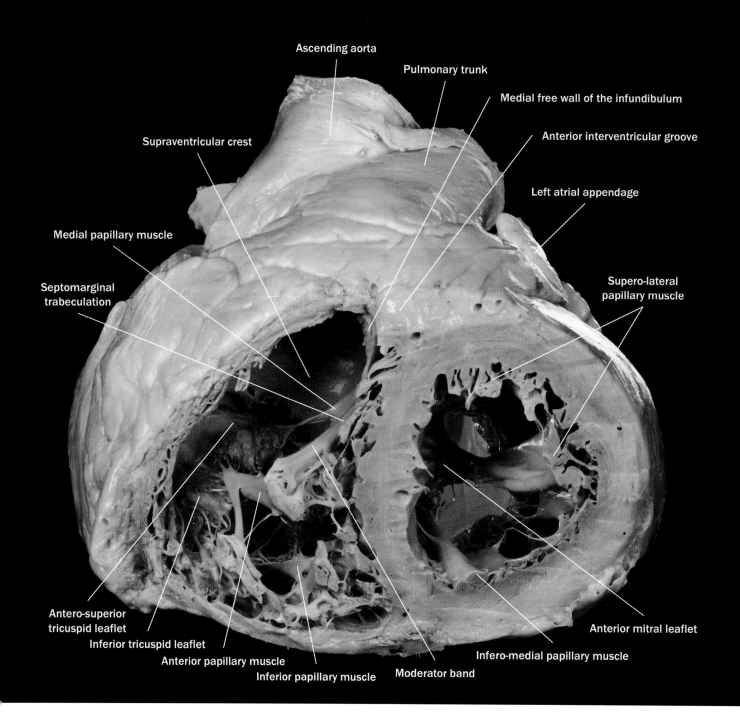

Figure 16 Progressive dissection images of the heart viewed from the left anterior oblique direction: Mid-ventricular level. 🔴🔵 Anaglyph 5.

In the right ventricle, the moderator band arises from the septomarginal trabeculation as it traverses toward the free wall. The anterior papillary muscle arises from both the moderator band and free wall trabeculations. The anterior papillary muscle anchors the commissure between the antero-superior and inferior tricuspid leaflets. The medial papillary muscle anchors the medial part of the antero-superior tricuspid leaflet. The inferior papillary muscle anchors the commissure between the inferior and septal tricuspid leaflets. Adjacent to the anterior interventricular groove, thin medial free wall

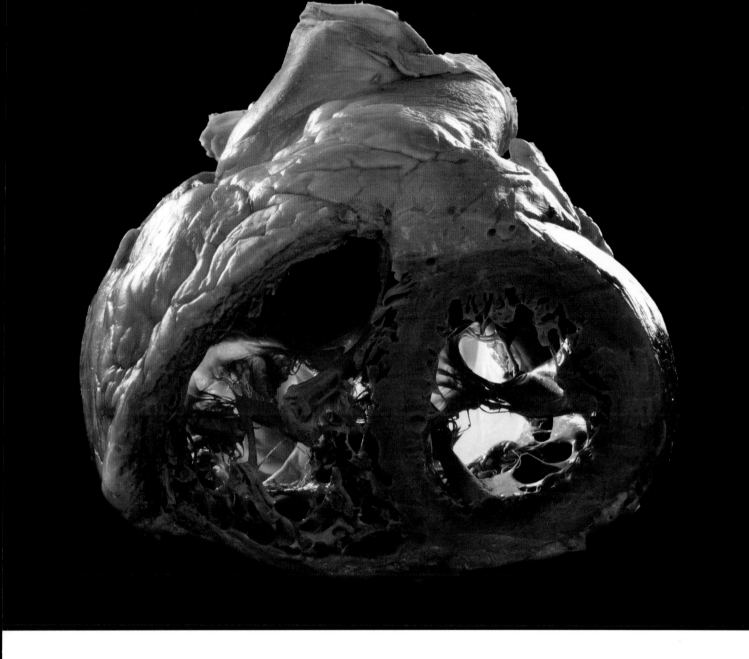

of the right ventricular outflow tract is observed. In the left ventricle, the bodies of the infero-medial and supero-lateral papillary muscles are sectioned. The predominant supero-lateral papillary muscle is located laterally, anchoring the middle part of the mitral leaflets. Another discrete small supero-lateral papillary muscle is located superior, anchoring the supero-lateral commissure. The infero-septal commissure is anchored by the infero-medial papillary muscle.

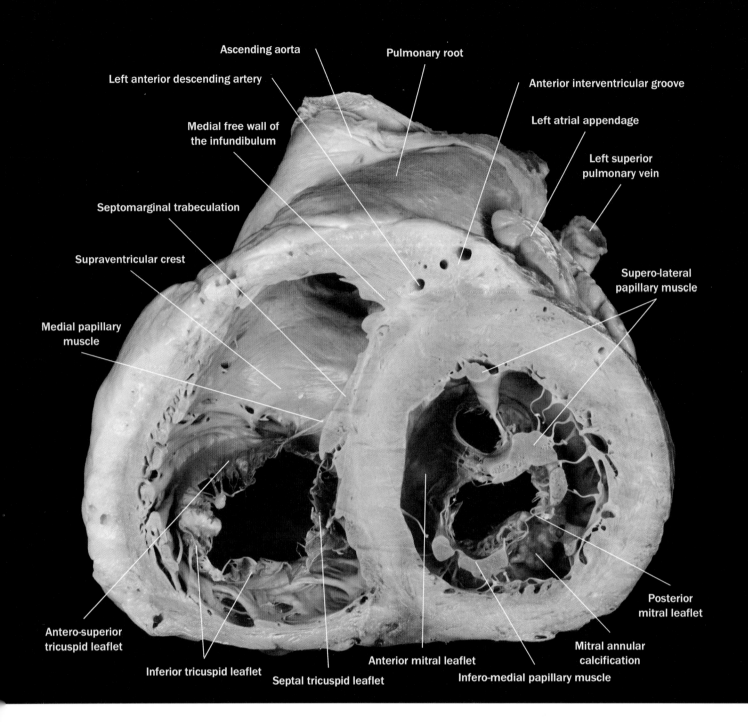

Ascending aorta

Pulmonary root

Left anterior descending artery

Anterior interventricular groove

Medial free wall of the infundibulum

Left atrial appendage

Left superior pulmonary vein

Septomarginal trabeculation

Supraventricular crest

Supero-lateral papillary muscle

Medial papillary muscle

Antero-superior tricuspid leaflet

Posterior mitral leaflet

Inferior tricuspid leaflet

Septal tricuspid leaflet

Anterior mitral leaflet

Mitral annular calcification

Infero-medial papillary muscle

Figure 17 Progressive dissection images of the heart viewed from the left anterior oblique direction: Basal ventricular level. Anaglyph 6.

In the right ventricle, *en face* view of the tricuspid valve can be seen. The chordae tendineae of the medial papillary muscle located at the inferior limb of the septomarginal trabeculation anchor the medial part of the antero-superior tricuspid leaflet. The septomarginal trabeculation is observed as the localized bulging of the superior ventricular septum toward the right ventricle. The chordae tendineae of the anterior papillary muscle anchor the commissure between the antero-superior and inferior tricuspid leaflets. The supraventricular crest, corresponding to the postero-lateral free wall of the right ventricular outflow tract or ventriculo-infundibular fold, lies along the superior margin of the tricuspid valve annulus. Thus, it is located perpendicular to the septomarginal trabeculation. Its surface is smooth without trabeculations. The medial part of the supraventricular crest lies anterior to the right coronary aortic sinus. The supraventricular crest is

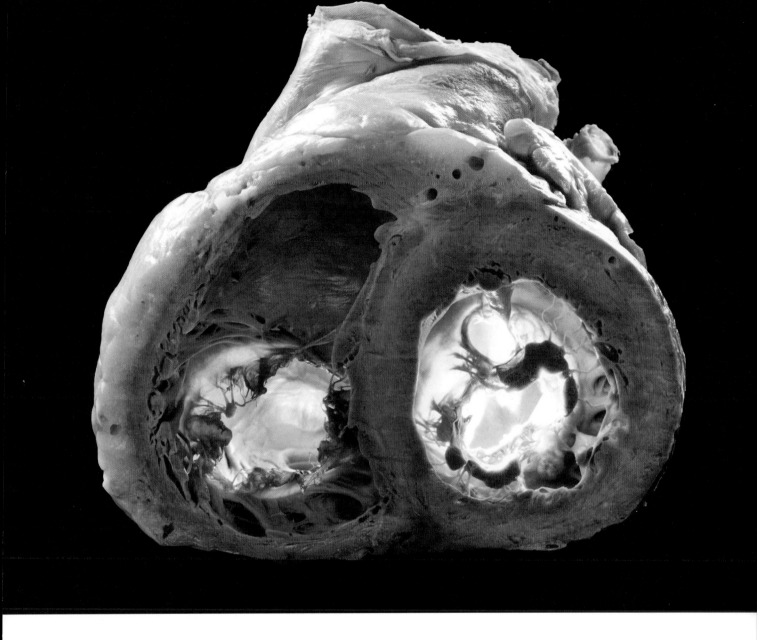

the part of inner curvature of the developing right heart. This separates the tricuspid valve from the pulmonary valve.[2] The medial part of the right ventricular outflow tract is not the septum, but the free wall adjacent to the left anterior descending artery running in the anterior interventricular groove. The apex of the left atrial appendage is adjacent to the pulmonary root, covering the superior to supero-lateral part of the basal left ventricle. In the left heart, multiple heads of the infero-medial and supero-lateral papillary muscles gives rise to chordae tendineae to infero-medial and supero-lateral halves of the both anterior and posterior mitral leaflets. The mitral annular calcification is observed at the attachment of the middle scallop of the posterior mitral leaflet.

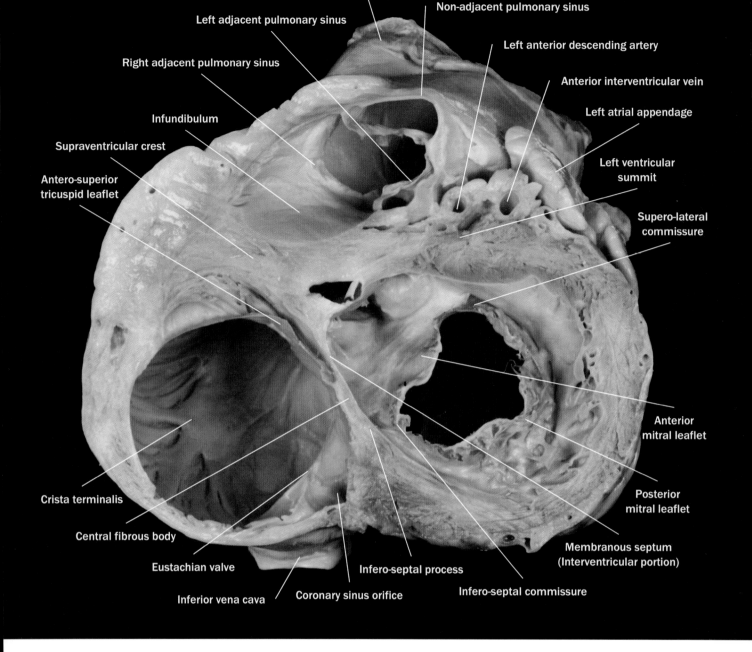

Non-adjacent pulmonary sinus

Left adjacent pulmonary sinus

Left anterior descending artery

Right adjacent pulmonary sinus

Anterior interventricular vein

Left atrial appendage

Infundibulum

Left ventricular summit

Supraventricular crest

Supero-lateral commissure

Antero-superior tricuspid leaflet

Anterior mitral leaflet

Crista terminalis

Posterior mitral leaflet

Central fibrous body

Membranous septum (Interventricular portion)

Eustachian valve

Infero-septal process

Inferior vena cava

Coronary sinus orifice

Infero-septal commissure

Figure 18 Progressive dissection images of the heart viewed from the left anterior oblique direction: Right atrioventricular junction level. 🔲🔳 Anaglyph 7.

As the tricuspid valve is located apical to the mitral valve, the right atrium is sectioned in this plane that shows the mitral valve annulus and basal left ventricle. In the right ventricle, the supraventricular crest is sectioned tangentially to show the right coronary aortic sinus located behind its medial part. The interventricular portion of the membranous septum separates the right ventricular inflow tracts from the left ventricular outflow tract. The infundibulum superior to the right coronary aortic sinus lacks trabeculations. The pulmonary root is located left antero-superior to the aortic root. The left adjacent pulmonary sinus is located most postero-inferior among the three pulmonary sinuses.[7] In the left ventricle, anterior and posterior mitral leaflets along with its infero-septal and supero-lateral commissures are observed. The interleaflet triangle between the left and non-coronary aortic sinuses is located central relative to the anterior mitral leaflet. Both commissures of the mitral leaflets do not reach the annulus. The aortic-to-mitral (aortomitral) continuity is the region between this interleaflet triangle and the hingeline of the anterior mitral leaflet, approximately corresponding to the line connecting both commissures. At the bilateral end of the aortic-to-mitral continuity, the right and left fibrous

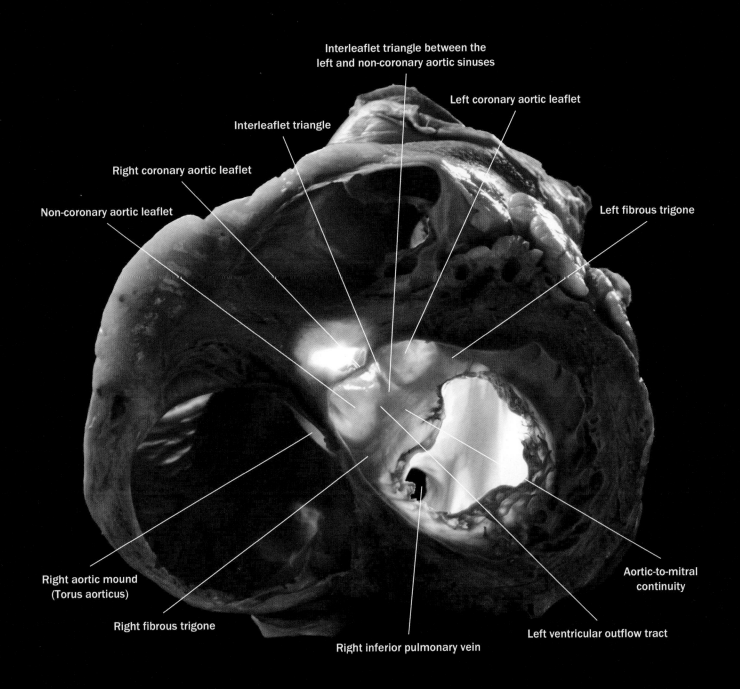

Interleaflet triangle between the
left and non-coronary aortic sinuses

Left coronary aortic leaflet

Interleaflet triangle

Right coronary aortic leaflet

Non-coronary aortic leaflet

Left fibrous trigone

Right aortic mound
(Torus aorticus)

Aortic-to-mitral
continuity

Right fibrous trigone

Right inferior pulmonary vein

Left ventricular outflow tract

trigones support the anterior mitral leaflet. The right and left fibrous trigones extend toward the infero-septal and supero-lateral commissures, respectively. Transillumination (right) shows the three coronary aortic sinuses/leaflets. Although the right and left coronary aortic sinuses are separated, this view is not appropriate to separate the non-coronary aortic sinus from the left and right coronary aortic sinuses.[8] The non-coronary aortic sinus is located most postero-inferior. Bulging of the non-coronary aortic sinus toward the right atrium is also transilluminated, which is referred to as the right aortic mound (torus aorticus).[9] The right aortic mound is, therefore, not the atrial septum, and it is located superior to the triangle of Koch. The basal superior part of the left ventricle supports the anterior half of the left coronary aortic sinus. The epicardial side is referred to as the left ventricular summit.[1,10] It is located superior to the supero-lateral commissure of the mitral valve. The left anterior descending artery and anterior interventricular vein is located within the epicardial adipose tissue on the left ventricular summit, covered by the left atrial appendage and pulmonary root.

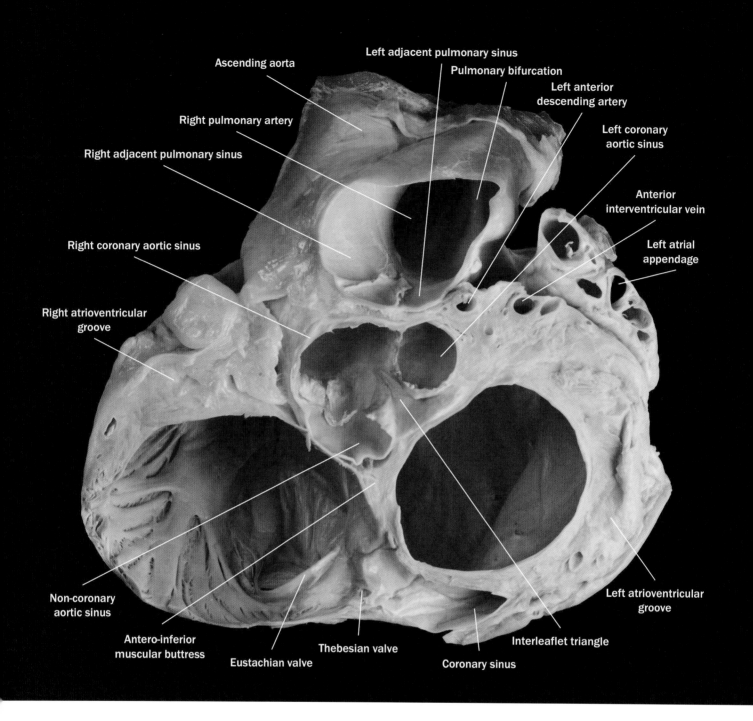

Figure 19 Progressive dissection images of the heart viewed from the left anterior oblique direction: Coronary sinus orifice level.

In the right atrium, the inferior end of the crista terminalis ramifies the pectinate muscles in fan-like fashion toward the Eustachian valve and right atrial vestibules. Due to the coronary sinus courses along the left atrioventricular groove inferior to the left atrium, the bottom of the left atrial vestibule is located superior relative to the bottom of the right atrial vestibule. The aortic root is located on the antero-superior interatrial groove. Thus, the non-coronary aortic sinus wedges between the both right and left atrial supero-medial free wall. The antero-inferior muscular buttress, also referred to as the anterior limbus of the fossa ovalis, is observed between the non-coronary aortic sinus and coronary sinus. This buttress is the true muscular atrial septum,[9] anchoring the primary septum at the floor of the fossa ovalis with the central fibrous body. The right and left coronary aortic sinuses are adjacent to the right and left adjacent pulmonary sinuses, respectively. The left anterior

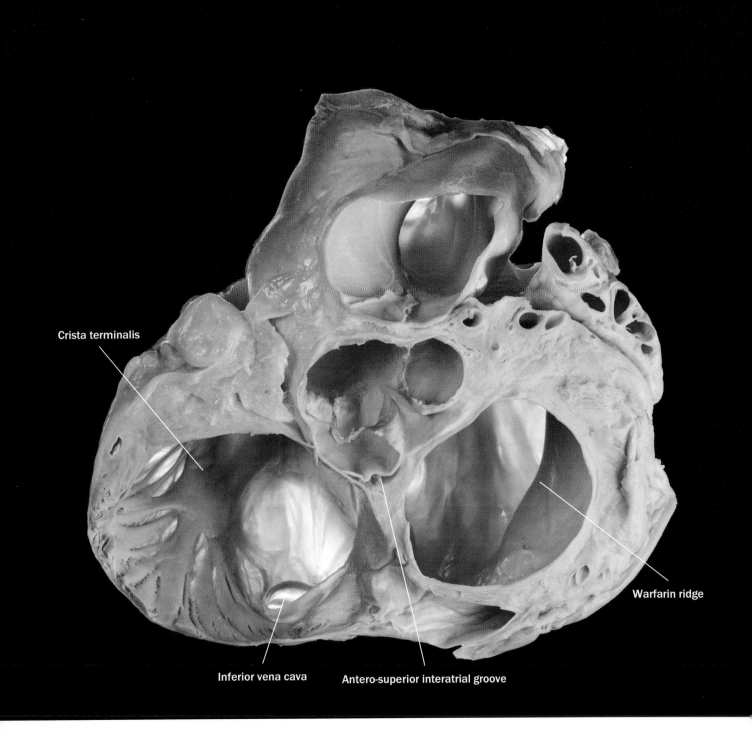

Crista terminalis

Inferior vena cava   Antero-superior interatrial groove

Warfarin ridge

descending artery is located adjacent to the left pulmonary aortic sinus overriding the aortic root. The Thebesian valve is located orthogonal to the Eustachian valve, guarding the orifice of the coronary sinus.[11] Transillumination (right) of the left atrial posterior wall enhances the existence of the warfarin ridge that is not transilluminated. This warfarin ridge, also referred to as the Coumadin ridge or left atrial ridge, is found between the left atrial appendage and the left pulmonary veins. The fold creating this ridge contains the vein of Marshall arising between the coronary sinus and the great cardiac vein. Transillumination reveals the paper-thin wall of the right atrial appendage between the pectinate muscles. Transillumination also reveals the thin posterior wall of the inferior sinus venarum (smooth) portion of the right atrium located superior to the orifice of the inferior vena cava.

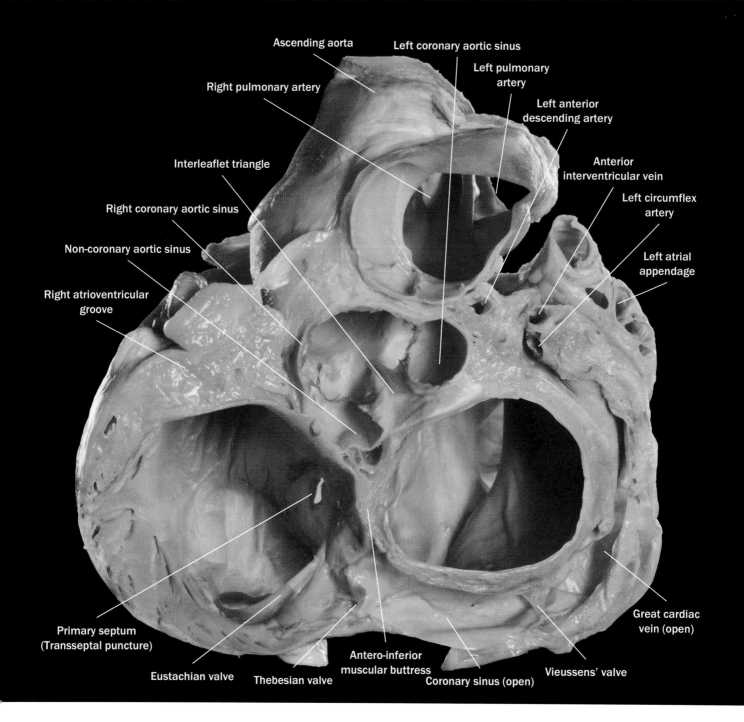

Figure 20 Progressive dissection images of the heart viewed from the left anterior oblique direction: Opening the coronary sinus and great cardiac vein. 🔲🟥 Anaglyph 8.

The hole created by transseptal puncture is observed at the superior part of the primary septum at the floor of the fossa ovalis. When the coronary sinus and great cardiac vein are open, the Vieussens' valve is observed at infero-lateral part of the left atrioventricular junction,[12] which demarcates the anatomical margin between the coronary sinus and the great cardiac vein. The orifice of the oblique vein (vein of Marshall) is located at the bottom of this valve.[13] As the coronary venous flow drains to the right atrium, the free margin of the valve is located at the coronary sinus side. Distal to the valve

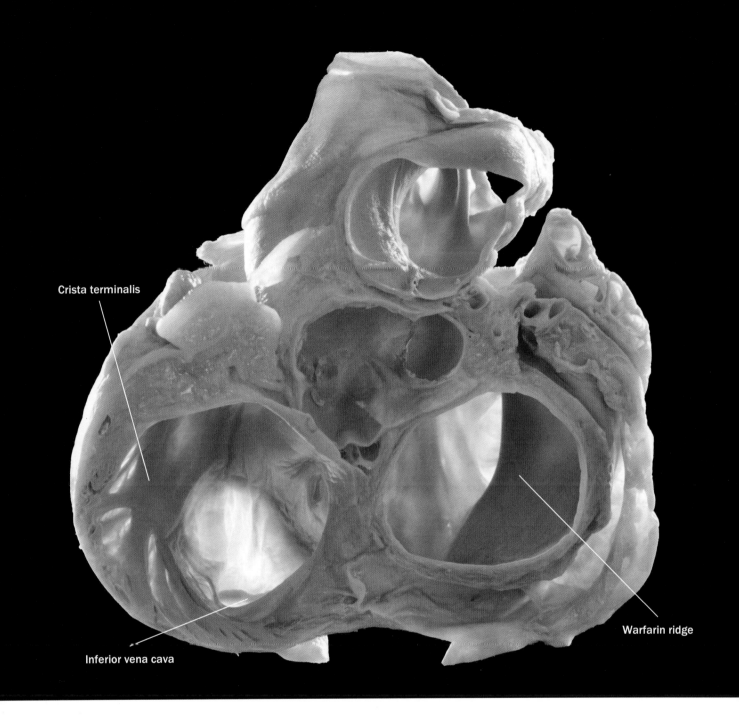

Crista terminalis

Inferior vena cava

Warfarin ridge

is the great cardiac vein. At the superior part of the left atrioventricular junction, inferior to the left atrial appendage, the vein runs inferior to the proximal circumflex artery, then overrides it from the atrial side. Then it becomes the anterior interventricular vein running toward the left ventricular summit along with the left anterior descending artery. Transillumination (right) shows the thin and smooth posterior wall of the inferior sinus venarum continuing to the orifice of the inferior vena cava.[14]

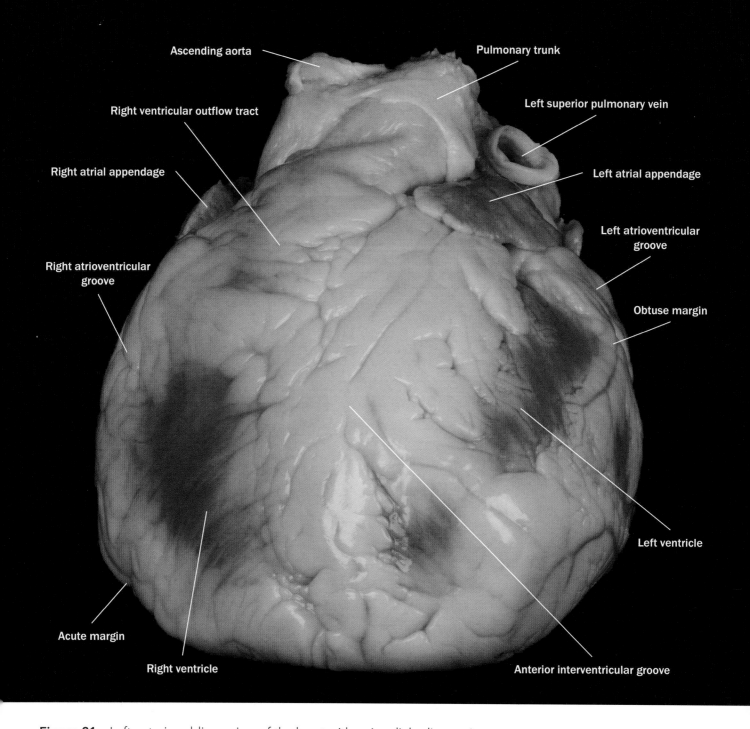

Figure 21 Left anterior oblique view of the heart with epicardial adipose tissue.

The right ventricular outflow tract crosses over the left ventricular outflow tract from the right antero-inferior direction to the left postero-superior direction. Rich epicardial adipose tissue is distributed along the coronary vessels, including the atrioventricular groove, anterior interventricular groove, and acute and obtuse margins. Localized regions in the right ventricular anterior free wall, left ventricular apical anterior wall, left ventricular basal-mid supero-lateral wall, and left ventricular basal-lateral wall lack the epicardial adipose tissue. The right and left atrial appendages are generally not covered by thick epicardial adipose tissue. Although the apex of the left atrial appendage is closely related to the basal superior left ventricle, it is independent of the adipose tissue of the left atrioventricular and anterior interventricular grooves, freely floating in the pericardial space.

References

1. McAlpine WA. Digitized collection of all the images created by Dr. McAlpine at UCLA. Copyright UCLA Cardiac Arrhythmia Center. Part of this collection appeared in *Heart and Coronary Arteries: An Anatomical Atlas for Clinical Diagnosis, Radiological Investigation, and Surgical Treatment*. New York: Springer-Verlag; 1975.
2. Mori S, Tretter JT, Spicer DE, et al. What is the real cardiac anatomy? *Clin Anat*. 2019;32:288–309.
3. Tretter JT, Sarwark AE, Anderson RH, et al. Assessment of the anatomical variation to be found in the normal tricuspid valve. *Clin Anat*. 2016;29:399–407.
4. Mori S, Fukuzawa K, Takaya T, et al. Clinical cardiac structural anatomy reconstructed within the cardiac contour using multi-detector-row computed tomography: Left ventricular outflow tract. *Clin Anat*. 2016;29:353–363.
5. Anderson RH, Spicer DE, Mori S. How best to describe the episcopal miter? *J Thorac Cardiovasc Surg*. 2017;154:1936–1937.
6. Mori S, Hanna P, Dacey MJ, et al. Comprehensive anatomy of the pericardial space and the cardiac hilum: Anatomical dissections with Intact pericardium. *JACC Cardiovasc Imaging*. 2021. DOI: 10.1016/j.jcmg.2021.04.016. Online ahead of print.
7. Mori S, Fukuzawa K, Takaya T, et al. Clinical cardiac structural anatomy reconstructed within the cardiac contour using multi-detector-row computed tomography: The arrangement and location of the cardiac valves. *Clin Anat*. 2016;29:364–370.
8. Mori S, Fukuzawa K, Takaya T, et al. Optimal angulations for obtaining an *en face* view of each coronary aortic sinus and the interventricular septum: Correlative anatomy around the left ventricular outflow tract. *Clin Anat*. 2015;28:494–505.
9. Mori S, Nishii T, Tretter JT, et al. Demonstration of living anatomy clarifies the morphology of interatrial communications. *Heart*. 2018;104:2003–2009.
10. Yamada T, McElderry HT, Doppalapudi H, et al. Idiopathic ventricular arrhythmias originating from the left ventricular summit: Anatomic concepts relevant to ablation. *Circ Arrhythm Electrophysiol*. 2010;3:616–623.
11. Katti K, Patil NP. The Thebesian valve: Gatekeeper to the coronary sinus. *Clin Anat*. 2012;25:379–385.
12. Zawadzki M, Pietrasik A, Pietrasik K, et al. Endoscopic study of the morphology of Vieussens' valve. *Clin Anat*. 2004;17: 318–321.
13. Marshall J. On the development of the great anterior veins in man and mammalia: Including an account of certain remnants of foetal structure found in the adult, a comparative view of these great veins in the different mammalia, and an analysis of their occasional peculiarities in the human subject. *Phil Trans R Soc Lond*. 1850;140:133–169.
14. Igawa O. Focus on the atrial structure: Useful anatomical information for catheter ablation. *J Arrhythm*. 2011;27:268–288.

4

The Heart in Relation to Electrocardiography

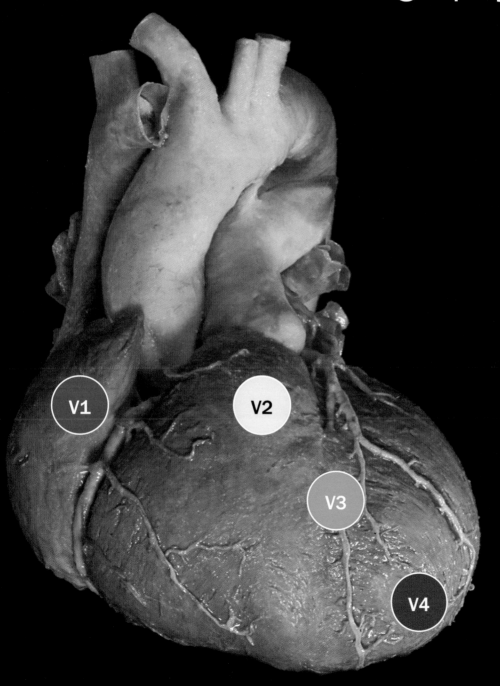

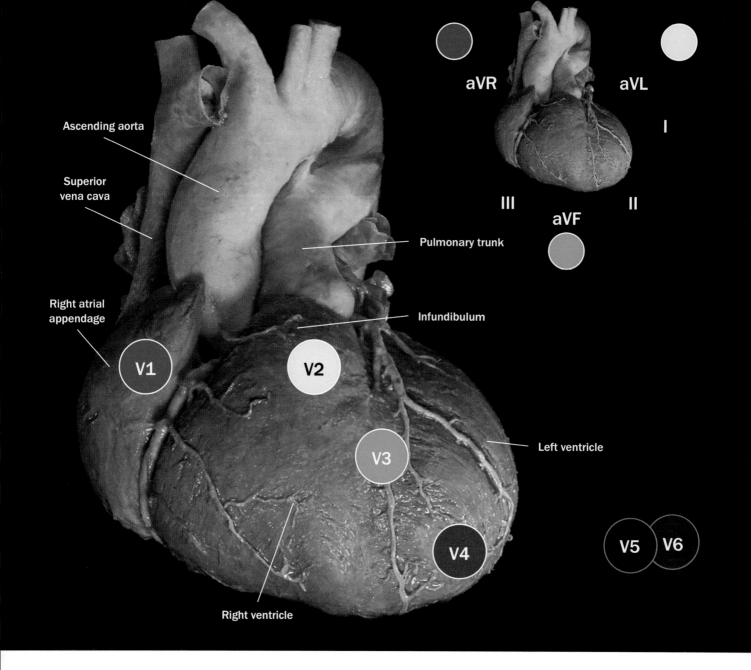

Figure 22 The heart and standard electrocardiographic electrodes viewed from the anterior direction.[1]

The standard limb (upper right) and precordial (left) electrodes are overlaid on the heart viewed from the anterior direction. Generally, the V1 and V2 electrodes are located anterior to the right atrial appendage and right ventricular outflow tract, respectively.[2] The V4 electrode is located left anterior to the cardiac apex. The limb leads I, II, and III are bipolar recordings using the right arm, right arm, and left arm as a negative, or reference, inputs, respectively. Bipolar recordings measure the difference in potential between two electrodes, showing the relative electrical potential as the vector. The precordial leads are unipolar recordings using the Wilson central terminal, the compound outputs of the left arm, right arm, and left leg, as a reference inputs. aVR, aVL, and aVF limb leads are augmented unipolar recordings using the compound outputs from left arm and leg, right arm and left leg, and left and right arm, as a negative inputs, respectively. Unipolar recordings measure absolute electrical potential at a single site relative to the potential at reference site that is deemed to be zero. Individually variable cardiac and thoracic anatomy are the major determinants to affect QRS complex, including the location of the heart, conduction tissue around the heart, shape of the heart, anatomy of the conduction system,[3] in addition to electrical features, including complicated propagation of the excitation[4] and cancellation of electrical forces.[5] Any simple frontal plane as well as horizontal or sagittal plane cannot precisely represent the three-dimensional anatomical axis of the ventricular mass directing from the right postero-superior direction toward the left antero-inferior direction. In addition, there are significant individual variations in the orientation of the heart[6] and its three-dimensional relationship between the electrodes. Therefore, three-dimensional anatomical axis does not necessarily show the good correlation with electrical QRS-axis evaluated on the selected frontal or horizontal planes.[7] Precise appreciation of individual three-dimensional anatomical relationship between the heart and electrodes is fundamental. However, considering significant individual variations in anatomy and complex three-dimensional electrical forces,[8] full understanding of the individual electrocardiogram still requires further sophisticated approach.

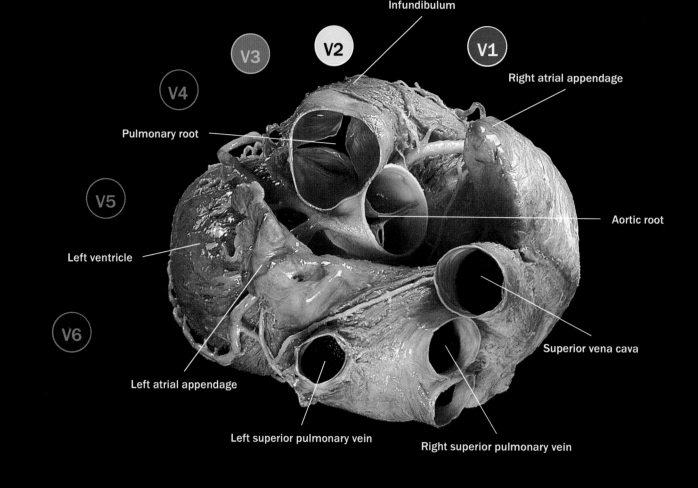

Infundibulum

V3 V2 V1

Right atrial appendage

Pulmonary root

Aortic root

V5

Left ventricle

V6

Superior vena cava

Left atrial appendage

Left superior pulmonary vein

Right superior pulmonary vein

Figure 23 The whole heart and precordial electrodes viewed from the superior direction.[1]

The precordial electrodes are overlaid on the heart viewed from the superior direction. Although this kind of horizontal two-dimensional image is frequently illustrated with all precordial electrodes, it is axiomatic that the electrodes are not located on the same flat horizontal plane. The plane involving the V3 electrode, the plane involving the V4–V6 electrodes are different from the plane involving the V1 and V2 electrodes. The V1, V2, and V4 electrodes are located anterior to the right atrial appendage, right ventricular outflow tract (infundibulum), and cardiac apex, respectively. The V5 and V6 electrodes are commonly distant from the heart with the left lung intervening.

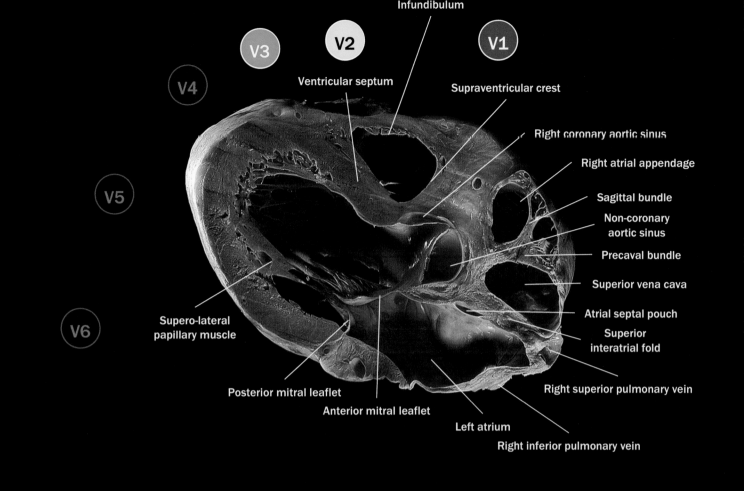

Figure 24 The heart and precordial electrodes: The horizontal plane at the level between the V1–V2 and V3 electrodes.[1]

The precordial electrodes are overlaid on the heart viewed from the superior direction. As this horizontal section shows the level between the V1–V2 and V3 electrodes, V4–V6 electrodes located inferior to this sectional plane are masked. The V1 and V2 electrodes are located anterior to the right atrial appendage and right ventricular outflow tract (infundibulum), respectively. The V3 electrode is located on the extending line of the superior ventricular septum. The right ventricular outflow tract is located anterior to the left ventricular outflow tract and left anterior to the aortic root. When viewing the left posterior direction from the V1, the basal-lateral wall of the right ventricular outflow tract is the closest, followed by the basal superior ventricular septum, and the supero-lateral free wall of the left ventricle. The supraventricular crest at the superior tricuspid annulus directs toward the V1 from the region anterior to the nadir of the right coronary aortic sinus. Similarly, when viewing the posterior direction from the V1, the right atrial appendage is the closest, followed by the pre-caval bundle, also referred to as the arcuate ridge, the superior vena cava, the superior interatrial fold superior to the fossa ovalis, and the right superior pulmonary vein.

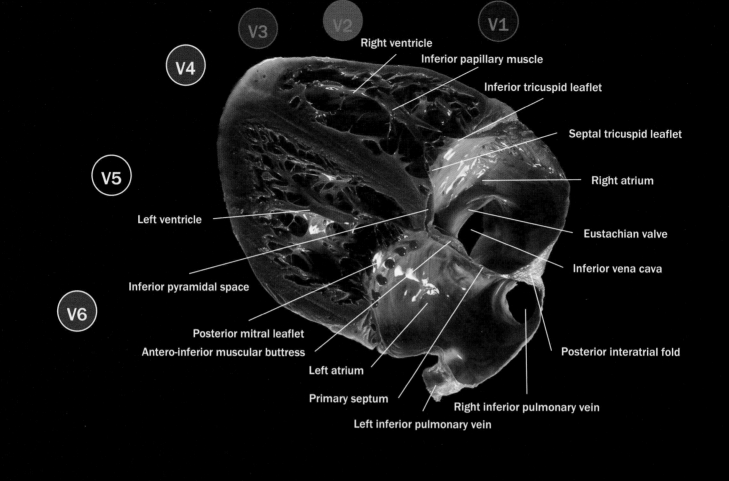

V3 V2 V1

V4

Right ventricle

Inferior papillary muscle

Inferior tricuspid leaflet

Septal tricuspid leaflet

V5

Right atrium

Left ventricle

Eustachian valve

Inferior vena cava

Inferior pyramidal space

V6

Posterior mitral leaflet

Antero-inferior muscular buttress

Posterior interatrial fold

Left atrium

Primary septum

Right inferior pulmonary vein

Left inferior pulmonary vein

Figure 25 The heart and precordial electrodes: The horizontal plane at the level of the V4–V6 electrodes.[1]

The heart shows an apical four-chamber image. The precordial electrodes are overlaid on the heart viewed from the superior direction. As this section is the level of the V4–V6 electrodes, V1–V3 electrodes located superior to this sectional plane are masked. The V4 electrode is located left anterior to the cardiac apex on the extending line of the inferior ventricular septum. Compared to V1 to V4 electrodes, the distance from the V5 and V6 electrodes to the heart is greater because of the intervening left lung. Generally, when considering the QRS-wave morphology of the ventricular arrhythmia, the difference in the vertical location between the V1–V2 and V4–V6 electrodes are not well appreciated and tend to be described as if they are located on the same flat plane in many simplified illustrations. However, this vertical difference matters as the electrical current should propagate three-dimensionally. For example, ventricular arrhythmia originating from the basal ventricular septum on this inferior plane,[9] corresponding to the infero-septal process[10] or infero-septal mitral annulus,[11] generally demonstrates R-wave predominance in every V1–V6 electrode as the region is distant from the V1–V6 electrodes. On the contrary, ventricular arrhythmia originating from the basal ventricular septum on the previous superior plane, corresponding to the septal left ventricular outflow tract[12] and the crest of the ventricular septum supporting the right coronary aortic sinus,[13] generally demonstrates S-wave predominance in V1 and V2 electrodes, as the focus gets closer to the V1 and V2 in the plane. To achieve R-wave predominance in every V1–V6 electrode on/above this superior plane, the arrhythmogenic foci need to be located away from the V1 and V2 electrodes toward the left posterior direction along the left ventricular outflow tract and mitral annulus. These foci correspond to the left ventricular basal superior free wall supporting the anterior half of the left coronary aortic sinus,[14] left ventricular summit,[15] and superior and supero-lateral mitral annulus;[11] all the regions are known to show precordial R-wave predominance. This focus shift from the basal superior ventricular septum toward the basal supero-lateral free wall has less effect on R-wave predominance observed in the V4–V6 electrodes, as the V4–V6 electrodes are located on the different inferior plane consistently distant from these superior foci. However, due to this focus shift from the basal superior ventricular septum toward the supero-lateral (left posterior) direction, the V5 and V6 electrodes show s waves combined with a decrease in R-wave amplitude.[16,17]

References

1. McAlpine WA. Digitized collection of all the images created by Dr. McAlpine at UCLA. Copyright UCLA Cardiac Arrhythmia Center. Part of this collection appeared in *Heart and Coronary Arteries: An Anatomical Atlas for Clinical Diagnosis, Radiological Investigation, and Surgical Treatment*. New York: Springer-Verlag; 1975.

2. Mori S, Izawa Y, Nishii T. Simple stereoscopic display of three-dimensional living heart anatomy relevant to electrophysiological practice. *JACC Clin Electrophysiol*. 2020;6:1473–1477.

3. Katz LN. Clinical electrocardiography—its present position and possible potentialities. *Circulation*. 1950;2:94–110.

4. Durrer D, van Dam RT, Freud GE, et al. Total excitation of the isolated human heart. *Circulation*. 1970;41:899–912.

5. Abildskov JA, Klein RM. Cancellation of electrocardiographic effects during ventricular excitation. *Sogo Rinsho*. 1962;11:247–251.

6. Fowler NO, Braunstein JR. Anatomic and electrocardiographic position of the heart. *Circulation*. 1951;3:906–910.

7. Engblom H, Foster JE, Martin TN, et al. The relationship between electrical axis by 12-lead electrocardiogram and anatomical axis of the heart by cardiac magnetic resonance in healthy subjects. *Am Heart J*. 2005;150:507–512.

8. Arntzenius AC. A Geometrical model of successive stages in excitation of the human heart; its value as a link between excitation and clinical vectorcardiography. *Cardiovasc Res*. 1969;3:198–208.

9. Liang JJ, Shirai Y, Briceño DF, et al. Electrocardiographic and electrophysiologic characteristics of idiopathic ventricular arrhythmias originating from the basal inferoseptal left ventricle. *JACC Clin Electrophysiol*. 2019;5:833–842.

10. Li A, Zuberi Z, Bradfield JS, et al. Endocardial ablation of ventricular ectopic beats arising from the basal inferoseptal process of the left ventricle. *Heart Rhythm*. 2018;15:1356–1362.

11. Tada H, Ito S, Naito S, et al. Idiopathic ventricular arrhythmia arising from the mitral annulus: a distinct subgroup of idiopathic ventricular arrhythmias. *J Am Coll Cardiol*. 2005;45:877–886.

12. Yokokawa M, Good E, Chugh A. Intramural idiopathic ventricular arrhythmias originating in the intraventricular septum: Mapping and ablation. *Circ Arrhythm Electrophysiol*. 2012;5:258–263.

13. Wang Y, Liang Z, Wu S, et al. Idiopathic ventricular arrhythmias originating from the right coronary sinus: Prevalence, electrocardiographic and electrophysiological characteristics, and catheter ablation. *Heart Rhythm*. 2018;15:81–89.

14. Lin D, Ilkhanoff L, Gerstenfeld E, et al. Twelve-lead electrocardiographic characteristics of the aortic cusp region guided by intracardiac echocardiography and electroanatomic mapping. *Heart Rhythm*. 2008;5:663–669.

15. Yamada T, McElderry HT, Doppalapudi H, et al. Idiopathic ventricular arrhythmias originating from the left ventricular summit: Anatomic concepts relevant to ablation. *Circ Arrhythm Electrophysiol*. 2010;3:616–623.

16. Kumagai K, Yamauchi Y, Takahashi A, et al. Idiopathic left ventricular tachycardia originating from the mitral annulus. *J Cardiovasc Electrophysiol*. 2005;16:1029–1036.

17. Yue-Chun L, Cheng Z, Jun H, et al. Catheter ablation of idiopathic premature ventricular contractions and ventricular tachycardias originating from the vicinity of endocardial and epicardial mitral annulus. *PLoS One*. 2013;8:e80777.

5

Sinus Venarum

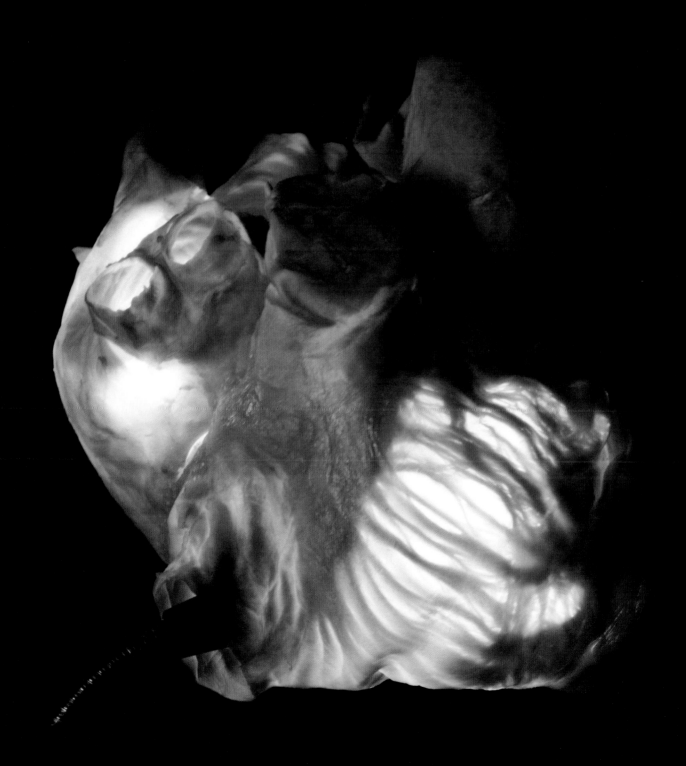

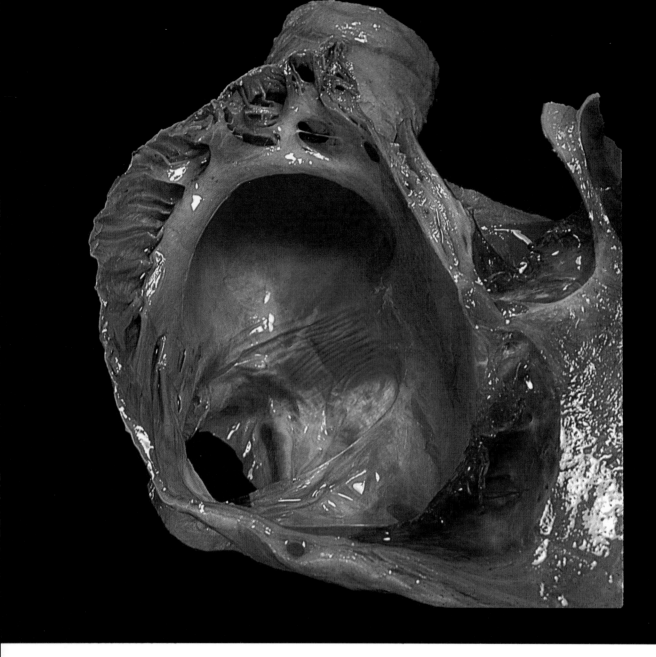

Figure 26 The internal aspect of the sinus venarum viewed from the right anterior oblique direction.[1]

The sinus venarum extends between the superior and inferior vena cava vertically. The crista terminalis is approximately 5 mm thick and 8 mm wide.[2] It demarcates the lateral margin of the sinus venarum, separated from the right atrial appendage. It shows a characteristic arcuate-shape anterior to the orifice of the superior vena cava.[3] This transverse part of the crista terminalis is referred to as the precaval bundle, or the arcuate ridge. The precaval bundle is then confluent with the Bachmann's bundle medially.[2] The Bachmann's bundle traverse on the anterior wall of the left atrium,[4] posterior to the

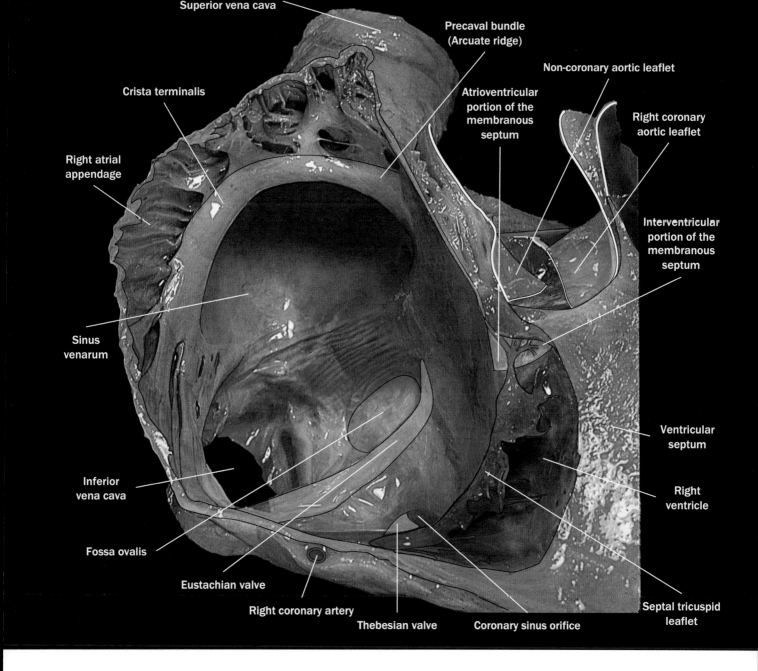

Superior vena cava

Precaval bundle
(Arcuate ridge)

Non-coronary aortic leaflet

Crista terminalis

Atrioventricular
portion of the
membranous
septum

Right coronary
aortic leaflet

Right atrial
appendage

Interventricular
portion of the
membranous
septum

Sinus
venarum

Ventricular
septum

Inferior
vena cava

Right
ventricle

Fossa ovalis

Eustachian valve

Septal tricuspid
leaflet

Right coronary artery

Thebesian valve

Coronary sinus orifice

aortic root and the transverse sinus. From the endocardial side, no discrete boarder is discerned to define the medial extent of the sinus venarum. The smooth endocardial surface of the sinus venarum continues toward the posterior rim of the fossa ovalis. The posterior rim of the fossa ovalis is not the septum but the posterior interatrial fold/groove, also referred to as the secondary septum. The anterior orifice of the inferior vena cava is guarded by the Eustachian valve.

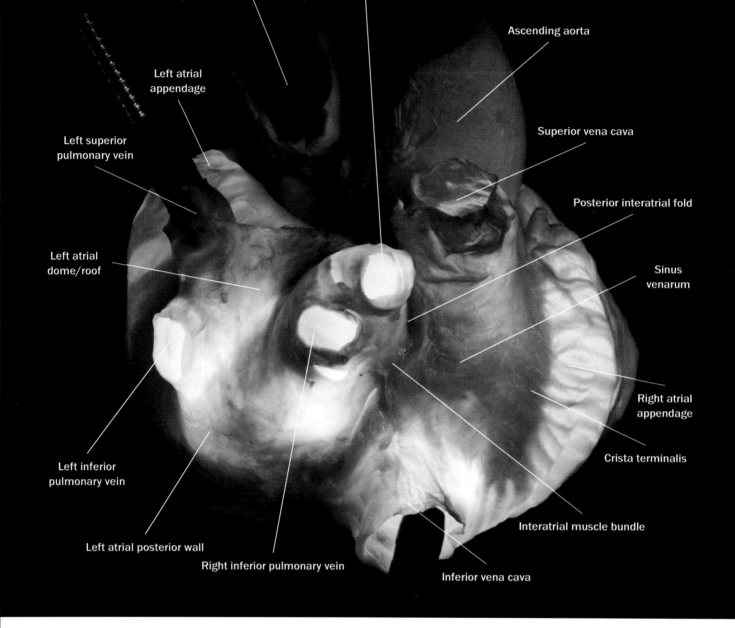

Left atrial
appendage

Left superior
pulmonary vein

Left atrial
dome/roof

Left inferior
pulmonary vein

Left atrial posterior wall

Right inferior pulmonary vein

Ascending aorta

Superior vena cava

Posterior interatrial fold

Sinus
venarum

Right atrial
appendage

Crista terminalis

Interatrial muscle bundle

Inferior vena cava

Figure 27 The external aspect of the sinus venarum visualized with transillumination.

The hearts are viewed from the right posterior (left) and right lateral (right) directions. The sinus venarum lacks pectinate muscle. It extends between the superior and inferior vena cava vertically. From the external side, the horizontal extent of the sinus venarum can be determined between the posterior interatrial fold/groove and terminal groove. Thus, the sinus venarum is a free wall. The superior and posterior interatrial fold is referred to as the Waterston's groove or Sondergaard's groove.[5] This groove is one of the access routes to the left atrium during mitral valve surgery without entering into the right atrium. This posterior interatrial fold is not exactly a vertical structure, but generally tilts toward the right atrium. Therefore, the left atrium leans against the right atrium. Thus, the orifice of the inferior vena cava is

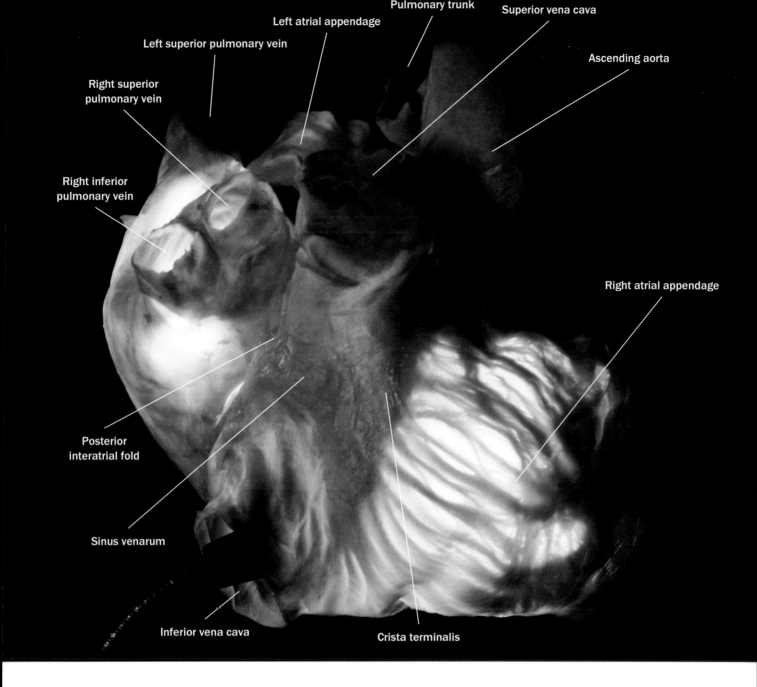

Pulmonary trunk

Left atrial appendage

Superior vena cava

Left superior pulmonary vein

Ascending aorta

Right superior pulmonary vein

Right inferior pulmonary vein

Right atrial appendage

Posterior interatrial fold

Sinus venarum

Inferior vena cava

Crista terminalis

located medial relative to the orifice of the superior vena cava. The thickness of the wall of the sinus venarum is not uniform. The wedge-shaped thinning region is observed superior to the orifice of the inferior vena cava.[6] The superior to middle part of the crista terminalis gives rise to multiple pectinate muscles running orthogonally toward the right atrial vestibule. Inferiorly, the crista terminalis ramifies into several pectinate muscles in a fan-like fashion. At the middle part of the sinus venarum, interatrial muscle bundle bridges the posterior interatrial fold. This epicardial bundle connects the sinus venarum with the anterior antrum of the right pulmonary veins.[7]

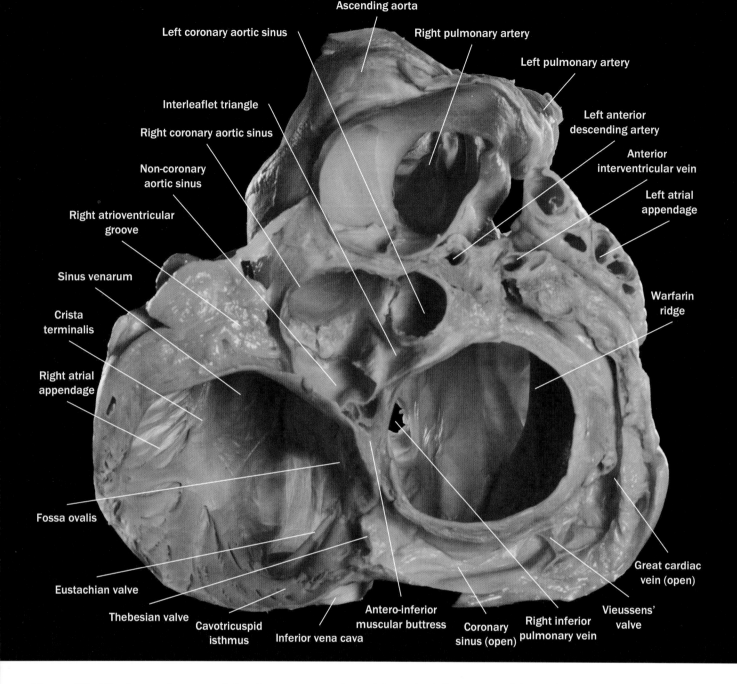

Ascending aorta

Left coronary aortic sinus

Right pulmonary artery

Left pulmonary artery

Interleaflet triangle

Right coronary aortic sinus

Non-coronary aortic sinus

Right atrioventricular groove

Sinus venarum

Crista terminalis

Right atrial appendage

Fossa ovalis

Eustachian valve

Thebesian valve

Cavotricuspid isthmus

Inferior vena cava

Antero-inferior muscular buttress

Coronary sinus (open)

Right inferior pulmonary vein

Vieussens' valve

Great cardiac vein (open)

Warfarin ridge

Left atrial appendage

Anterior interventricular vein

Left anterior descending artery

Figure 28   The internal aspect of the sinus venarum viewed from the left anterior oblique direction.

From this direction, the *en face* view of the sinus venarum extending between the crista terminalis and posterior interatrial fold is observed. Superior to the orifice of the inferior vena cava, the right posterior wall of the sinus venarum shows a wedge-shaped thinning where it is transilluminated. Laterally, the crista terminalis descends and ramifies into multiple fan-like pectinate muscles toward the infero-lateral to infero-medial right atrial vestibule. Therefore, the pectinate muscles run within the cavotricuspid isthmus in an oblique fashion. This alignment creates non-uniform feature of the isthmus,[5] in terms of direction of pectinate muscles and wall thickness. The orifice of the inferior vena cava is located medial just next to the atrial septum. It is guarded by the Eustachian valve anteriorly. The atrial septum tilts toward the right atrium.

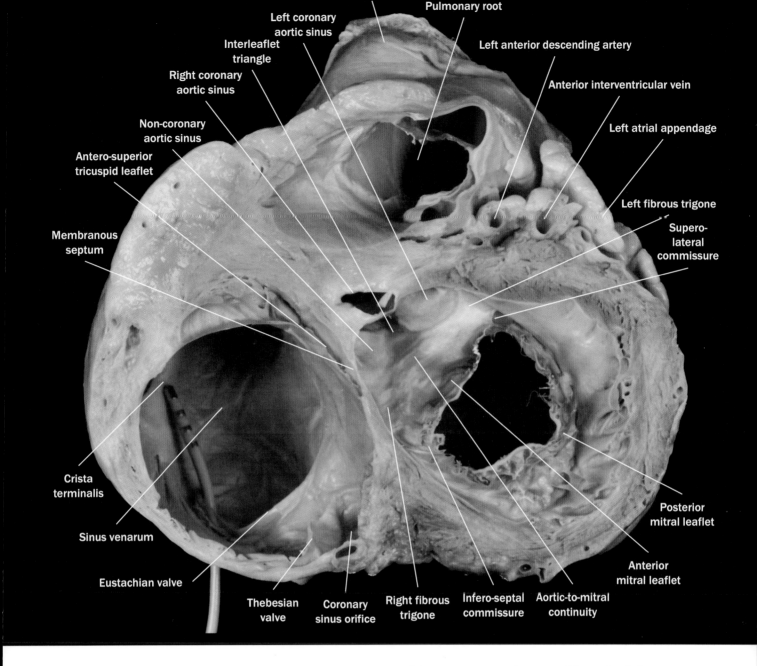

Figure 29 The ablation catheter placed on the middle part of the crista terminalis viewed from the left anterior oblique direction.

The catheter is placed on the middle part of the crista terminalis running vertically at the lateral margin of the sinus venarum. The crista terminalis, when viewed and mapped using this direction, is located medial relative to the lateral border of the cardiac silhouette, with the tip directing away from the observer. From the right atrial appendage, counterclockwise rotation torque of the catheter is necessary to reach the crista terminalis.[8] Further torque enables one to trace the right posterior wall of the sinus venarum, when using transfemoral venous approach. When ablating the lateral to posterior sinus venarum, care for the phrenic nerve is necessary.[9] The right phrenic nerve generally descends on the pericardium close to the crista terminalis and sinus venarum, anterior to the right pulmonary hilum.[10]

References

1. McAlpine WA. Digitized collection of all the images created by Dr. McAlpine at UCLA. Copyright UCLA Cardiac Arrhythmia Center. Part of this collection appeared in *Heart and Coronary Arteries: An Anatomical Atlas for Clinical Diagnosis, Radiological Investigation, and Surgical Treatment.* New York: Springer-Verlag; 1975.

2. Sánchez-Quintana D, Anderson RH, Cabrera JA, et al. The terminal crest: Morphological features relevant to electrophysiology. *Heart.* 2002;88:406–411.

3. Farré J, Anderson RH, Cabrera JA, et al. Fluoroscopic cardiac anatomy for catheter ablation of tachycardia. *Pacing Clin Electrophysiol.* 2002;25:76–94.

4. Pashakhanloo F, Herzka DA, Ashikaga H, et al. Myofiber architecture of the human atria as revealed by submillimeter diffusion tensor imaging. *Circ Arrhythm Electrophysiol.* 2016;9:e004133.

5. Ho SY, Anderson RH, Sánchez-Quintana D. Atrial structure and fibres: Morphologic bases of atrial conduction. *Cardiovasc Res.* 2002;54:325–336.

6. Igawa O. Focus on the atrial structure: Useful anatomical information for catheter ablation. *J Arrhythm.* 2011;27:268–288.

7. Ho SY, Cabrera JA, Sánchez-Quintana D. Left atrial anatomy revisited. *Circ Arrhythm Electrophysiol.* 2012;5:220–228.

8. Marchlinski FE, Ren JF, Schwartzman D, et al. Accuracy of fluoroscopic localization of the crista terminalis documented by intracardiac echocardiography. *J Interv Card Electrophysiol.* 2000;4:415–421.

9. Misher J, Zeitlin J, Khan M, et al. Novel technique to avoid diaphragmatic paralysis during focal ablation of a non-pulmonary vein trigger mapped to the crista terminalis. *Heart Rhythm Case Rep.* 2017;3:536–538.

10. Mori S, Hanna P, Dacey MJ, et al. Comprehensive anatomy of the pericardial space and the cardiac hilum: Anatomical dissections with intact pericardium. *JACC Cardiovasc Imaging.* 2021. DOI: 10.1016/j.jcmg.2021.04.016. Online ahead of print.

6

Fossa Ovalis

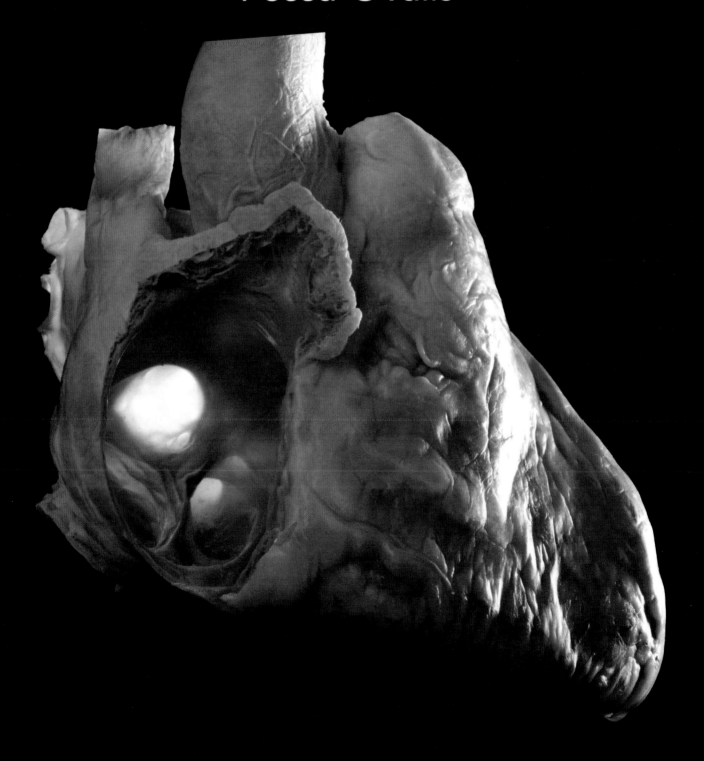

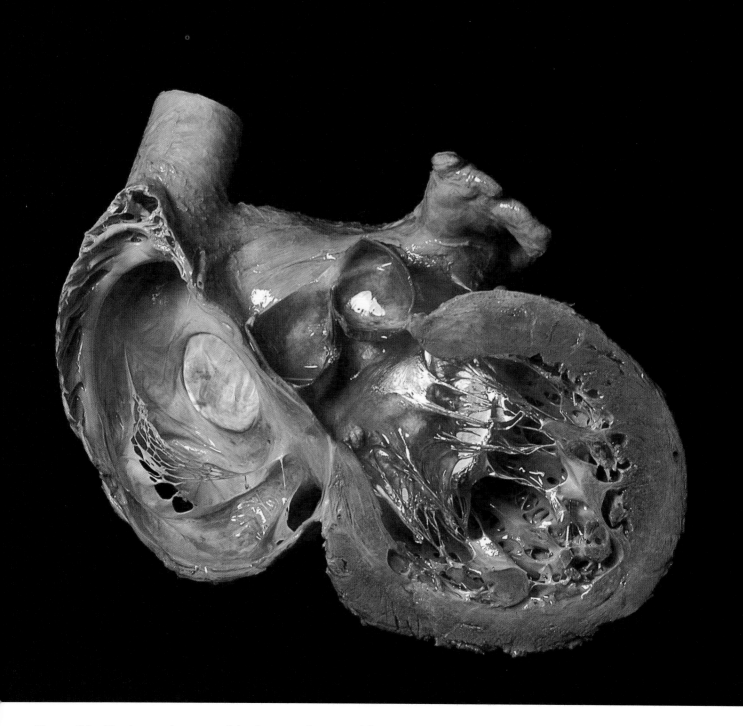

Figure 30 The internal aspect of the fossa ovalis viewed from the anterior direction.[1]

The primary septum is located at the floor of the fossa ovalis. The atrial septum physiologically tilts toward the right atrium. The extent of this tilting is affected by the multiple factors, including age, body shape, size of the left atrium, tilting of the aortic root, shape of the heart, and rotation of the heart along its longitudinal axis. Generally, young and lean patients with vertical hearts show less tilting, compared to elderly and obese patients with horizontal hearts. This physiological tilt brings the fossa ovalis superior to the orifice of the inferior vena cava like a roof. However, as this roof is not horizontal but oblique, the majority of the transseptal punctures are eventually created at the site near the superior rim of the fossa ovalis.[2] The pushing force applied to the system causes the needle tip to slip superiorly, when using conventional needle via transfemoral venous approach. A less-tilted primary septum increases the difficulty of the puncture. In that case, it requires additional curve to the needle to prevent superior slip of the system. The radiofrequency needle is a promising alternative to avoid the superior shift of the puncture site and facilitate safe and smooth procedure.[3] The primary septum at the floor of the fossa

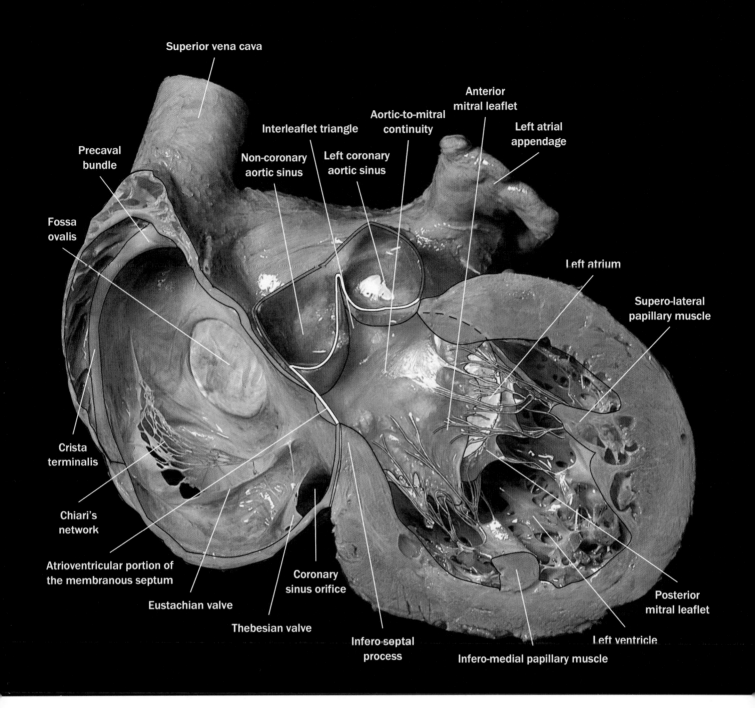

Superior vena cava

Precaval
bundle

Fossa
ovalis

Interleaflet triangle

Non-coronary
aortic sinus

Left coronary
aortic sinus

Aortic-to-mitral
continuity

Anterior
mitral leaflet

Left atrial
appendage

Left atrium

Supero-lateral
papillary muscle

Crista
terminalis

Chiari's
network

Atrioventricular portion of
the membranous septum

Eustachian valve

Thebesian valve

Coronary
sinus orifice

Infero-septal
process

Infero-medial papillary muscle

Posterior
mitral leaflet

Left ventricle

ovalis is surrounded by the interatrial fold, except the anterior limbus. This anterior limbus is a muscular component of the atrial septum, referred to as the antero-inferior muscular buttress derived from the vestibular spine.[4] The buttress connects the primary septum to the central fibrous body at the bottom of the non-coronary aortic sinus. This antero-inferior muscular buttress and the primary septum at the floor of the fossa ovalis are the only anatomical true atrial septum, defined as the non-folding single partition between both atria.[5] Chiari's network is observed in continuity with the Eustachian valve. It is found in approximately one-tenth of the dissected hearts.[6] The non-coronary aortic sinus is located left anterior to the fossa ovalis. Therefore, conventionally, the pig-tail catheter placed in the non-coronary aortic sinus[7] or His catheter[8] can be used as a good indicator to facilitate safe transseptal puncture. However, the relationship between the fossa ovalis and the aortic root varies according to the extent of wedging of the aortic root.[9] The paired section of this image is Figure 122.

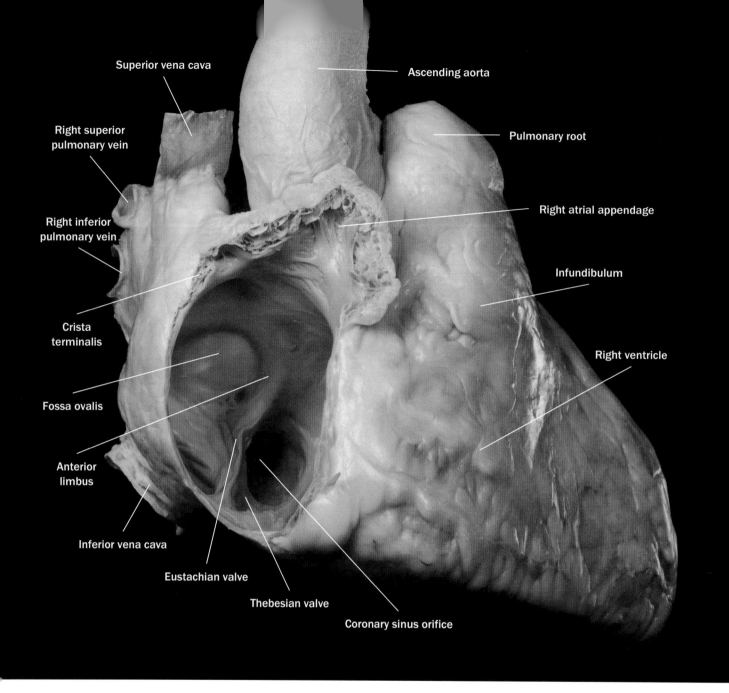

Figure 31   The medial aspect of the right atrium viewed from the right anterior oblique direction. 👓 Anaglyph 9.

The lateral wall of the right atrial appendage is removed. The right posterior edge of this sectional line corresponds to the anterior margin of the crista terminalis. Nearly *en face* views of the fossa ovalis,[10] the orifice of the coronary sinus, and Thebesian valve are observed; although, the fossa ovalis tilts inferior. The fossa ovalis is built up like an oblique roof against the orifice of the inferior vena cava. In contrast, the Eustachian valve/ridge is seen tangentially guarding the anterior orifice of the inferior vena cava. The light source from the left atrium (right) transilluminates the primary septum, antero-inferior muscular buttress, coronary sinus, and floor of the triangle of Koch. The right aortic mound

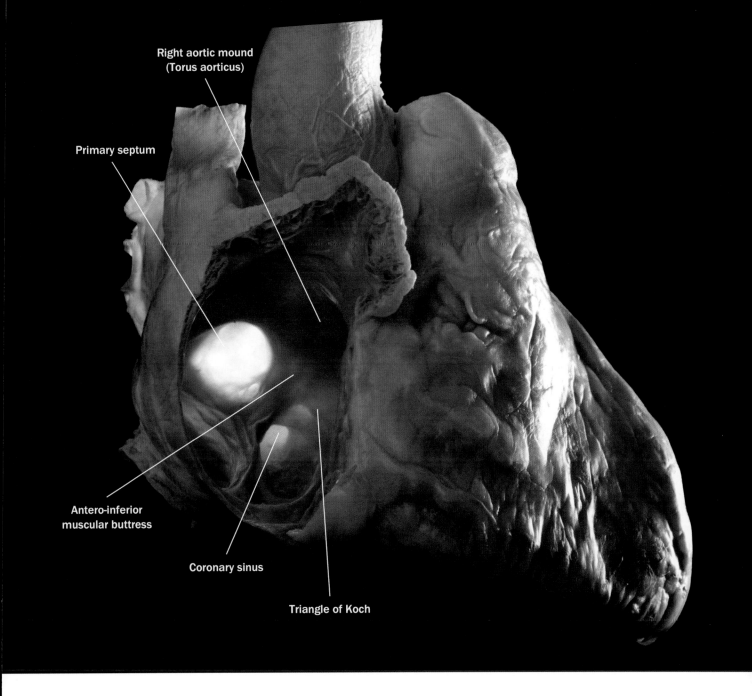

Right aortic mound
(Torus aorticus)

Primary septum

Antero-inferior
muscular buttress

Coronary sinus

Triangle of Koch

shows a negative transillumination left anterior to the fossa ovalis and superior to the coronary sinus orifice. As it is the imprint of the anterior half of the non-coronary aortic sinus bulging into the right atrium, this medial free wall of the right atrial appendage should not be deemed as the high atrial septum. The proximity of the fossa ovalis and this aortic mound is important to estimate the potential risk of injuring the aortic root during the implantation of an occlusion device to the *ostium secundum* defect or patent foramen ovale.[11,12] Refer to Figure 10.

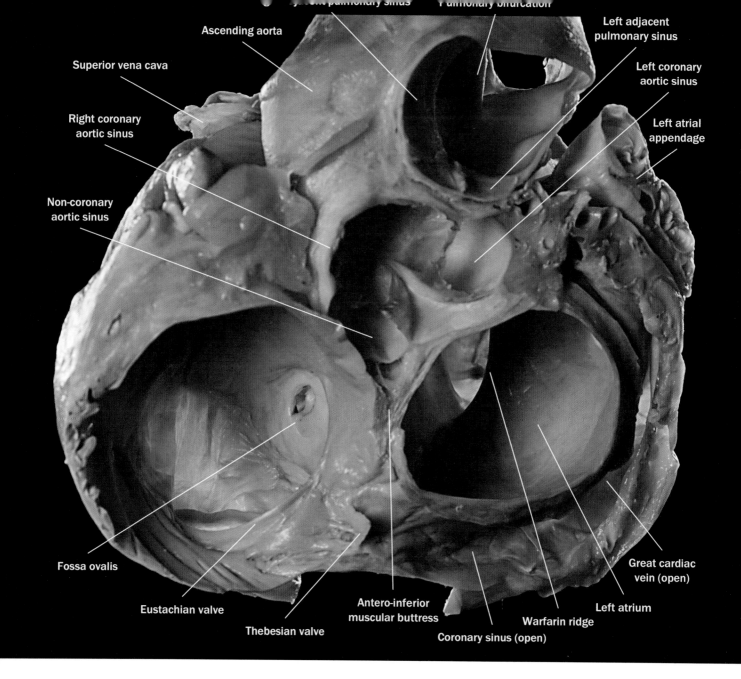

Superior vena cava

Right coronary aortic sinus

Non-coronary aortic sinus

Ascending aorta

Left adjacent pulmonary sinus

Left coronary aortic sinus

Left atrial appendage

Fossa ovalis

Eustachian valve

Thebesian valve

Antero-inferior muscular buttress

Coronary sinus (open)

Warfarin ridge

Left atrium

Great cardiac vein (open)

Figure 32   The fossa ovalis viewed from the left anterior oblique direction.

The heart is cut at the level of the left atrioventricular junction. Transillumination (right) enhances the thin wall of the inferior sinus venarum/inferior vena cava that is adjacent to the inferior rim of the fossa ovalis. Thus, any approaches inferior to the fossa ovalis is not dealing with the left atrium; rather it is accessing into the epicardial adipose tissue within the

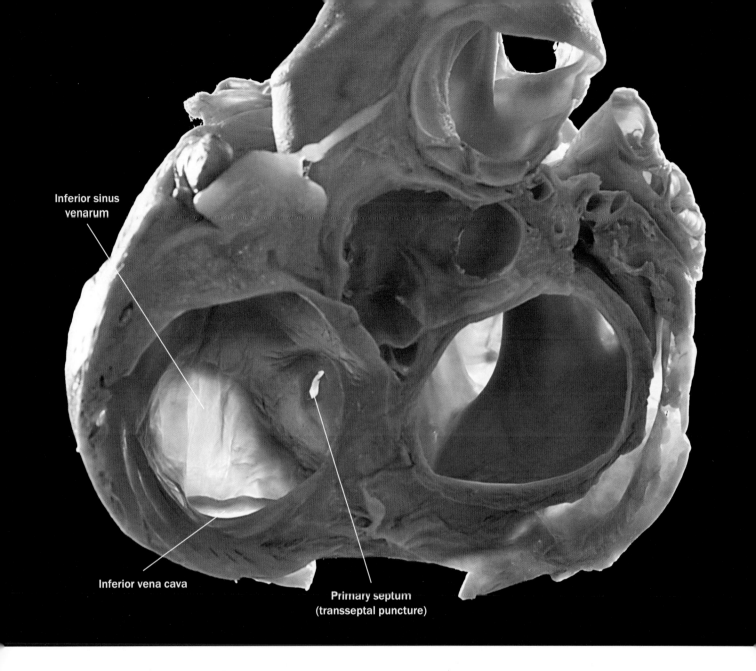

Inferior sinus
venarum

Inferior vena cava

Primary septum
(transseptal puncture)

inferior interatrial groove. In some patients with aortic elongation, the descending aorta runs close to this region.[12] The hole created by transseptal puncture is observed at the superior part of the primary septum at the floor of the fossa ovalis.

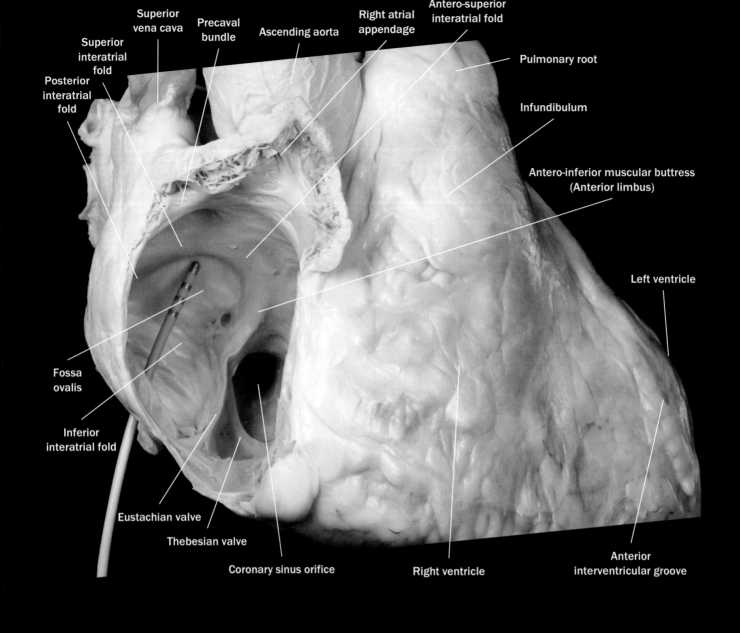

Figure 33 The ablation catheter placed on the primary septum close to the superior rim of the fossa ovalis.

The fossa ovalis is surrounded by the interatrial fold/groove antero-superior, superior, posterior, and inferior. Only the primary septum at the floor of the fossa ovalis and anterior limbus, also referred to as the antero-inferior muscular buttress, is the true atrial septum.[5] Thus, the wall inferior to the fossa ovalis and posterior to the Eustachian ridge is not the true atrial septum, even if it is referred to as the lower atrial septum.[13] On the contrary, it is the medial thin free wall of the sinus venarum/inferior vena cava itself facing to the inferior interatrial groove.[12] The antero-inferior buttress is the muscular component of the true atrial septum. It anchors the primary septum to the central fibrous body. As the fossa ovalis tilts inferior, it is located supero-medial relative to the orifice of the inferior vena cava. When using the transfemoral venous approach, the common location of the transseptal puncture is close to the superior rim of the fossa ovalis as the pushing force makes the centrally placed tip slip superiorly within the area of the primary septum. Common location of the patent foramen ovale is the antero-superior margin of the fossa ovalis,[14] found in one-sixth[15] to one-fourth of the dissected hearts.[16] Refer to Figure 9.

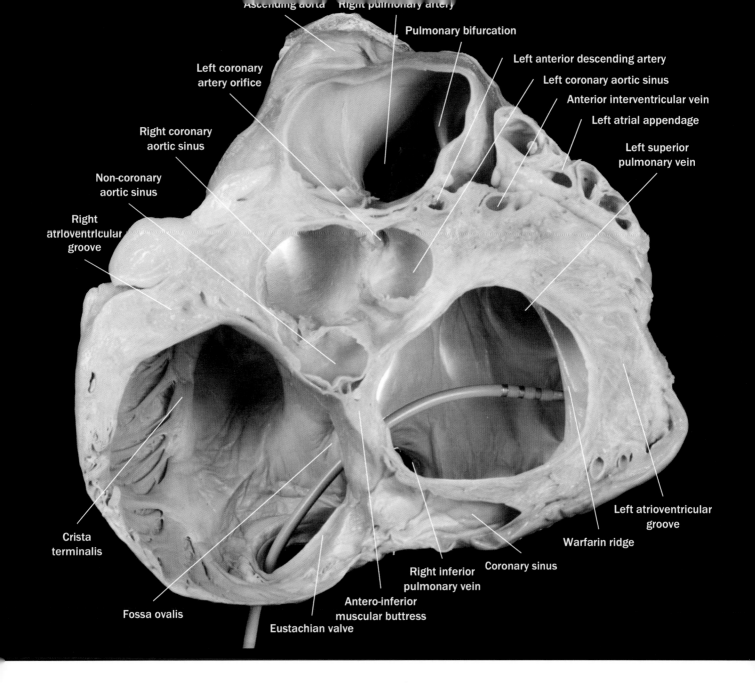

Figure 34 Transseptal approach viewed from the left anterior oblique direction.

The image is displayed from the left anterior oblique direction to obtain the short axis image of the heart cut at the level of the left atrioventricular junction. The puncture site at the fossa ovalis is located right postero-superior to the coronary sinus orifice, posterior to the antero-inferior muscular buttress, and right postero-inferior to the non-coronary aortic sinus. The tip is placed on the posterior surface of the warfarin (Coumadin) ridge.

References

1. McAlpine WA. Digitized collection of all the images created by Dr. McAlpine at UCLA. Copyright UCLA Cardiac Arrhythmia Center. Part of this collection appeared in *Heart and Coronary Arteries: An Anatomical Atlas for Clinical Diagnosis, Radiological Investigation, and Surgical Treatment.* New York: Springer-Verlag; 1975.

2. Hanaoka T, Suyama K, Taguchi A, et al. Shifting of puncture site in the fossa ovalis during radiofrequency catheter ablation: Intracardiac echocardiography-guided transseptal left heart catheterization. *Jpn Heart J.* 2003;44:673–680.

3. Bidart C, Vaseghi M, Cesario DA, et al. Radiofrequency current delivery via transseptal needle to facilitate septal puncture. *Heart Rhythm.* 2007;4:1573–1576.

4. Kim JS, Virágh S, Moorman AF, et al. Development of the myocardium of the atrioventricular canal and the vestibular spine in the human heart. *Circ Res.* 2001;88:395–402.

5. Mori S, Nishii T, Tretter JT, et al. Demonstration of living anatomy clarifies the morphology of interatrial communications. *Heart.* 2018;104:2003–2009.

6. Bhatnagar KP, Nettleton GS, Campbell FR, et al. Chiari anomalies in the human right atrium. *Clin Anat.* 2006;19:510–516.

7. Gonzalez MD, Otomo K, Shah N, et al. Transseptal left heart catheterization for cardiac ablation procedures. *J Interv Card Electrophysiol.* 2001;5:89–95.

8. De Ponti R, Zardini M, Storti C, et al. Trans-septal catheterization for radiofrequency catheter ablation of cardiac arrhythmias. Results and safety of a simplified method. *Eur Heart J.* 1998;19:943–950.

9. Mori S, Anderson RH, Takaya T, et al. The association between wedging of the aorta and cardiac structural anatomy as revealed using multidetector-row computed tomography. *J Anat.* 2017;231:110–120.

10. Walmsley R, Watson H. The medial wall of the right atrium. *Circulation.* 1966;34:400–411.

11. Chun DS, Turrentine MW, Moustapha A, et al. Development of aorta-to-right atrial fistula following closure of secundum atrial septal defect using the amplatzer septal occluder. *Catheter Cardiovasc Interv.* 2003;58:246–251.

12. Mori S, Fukuzawa K, Takaya T, et al. Clinical cardiac structural anatomy reconstructed within the cardiac contour using multi-detector-row computed tomography: Atrial septum and ventricular septum. *Clin Anat.* 2016;29:342–352.

13. Acosta H, Viafara LM, Izquierdo D, et al. Atrial lead placement at the lower atrial septum: A potential strategy to reduce unnecessary right ventricular pacing. *Europace.* 2012;14:1311–1316.

14. Ho SY, Cabrera JA, Sánchez-Quintana D. Left atrial anatomy revisited. *Circ Arrhythm Electrophysiol.* 2012;5:220–228.

15. Kuramoto J, Kawamura A, Dembo T, et al. Prevalence of patent foramen ovale in the Japanese population—autopsy study. *Circ J.* 2015;79:2038–2042.

16. Hagen PT, Scholz DG, Edwards WD. Incidence and size of patent foramen ovale during the first 10 decades of life: An autopsy study of 965 normal hearts. *Mayo Clin Proc.* 1984;59:17–20.

7

Coronary Sinus Orifice

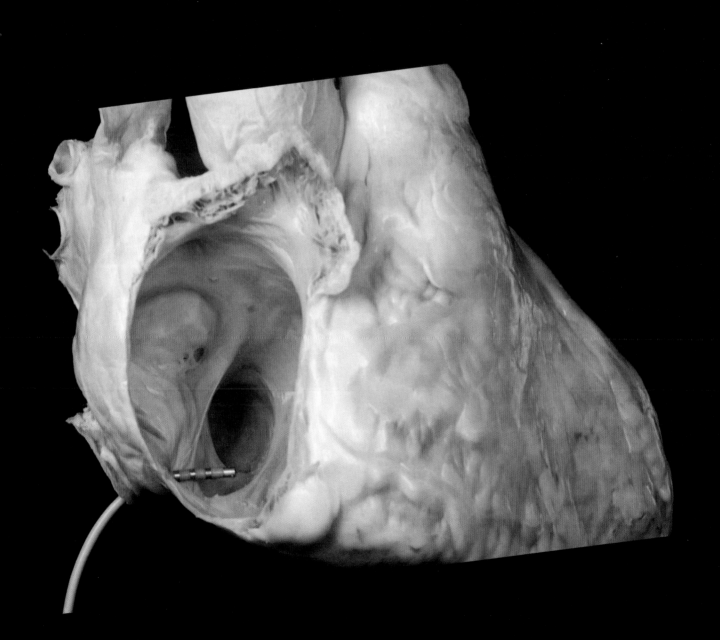

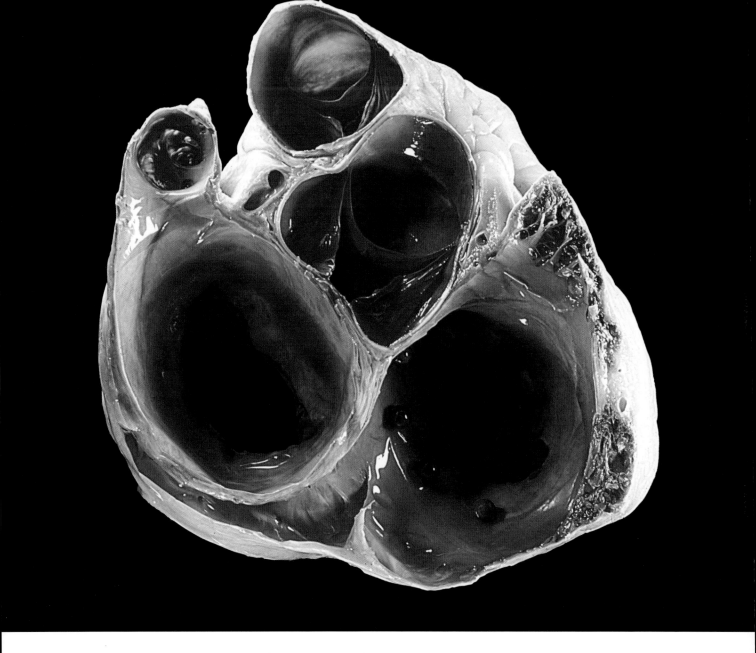

Figure 35   The coronary sinus viewed from the atrial side.[1]

The coronary sinus is located inferior to the left atrial vestibule around the attachment of the posterior mitral leaflet. The inferior half of the coronary sinus orifice is guarded by the Thebesian valve. The Thebesian valve is found in the nine-tenths of the dissected hearts,[2] and it covers more than 50% of the coronary sinus orifice in one-third of the dissected hearts[3] with various morphologies.[4] The non-coronary aortic sinus wedges on the antero-superior interatrial groove between the supero-medial wall of the right and left atrium. This wedging of the non-coronary aortic sinus creates the left and right

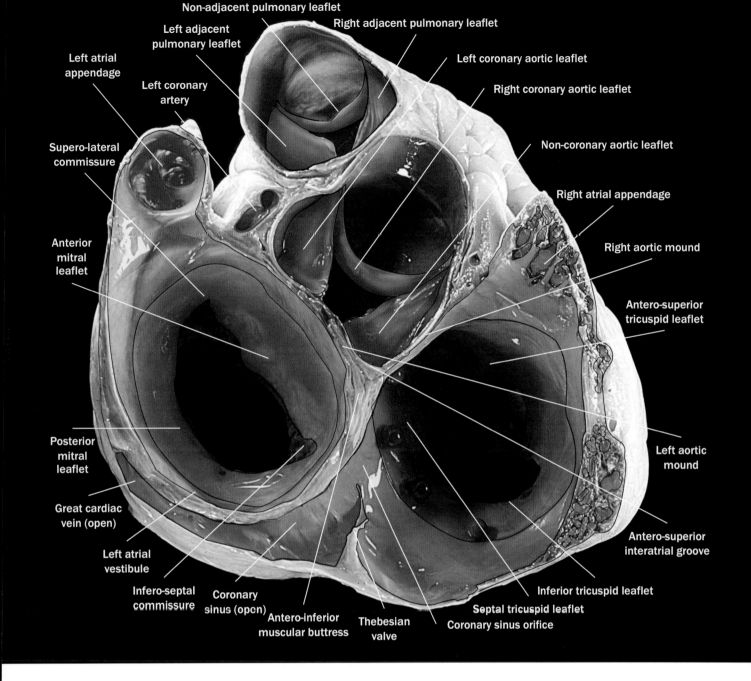

Non-adjacent pulmonary leaflet

Left adjacent pulmonary leaflet

Right adjacent pulmonary leaflet

Left atrial appendage

Left coronary artery

Left coronary aortic leaflet

Right coronary aortic leaflet

Supero-lateral commissure

Non-coronary aortic leaflet

Right atrial appendage

Anterior mitral leaflet

Right aortic mound

Antero-superior tricuspid leaflet

Posterior mitral leaflet

Left aortic mound

Great cardiac vein (open)

Antero-superior interatrial groove

Left atrial vestibule

Inferior tricuspid leaflet

Infero-septal commissure

Coronary sinus (open)

Septal tricuspid leaflet

Coronary sinus orifice

Antero-inferior muscular buttress

Thebesian valve

aortic mound into each atrium, the imprint of the aortic root bulging into the atria. Between the orifice of the coronary sinus and the non-coronary aortic sinus, the antero-inferior muscular buttress (also referred to as the anterior limbus of the fossa ovalis) is working as the muscular component of the true atrial septum. The paired section of this image is Figure 41.

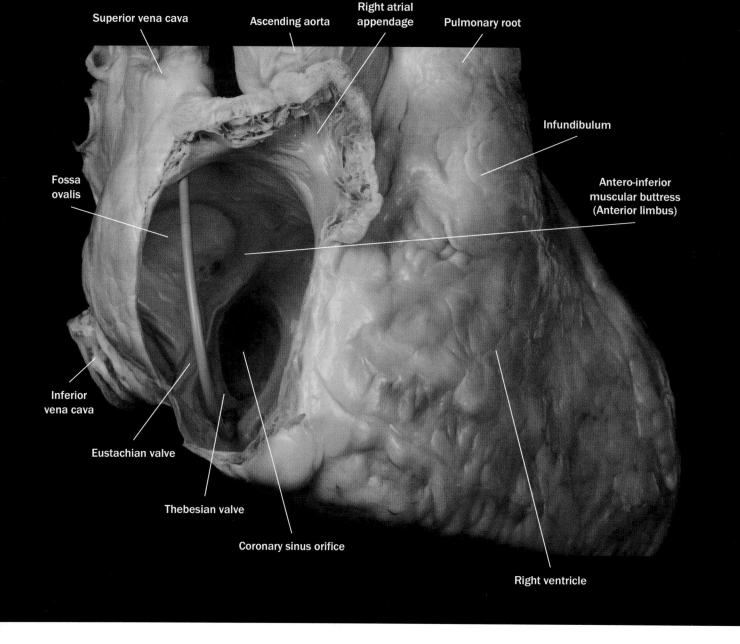

Superior vena cava

Ascending aorta

Right atrial appendage

Pulmonary root

Infundibulum

Antero-inferior muscular buttress (Anterior limbus)

Fossa ovalis

Inferior vena cava

Eustachian valve

Thebesian valve

Coronary sinus orifice

Right ventricle

Figure 36 The ablation catheter trapped by the Thebesian valve. Anaglyph 10.

When the Thebesian valve is prominent, it can work as the anatomical obstacle to the procedure related to the coronary venous system.[5] Right anterior oblique (left) and left anterior oblique (right) views show further

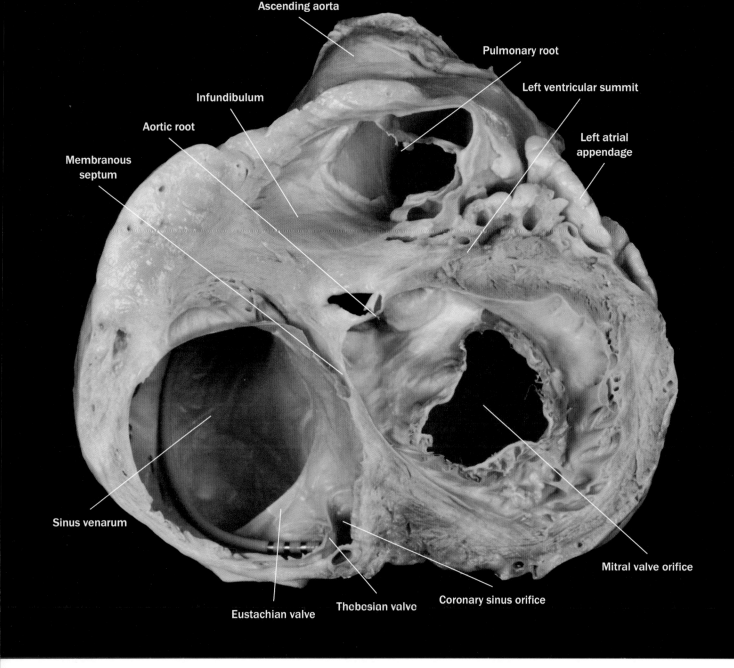

Ascending aorta

Pulmonary root

Infundibulum

Left ventricular summit

Aortic root

Left atrial
appendage

Membranous
septum

Sinus venarum

Mitral valve orifice

Eustachian valve

Thebesian valve

Coronary sinus orifice

forced pushing maneuvers do not resolve this situation to insert the catheter into the coronary sinus. Refer to Figure 37.

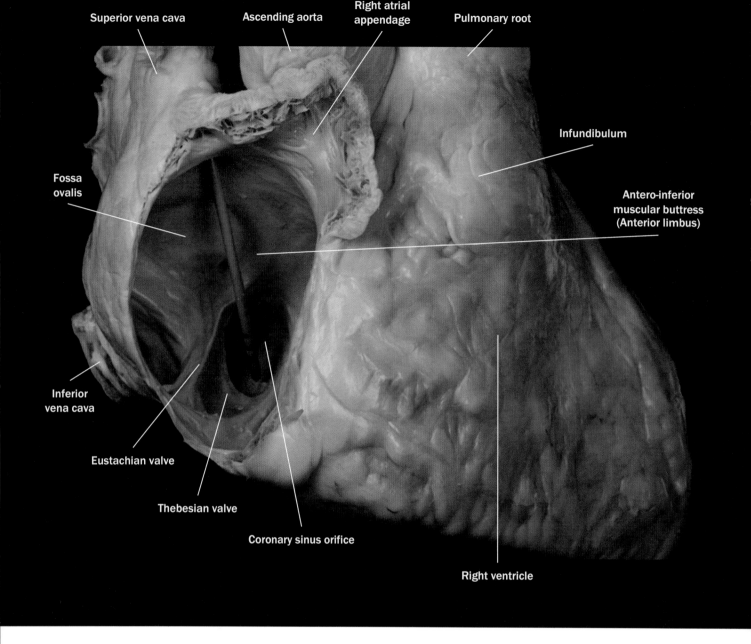

Superior vena cava

Ascending aorta

Right atrial
appendage

Pulmonary root

Infundibulum

Fossa
ovalis

Antero-inferior
muscular buttress
(Anterior limbus)

Inferior
vena cava

Eustachian valve

Thebesian valve

Coronary sinus orifice

Right ventricle

Figure 37   The ablation catheter avoiding the Thebesian valve. 🕶 Anaglyph 11.

Right anterior oblique (left) and left anterior oblique (right) views show the optimal curve and course of the catheter to avoid entrapment by the Thebesian valve guarding the inferior orifice of the coronary sinus. Unless the patients have coronary sinus atresia, the catheter can be slid from the superior side of the coronary sinus orifice, with the catheter tip

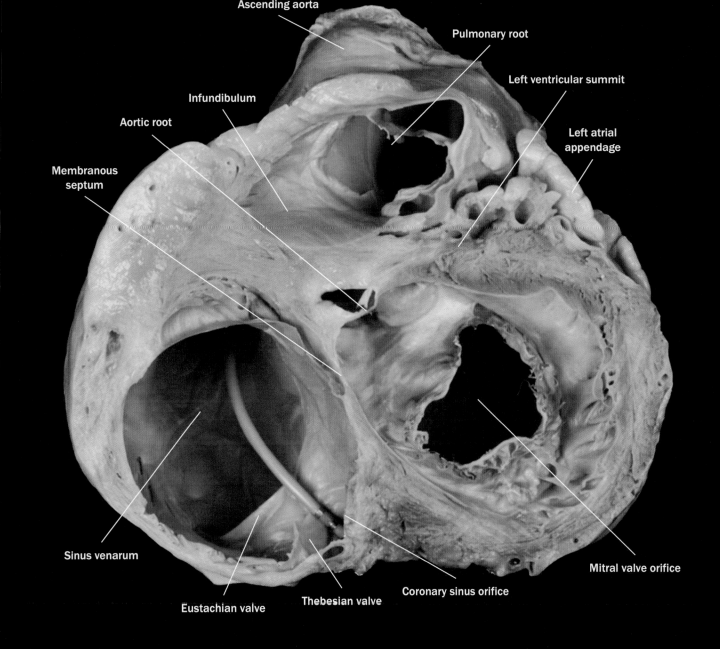

Ascending aorta

Pulmonary root

Left ventricular summit

Left atrial appendage

Infundibulum

Aortic root

Membranous septum

Sinus venarum

Eustachian valve

Thebesian valve

Coronary sinus orifice

Mitral valve orifice

scanning the supero-medial direction. The right image also shows that the height of the Eustachian ridge becomes prominent in the medial portion. From the superior approach, clockwise torque makes the catheter tip direct toward anterior wall of the coronary sinus and vice versa. Refer to Figure 36.

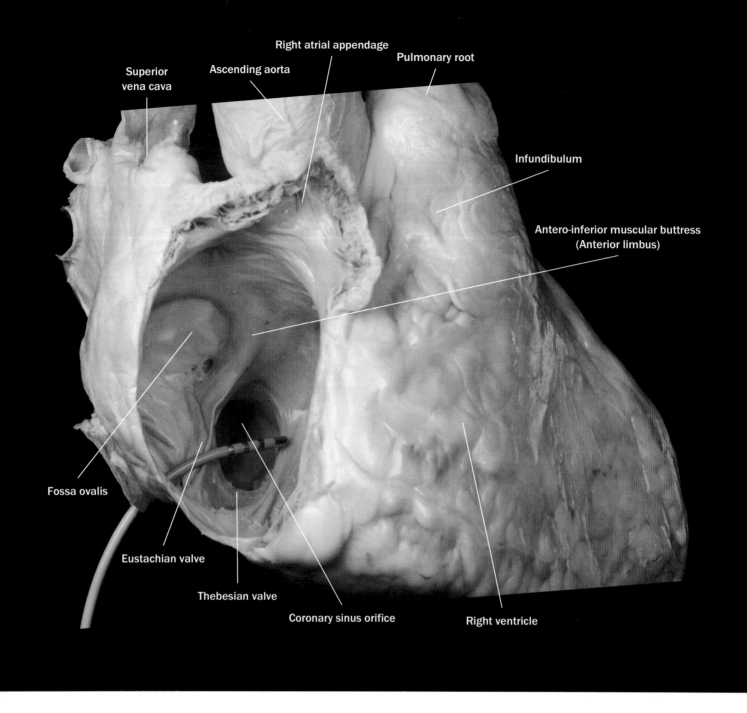

Superior
vena cava

Ascending aorta

Right atrial appendage

Pulmonary root

Infundibulum

Antero-inferior muscular buttress
(Anterior limbus)

Fossa ovalis

Eustachian valve

Thebesian valve

Coronary sinus orifice

Right ventricle

Figure 38   The ablation catheter located at the septal isthmus viewed from the right anterior oblique direction: Right atrial image.

The left image shows the catheter tip location during a slow pathway modification at the septal isthmus just anterior to the coronary sinus orifice. The septal isthmus is the potential location of the right inferior nodal extension.[6] In some cases, with left variant atrioventricular nodal reentrant tachycardia using the left inferior nodal extension, an intra-coronary sinus approach is required (right) to ablate anterior wall of the coronary sinus.[7] When viewing from the right anterior oblique direction, the septal isthmus and anterior wall of the coronary sinus orifice is not a simple flat plane facing to the operator

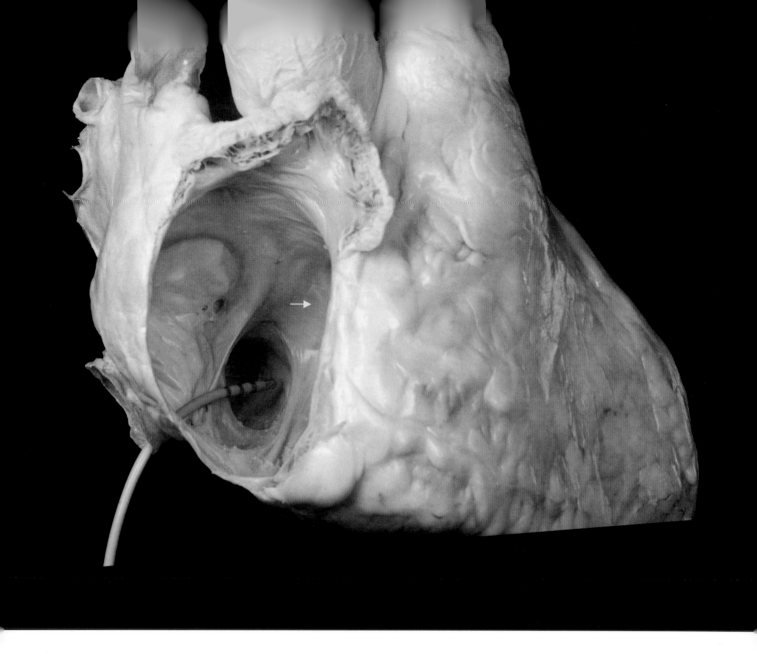

as shown by some illustrations. Rather, the septal isthmus shows a funnel-shaped slope leaning away from the observer toward the coronary sinus orifice.[8] Optimal contact and fixation of the tip requires fine torque adjustments of the catheter to trace this funnel shaped anatomy, in addition to push/pull maneuvers. Left anterior oblique view is useful to adjust the clockwise/counterclockwise torque, as well as to estimate the proximity to the mid-septum region to avoid inadvertent injury to the compact atrioventricular node (yellow arrow). Refer to Figure 39.

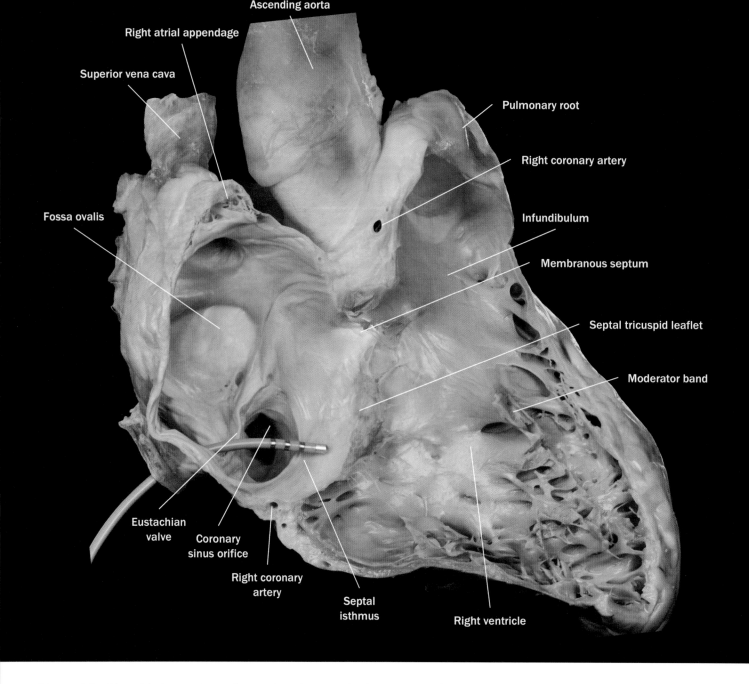

Ascending aorta

Right atrial appendage

Superior vena cava

Pulmonary root

Right coronary artery

Fossa ovalis

Infundibulum

Membranous septum

Septal tricuspid leaflet

Moderator band

Eustachian valve

Coronary sinus orifice

Right coronary artery

Septal isthmus

Right ventricle

Figure 39   The ablation catheter located at the septal isthmus viewed from the right anterior oblique direction: Open heart image.

The left image shows the common location of the slow pathway modification, corresponding to the right inferior nodal extension. The membranous septum is transilluminated. The right image shows the deeper section with the removal of the muscular ventricular septum, showing the close relationship between the anterior wall of the coronary sinus orifice and the left ventricular basal infero-medial wall, referred to as the infero-septal process. Epicardial ablation via the coronary sinus[9]

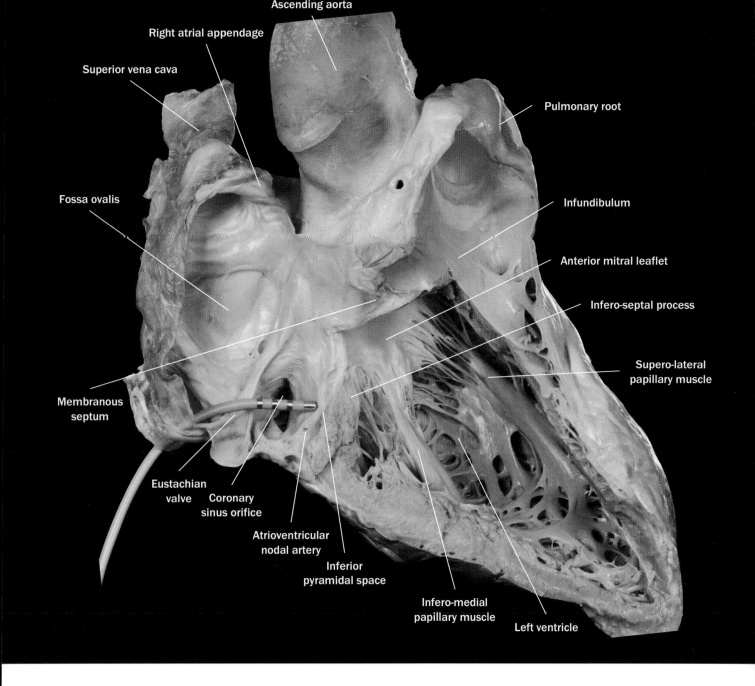

Ascending aorta

Right atrial appendage

Superior vena cava

Pulmonary root

Fossa ovalis

Infundibulum

Anterior mitral leaflet

Infero-septal process

Supero-lateral
papillary muscle

Membranous
septum

Eustachian
valve   Coronary
sinus orifice

Atrioventricular
nodal artery

Inferior
pyramidal space

Infero-medial
papillary muscle

Left ventricle

is an alternative approach to the transaortic retrograde or transseptal antegrade approaches to treat the ventricular arrhythmia originating from the infero-septal process.[10] At this region, thin epicardial fibro-adipose tissue containing the atrioventricular nodal artery, referred to as the inferior pyramidal space, intervenes between the right atrium and the left ventricle.[8] Refer to Figure 38.

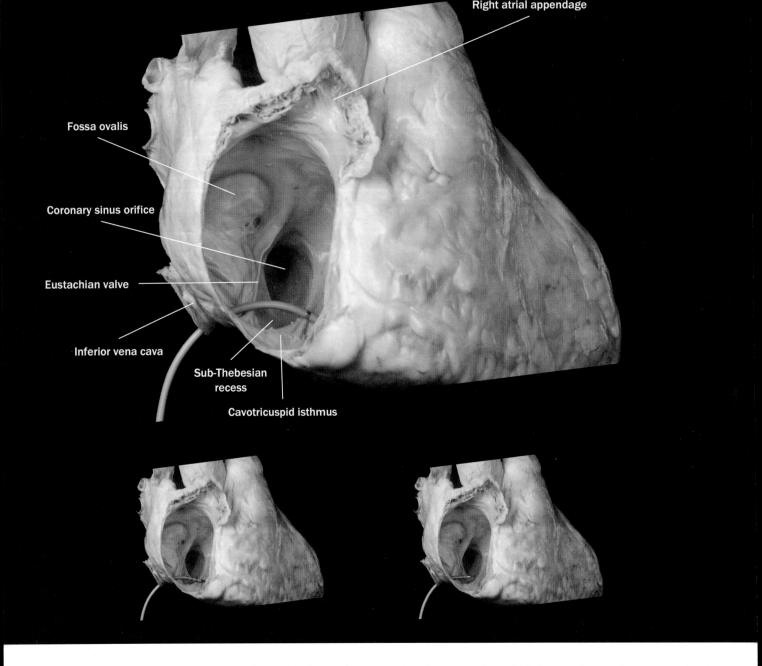

Right atrial appendage

Fossa ovalis

Coronary sinus orifice

Eustachian valve

Inferior vena cava

Sub-Thebesian recess

Cavotricuspid isthmus

Figure 40 The sequential images of the ablation catheter tracing the cavotricuspid isthmus viewed from the right anterior oblique direction: Right atrial image.

The ablation catheter is pulled back from the tricuspid annulus to the inferior vena cava. The surface of the cavotricuspid isthmus is irregular due to the variable course and thickness of the pectinate muscles,[11] sub-Thebesian recess, also referred to as the sub-Eustachian pouch[12] and Eustachian valve. These structures are the anatomical obstacles that prevent optimal attachment of the catheter tip to the isthmus floor. The prominent Eustachian valve acts as a fulcrum for the catheter

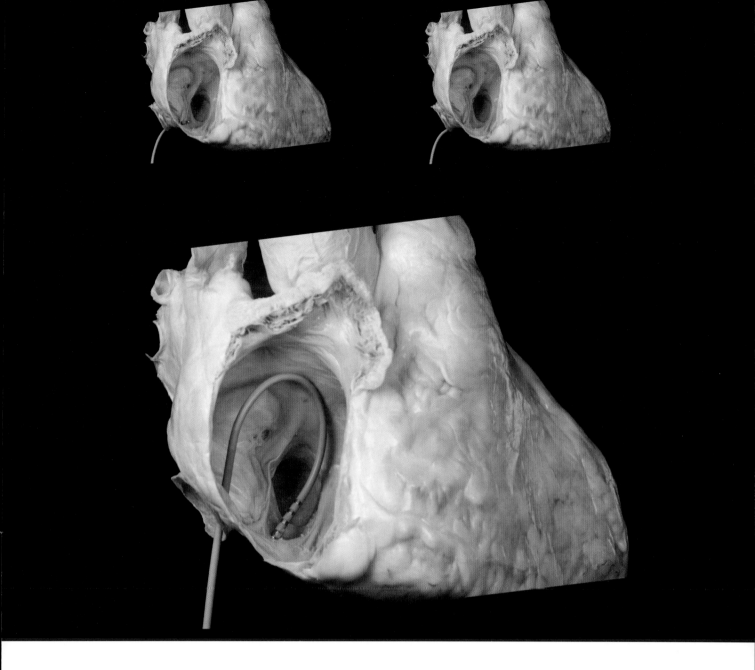

(lower right image on the left page and upper left image on the right page), preventing the tip from optimal contact to the region even if full deflection is applied.[11] The lower image on the right page shows the U-turn approach to reach the potential lesion gaps. To secure the optimal contact, use of the deflectable long sheath, or lateral shift of the ablation line is also effective as the Eustachian ridge becomes less prominent in the lateral portion. Refer to Figure 37.

References

1. McAlpine WA. Digitized collection of all the images created by Dr. McAlpine at UCLA. Copyright UCLA Cardiac Arrhythmia Center. Part of this collection appeared in *Heart and Coronary Arteries: An Anatomical Atlas for Clinical Diagnosis, Radiological Investigation, and Surgical Treatment.* New York: Springer-Verlag; 1975.
2. Katti K, Patil NP. The Thebesian valve: Gatekeeper to the coronary sinus. *Clin Anat.* 2012;25:379–385.
3. Felle P, Bannigan JG. Anatomy of the valve of the coronary sinus (Thebesian valve). *Clin Anat.* 1994;7:10–12.
4. Hołda MK, Klimek-Piotrowska W, Koziej M, et al. Anatomical variations of the coronary sinus valve (Thebesian valve): Implications for electrocardiological procedures. *Europace.* 2015;17:921–927.
5. Cao M, Chang P, Garon B, et al. Cardiac resynchronization therapy: Double cannulation approach to coronary venous lead placement via a prominent thebesian valve. *Pacing Clin Electrophysiol.* 2013;36:e70–e73.
6. Inoue S, Becker AE. Posterior extensions of the human compact atrioventricular node: A neglected anatomic feature of potential clinical significance. *Circulation.* 1998;97:188–193.
7. Otomo K, Okamura H, Noda T, et al. "Left-variant" atypical atrioventricular nodal reentrant tachycardia: Electrophysiological characteristics and effect of slow pathway ablation within coronary sinus. *J Cardiovasc Electrophysiol.* 2006;17:1177–1183.
8. Mori S, Fukuzawa K, Takaya T, et al. Clinical structural anatomy of the Inferior pyramidal space reconstructed within the cardiac contour using multidetector-row computed tomography. *J Cardiovasc Electrophysiol.* 2015;26:705–712.
9. Tavares L, Dave A, Valderrábano M. Successful ablation of premature ventricular contractions originating from the inferoseptal process of the left ventricle using a coronary sinus approach. *Heart Rhythm Case Rep.* 2018;4:371–374.
10. Li A, Zuberi Z, Bradfield JS, et al. Endocardial ablation of ventricular ectopic beats arising from the basal inferoseptal process of the left ventricle. *Heart Rhythm.* 2018;15:1356–1362.
11. Asirvatham SJ. Correlative anatomy and electrophysiology for the interventional electrophysiologist: Right atrial flutter. *J Cardiovasc Electrophysiol.* 2009;20:113–122.
12. Mori S, Tretter JT, Spicer DE, et al. What is the real cardiac anatomy? *Clin Anat.* 2019;32:288–309.

8

Right Atrial Appendage

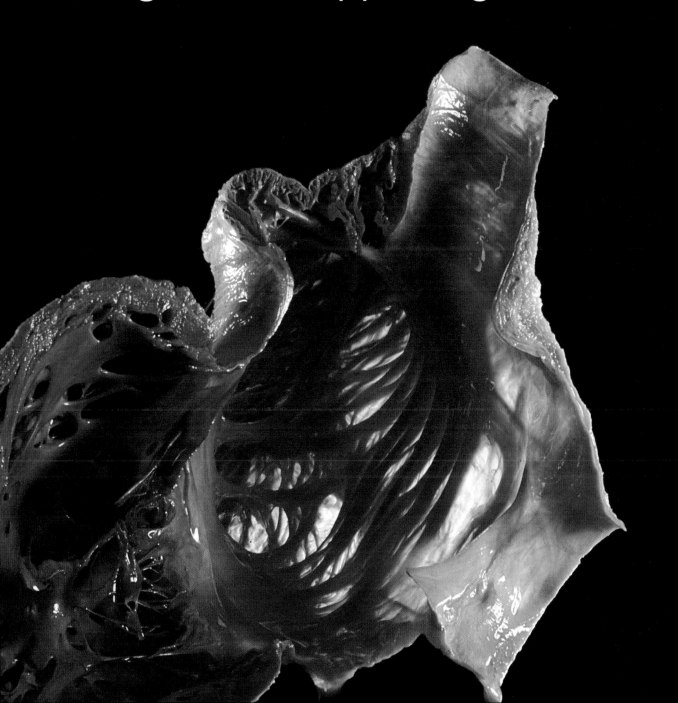

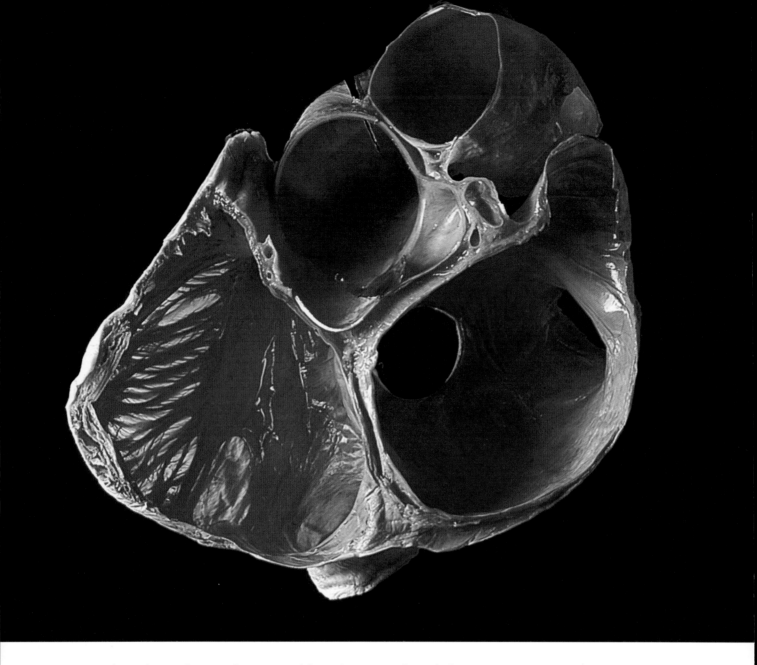

Figure 41 The right atrial appendage viewed from the ventricular side.[1]

The pectinate muscles originate from the crista terminalis and direct toward the right atrial vestibule running on the lateral and inferior free wall of the right atrial appendage. The arrangement of the pectinate muscles is variable and non-uniform, especially around the cavotricuspid isthmus.[2] At its inferior end, the crista terminalis ramifies into several pectinate muscles. The wall of the right atrial appendage between the pectinate muscle is paper thin. The medial part of the right atrial

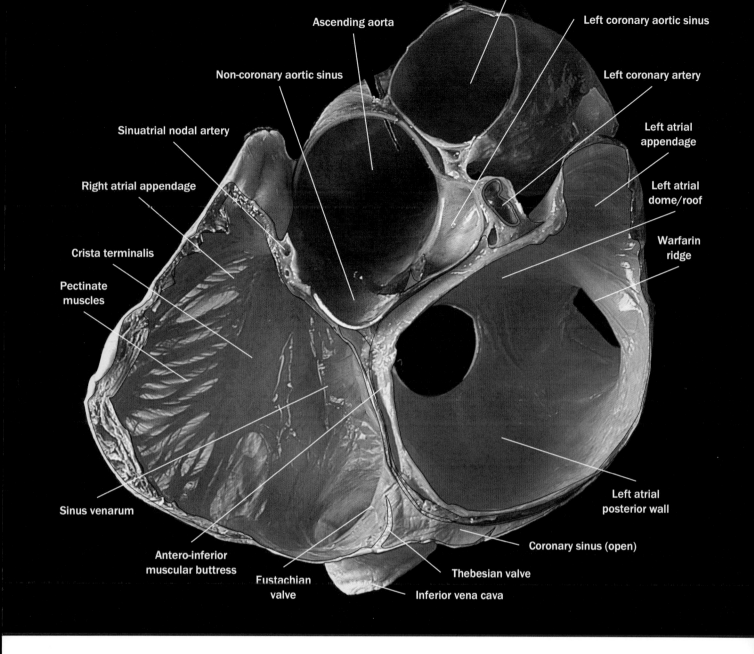

Ascending aorta

Left coronary aortic sinus

Non-coronary aortic sinus

Left coronary artery

Sinuatrial nodal artery

Left atrial appendage

Right atrial appendage

Left atrial dome/roof

Crista terminalis

Warfarin ridge

Pectinate muscles

Sinus venarum

Left atrial posterior wall

Antero-inferior muscular buttress

Coronary sinus (open)

Eustachian valve

Thebesian valve

Inferior vena cava

appendage faces to the aortic root intervened by the right-side transverse sinus. The sinuatrial nodal artery originating from the proximal right coronary artery runs on the epicardial side of the medial right atrial appendage.[3] The paired section of this image is Figure 35.

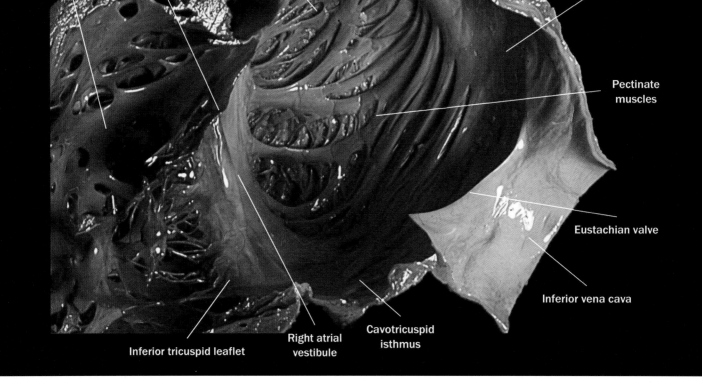

Pectinate muscles

Eustachian valve

Inferior vena cava

Inferior tricuspid leaflet

Right atrial vestibule

Cavotricuspid isthmus

Figure 42　The free wall of the right atrial appendage viewed from the medial direction.[1]

The superior part of the crista terminalis continues to the precaval bundle, also referred to as the arcuate ridge. Multiple pectinate muscles originate from the crista terminalis directing toward the right arial vestibule. The right atrial vestibule has the smooth endocardial surface, continuing to the tricuspid annulus. The crista terminalis does not extend to reach the orifice of the inferior vena cava, but it splits into several pectinate muscles radiating toward the Eustachian valve and cavo-tricuspid isthmus. Some pectinate muscles have a uniform parallel arrangement, whereas others show irregular crossover

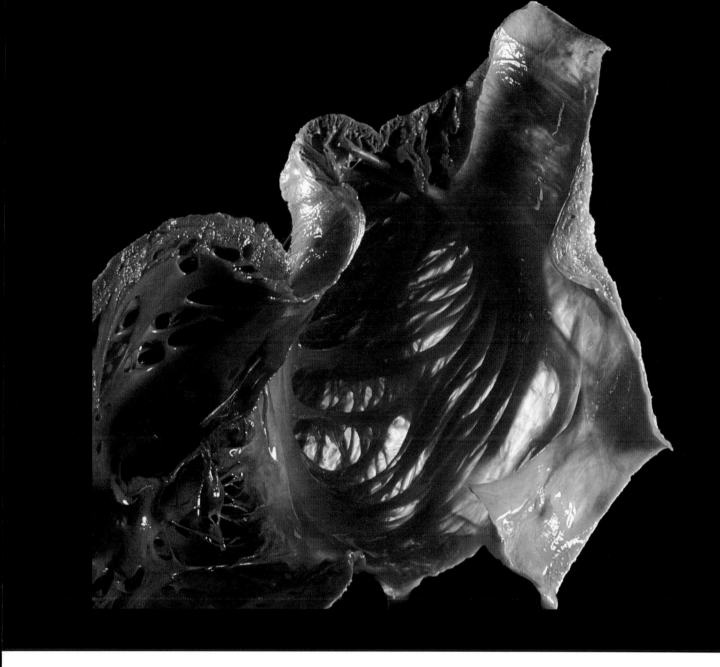

patterns.[2] From the precaval bundle, the sagittal bundle (also referred to as the septum spurium) originates running anterior across the body of the right atrial appendage from the medial to lateral side.[2] Superior to this sagittal bundle, at the middle portion on the superior ridge of the right atrial appendage, the saddle-like bend is created.[4] Transillumination (right) shows the paper-thin free wall of the right atrial appendage between the pectinate muscles. The trabeculations on the right ventricular free wall extends to the level of the atrioventricular junction.

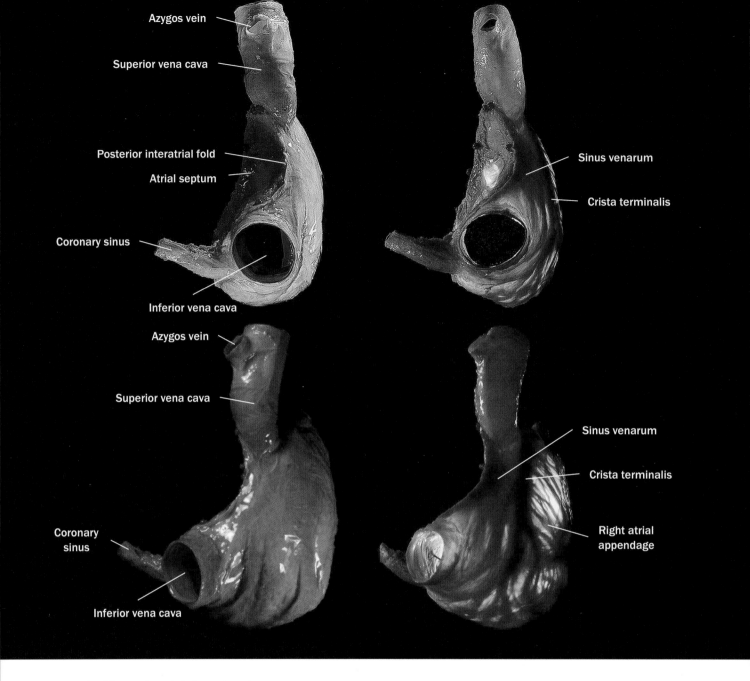

Figure 43 The isolated right atrium.[1]

The upper and lower pairs of images are viewed from the right posterior and right lateral directions, respectively. The sinus venarum is not a straight structure. The proximal superior and inferior vena cava are aligned in an angled fashion to each other, with the axis of the inferior vena cava directing toward the left antero-superior direction. In contrast, the axis of the superior vena cava is nearly vertical. Therefore, the catheter inserted from the inferior vena cava in parallel fashion to its axis is delivered into the apex of the right atrial appendage. Transillumination (right) enhances the crista terminalis and pectinate muscles. The inferior part of the crista terminalis ramifies into multiple pectinate muscles in fan-like fashion. One of those pectinate muscles runs along the Eustachian valve from lateral to medial side. Others running into the cavotricuspid isthmus in oblique fashion. In addition to the free wall of the right atrial appendage between the pectinate muscles, the infero-posterior wall of the sinus venarum is thin[4] and also transilluminated.

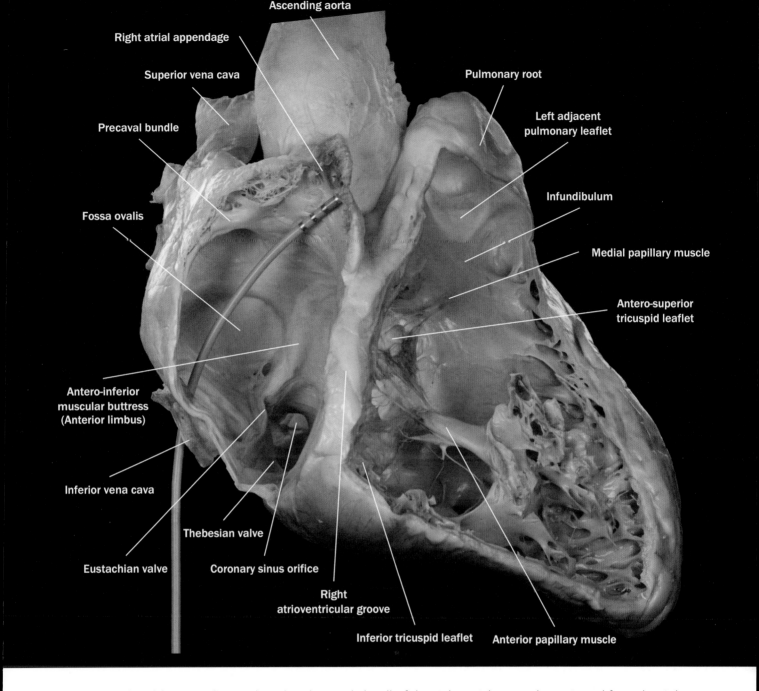

Figure 44   The ablation catheter placed at the medial wall of the right atrial appendage viewed from the right anterior oblique direction.

This site is adjacent to the aortic root/ascending aorta intervened by the right-side transverse sinus. On the medial epicardial surface of this site, right sinuatrial nodal artery may run toward superior terminal groove in two-thirds of cases.[5] This medial free wall of the right atrial appendage should not be deemed as the high atrial septum. Intervention around this region has a potential risk to injure the right sinuatrial nodal artery and aortic root/ascending aorta.[6]

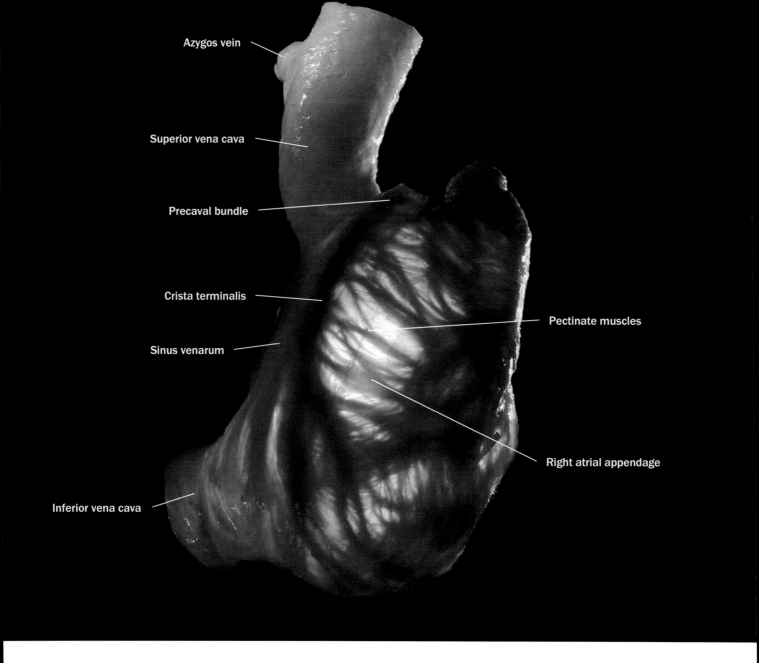

Azygos vein

Superior vena cava

Precaval bundle

Crista terminalis

Sinus venarum

Inferior vena cava

Pectinate muscles

Right atrial appendage

Figure 45   The transilluminated right atrium in isolation[1] and *in situ.*

The right atrium is viewed from the right anterior oblique direction (left) and right superior direction (right). Ramification of the pectinate muscles from the crista terminalis and paper-thin free wall of the right atrial appendage are observed. The superior part of the crista terminalis continues to the precaval bundle, also referred to as the arcuate ridge. From the precaval bundle, the sagittal bundle runs toward the lateral wall of the right atrial appendage. Superior to the sagittal bundle, the saddle-like bend is created at the middle portion at the superior ridge of the right atrial appendage.[4] The aortic root is deeply wedged into the center of the heart, surrounded by the left atrium, right atrial

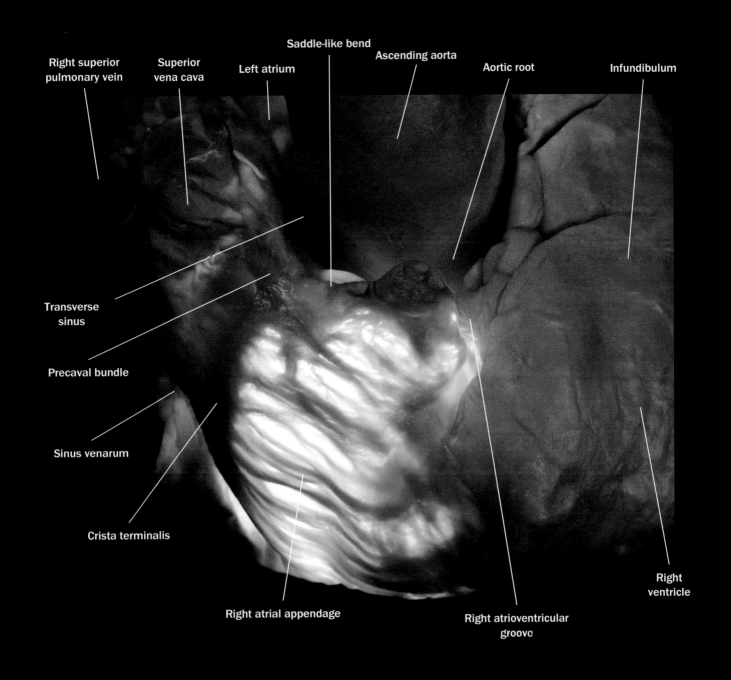

Right superior pulmonary vein

Superior vena cava

Left atrium

Saddle-like bend

Ascending aorta

Aortic root

Infundibulum

Transverse sinus

Precaval bundle

Sinus venarum

Crista terminalis

Right atrial appendage

Right atrioventricular groove

Right ventricle

appendage, and right ventricular outflow tract (infundibulum). The apex of the right atrial appendage covers the proximal aorta and the right atrioventricular groove, intervened by the right-side transverse sinus. Since the apex of the right atrial appendage is a free structure, the right-side entrance/exit of the transverse sinus can be approached either antero-medially from the medial side of the apex of the right atrial appendage, or postero-laterally over the superior ridge of the right atrial appendage.[7]

References

1. McAlpine WA. Digitized collection of all the images created by Dr. McAlpine at UCLA. Copyright UCLA Cardiac Arrhythmia Center. Part of this collection appeared in *Heart and Coronary Arteries: An Anatomical Atlas for Clinical Diagnosis, Radiological Investigation, and Surgical Treatment*. New York: Springer-Verlag; 1975.

2. Sánchez-Quintana D, Anderson RH, Cabrera JA, et al. The terminal crest: Morphological features relevant to electrophysiology. *Heart*. 2002;88:406–411.

3. Pardo Meo J, Scanavacca M, Sosa E, et al. Atrial coronary arteries in areas involved in atrial fibrillation catheter ablation. *Circ Arrhythm Electrophysiol*. 2010;3:600–605.

4. Igawa O. Focus on the atrial structure: Useful anatomical information for catheter ablation. *J Arrhythm*. 2011;27:268–288.

5. Saremi F, Abolhoda A, Ashikyan O, et al. Arterial supply to sinuatrial and atrioventricular nodes: Imaging with multidetector CT. *Radiology*. 2008;246:99–107.

6. Aligeti VR, South HL, Hirsh JB, et al. Aorto-right atrial fistula following transseptal catheterization and catheter ablation for atrial fibrillation. *J Cardiovasc Electrophysiol*. 2012;23:659–661.

7. Mori S, Hanna P, Dacey MJ, et al. Comprehensive anatomy of the pericardial space and the cardiac hilum: Anatomical dissections with Intact pericardium. *JACC Cardiovasc Imaging*. 2021. DOI: 10.1016/j.jcmg.2021.04.016. Online ahead of print.

9

Tricuspid Valve, Right Ventricular Inflow

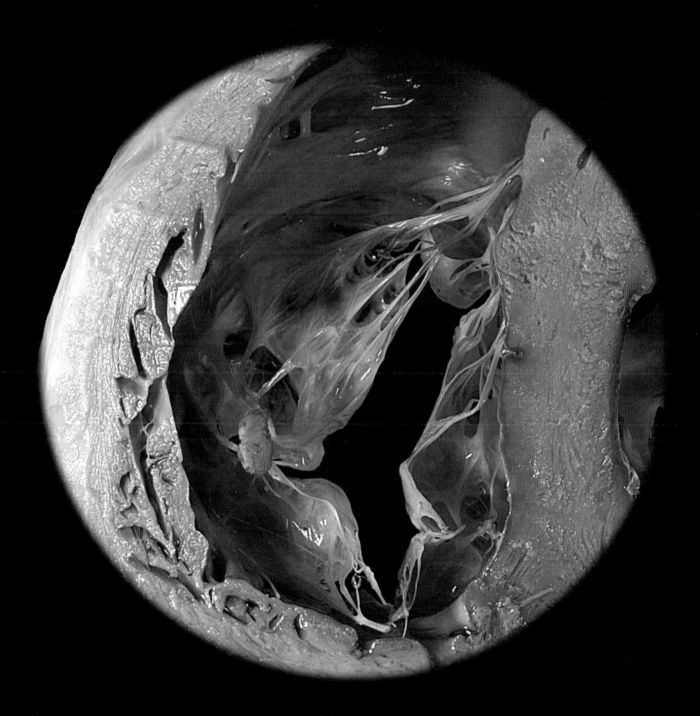

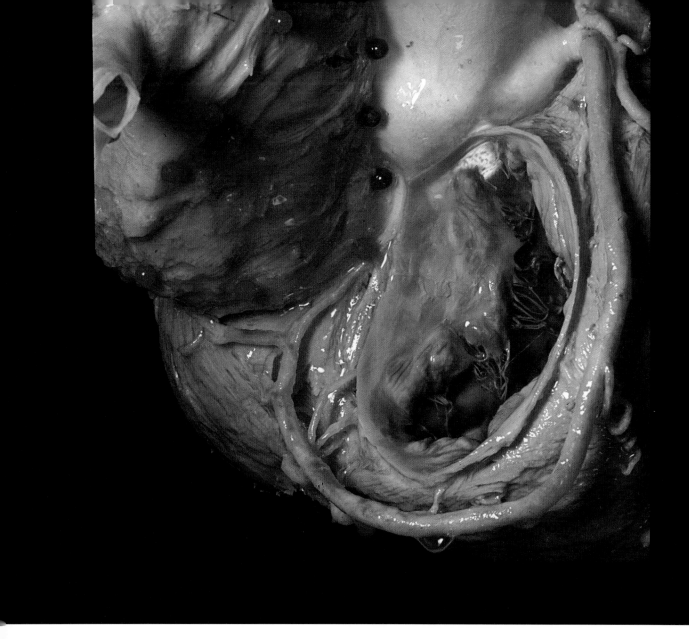

Figure 46   The tricuspid annulus viewed from the right lateral direction.[1]

The right atrium, coronary sinus, and epicardial adipose tissue of the atrioventricular groove and inferior pyramidal space are removed. The red and blue beads demarcate the atrial septum, involving the area surrounded by the interatrial fold. The septal tricuspid leaflet divides the membranous septum into the atrioventricular and interventricular portions. The septal tricuspid leaflet is directly anchored to the ventricular septum by multiple chordae tendineae. The firm and thick fibrous tissue at the bottom of the non-coronary aortic sinus, referred to as the right fibrous trigone,[1,2] connects the aortic root, atrial septum, ventricular septum, and infero-septal process. The membranous septum, septal tricuspid leaflet, and anterior mitral leaflet is in fibrous continuity with the right fibrous trigone.[1] The right fibrous trigone itself is also referred to as the central fibrous body.[1,2] Sometimes, the central fibrous body is used to indicate both the right fibrous trigone and the adjacent atrioventricular portion of the membranous septum,[3,4] as it is hard to define distinct boundary between them. The central fibrous body is the central piece of the cardiac skeleton[3] and the key structure to locate the atrioventricular conduction axis. The medial tricuspid annulus is located apical to the mitral annulus, allowing the triangular shaped offset

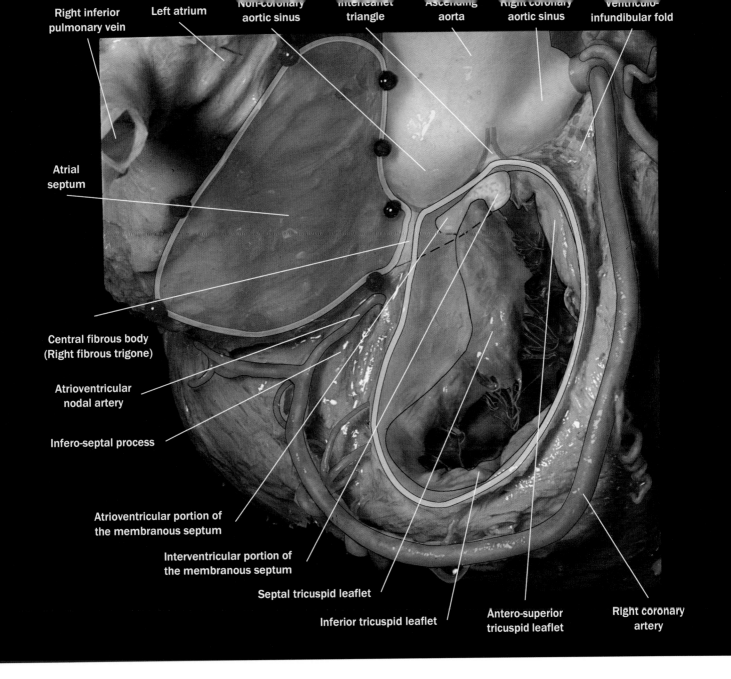

Right inferior pulmonary vein

Left atrium

Non-coronary aortic sinus

Interleaflet triangle

Ascending aorta

Right coronary aortic sinus

Ventriculo-infundibular fold

Atrial septum

Central fibrous body (Right fibrous trigone)

Atrioventricular nodal artery

Infero-septal process

Atrioventricular portion of the membranous septum

Interventricular portion of the membranous septum

Septal tricuspid leaflet

Inferior tricuspid leaflet

Antero-superior tricuspid leaflet

Right coronary artery

of the left ventricular base, referred to as the infero-septal process. At this region, the epicardial side of the infero-septal process faces the right atrium at the floor of the triangle of Koch. This infero-septal process is covered by the wedging epicardial adipose tissue referred to as the inferior pyramidal space, containing the atrioventricular nodal artery.[4] The atrioventricular nodal artery ascends toward the central fibrous body. On the apex of the inferior pyramidal space, the atrioventricular node is located on the right side of the central fibrous body. Thus, the atrioventricular node is sandwiched between the central fibrous body and the medial right atrium at the apex of the triangle of Koch.[5] Therefore, the atrioventricular node is an epicardial structure.[6] To enter into the heart, the penetrating bundle corresponding to the bundle of His needs to penetrate the central fibrous body from the right posterior side at the postero-inferior part of the atrioventricular portion of the membranous septum. Then, the axis emerges at the inferior margin of the membranous septum on the crest of the ventricular septum. Refer to Figure 67.

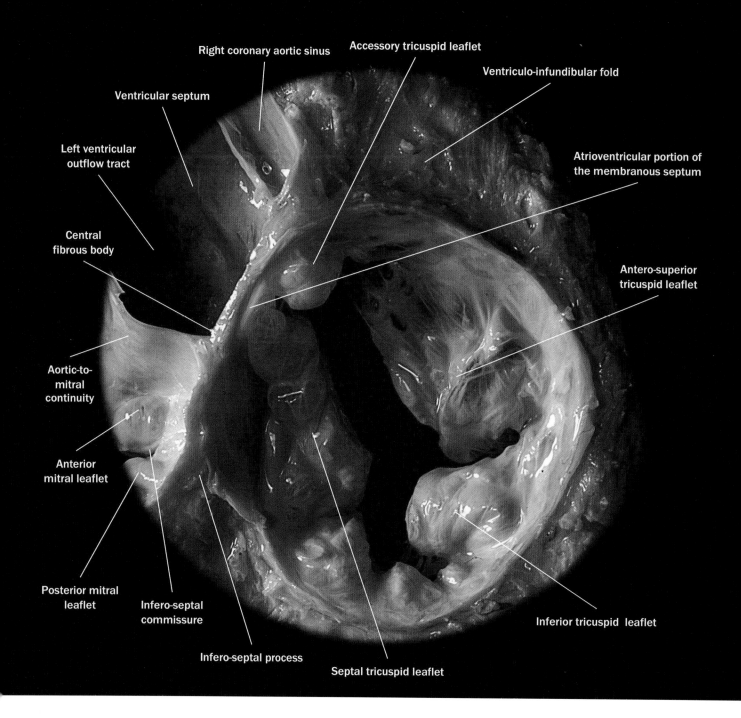

Figure 47   The tricuspid valve viewed from the atrial and ventricular direction.[1]

The tricuspid valve is demonstrated from the atrial (left) and ventricular (right) side. The septal, antero-superior, and inferior tricuspid leaflets are shown with an accessory leaflet at the commissure between the septal and antero-superior tricuspid leaflets. The septal tricuspid leaflet divides the membranous septum into atrioventricular and interventricular portions. The septal tricuspid leaflet is anchored by multiple chordae tendineae on the ventricular septum. The accessory leaflet and medial part of the antero-superior tricuspid leaflet are anchored by the chordae tendineae originating from the medial papillary muscle located on the inferior limb of the septomarginal trabeculation. The commissure between the antero-superior and inferior tricuspid leaflets is anchored by the chordae tendineae originating from the anterior papillary

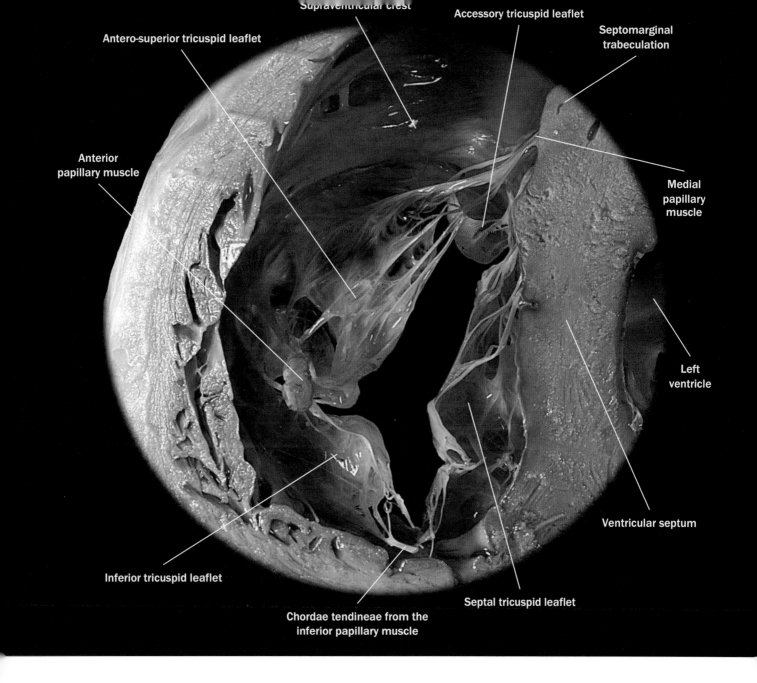

Supraventricular crest

Antero-superior tricuspid leaflet

Accessory tricuspid leaflet

Septomarginal trabeculation

Anterior papillary muscle

Medial papillary muscle

Left ventricle

Ventricular septum

Inferior tricuspid leaflet

Chordae tendineae from the inferior papillary muscle

Septal tricuspid leaflet

muscle. The commissure between the inferior and septal tricuspid leaflet is anchored by the chordae tendineae originating from the inferior papillary muscle. The relationships between these papillary muscles and leaflets are not consistent, but are rather variable.[7] The superior and ventricular parts of the tricuspid annulus is the supraventricular crest corresponding to the postero-lateral free wall of the right ventricular outflow tract located anterior to the right atrioventricular groove and the right coronary aortic sinus. This structure is also referred to as the ventriculo-infundibular fold.

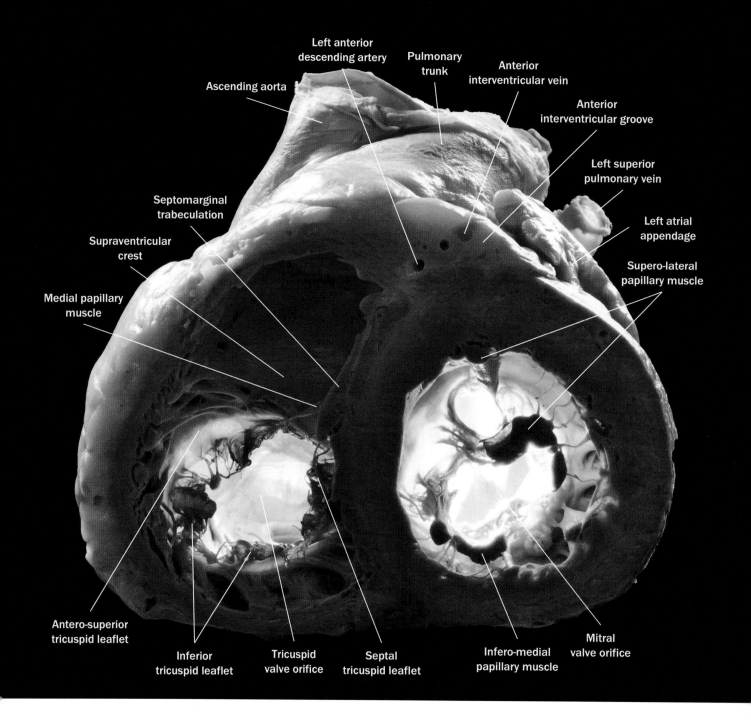

Left anterior
descending artery

Pulmonary
trunk

Anterior
interventricular vein

Ascending aorta

Anterior
interventricular groove

Left superior
pulmonary vein

Septomarginal
trabeculation

Left atrial
appendage

Supraventricular
crest

Supero-lateral
papillary muscle

Medial papillary
muscle

Antero-superior
tricuspid leaflet

Inferior
tricuspid leaflet

Tricuspid
valve orifice

Septal
tricuspid leaflet

Infero-medial
papillary muscle

Mitral
valve orifice

Figure 48 The atrioventricular valves viewed from the ventricular side.

The orifice of the tricuspid valve shows a characteristic morphology as if the medial corner of the orifice is pulled up toward the superior septal direction. This is because the medial part of the antero-superior tricuspid leaflet is anchored by the chordae tendineae originating from the medial papillary muscle. The medial papillary muscle originates from the septomarginal trabeculation that is located at the superior septum. The chordae tendineae of the anterior papillary muscle anchor the commissure between the antero-superior and inferior tricuspid leaflets. The medial part of the supraventricular crest, the postero-lateral free wall of the right ventricular outflow tract, is located in front of the right coronary aortic sinus. Compared to the endocardial surface of this supraventricular crest and the right-side ventricular septum, the lateral and inferior free wall of the basal right ventricle has rich trabeculations extending to the level of the tricuspid valve attachment.

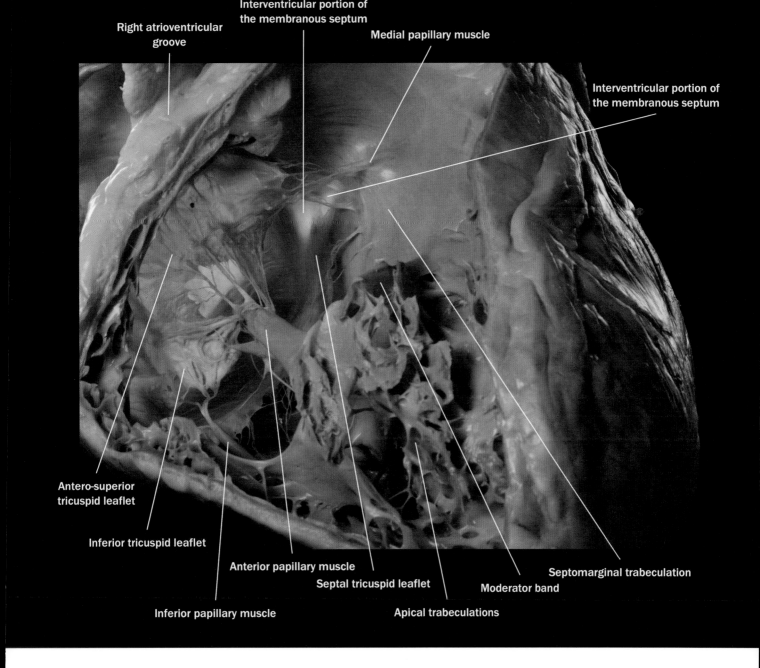

Right atrioventricular groove

Interventricular portion of the membranous septum

Medial papillary muscle

Interventricular portion of the membranous septum

Antero-superior tricuspid leaflet

Inferior tricuspid leaflet

Anterior papillary muscle

Septal tricuspid leaflet

Septomarginal trabeculation

Moderator band

Inferior papillary muscle

Apical trabeculations

Figure 49 The tricuspid valve viewed from the anterior direction. 🔴🔵 Anaglyph 12.

The membranous septum is transilluminated. The medial part of the antero-superior tricuspid leaflet is anchored by the chordae tendineae arising from the medial papillary muscle. The chordae tendineae from the anterior papillary muscle anchors the commissure between the antero-superior and inferior tricuspid leaflets. The chordae tendineae from the inferior papillary muscle anchor the inferior tricuspid leaflet. The septal tricuspid leaflet is anchored by the multiple septal chordae tendineae. The septal tricuspid leaflet divides the membranous septum into the atrioventricular and interventricular portions.

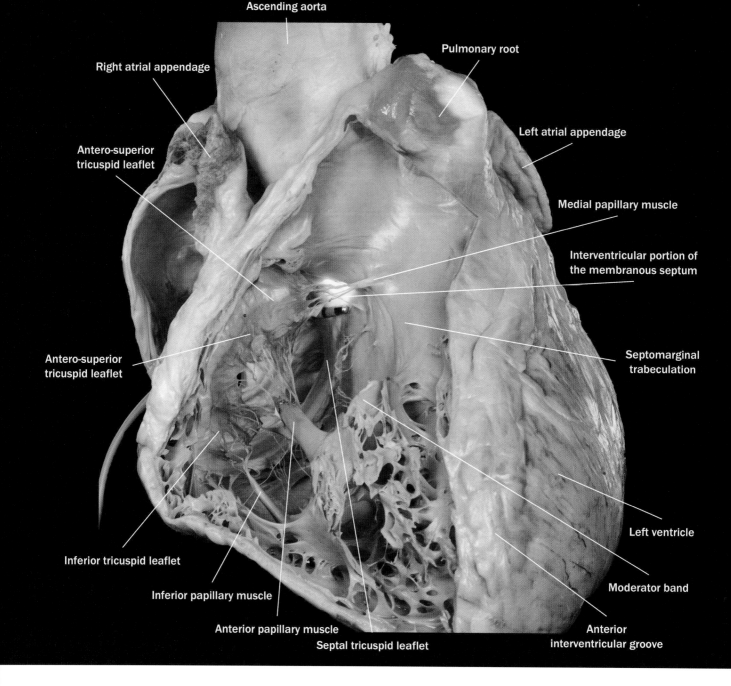

Ascending aorta

Pulmonary root

Right atrial appendage

Left atrial appendage

**Antero-superior
tricuspid leaflet**

Medial papillary muscle

**Interventricular portion of
the membranous septum**

**Antero-superior
tricuspid leaflet**

**Septomarginal
trabeculation**

Inferior tricuspid leaflet

Left ventricle

Inferior papillary muscle

Moderator band

Anterior papillary muscle

**Anterior
interventricular groove**

Septal tricuspid leaflet

Figure 50 The catheter placed at the inferior margin of the membranous septum. [⬜⬜] Anaglyph 13.

The left image is viewed from the anterior direction, and the right image is viewed from the left anterior oblique direction. The membranous septum is transilluminated (left). The membranous septum tilts toward the right anterior direction along with the tilting of the aortic root. The catheter is fixed at the angle created by this tilting at the inferior margin of the membranous septum, where is the location of the bundle of His. Refer to Figure 5. The location is close to the commissure between the septal and antero-superior tricuspid leaflets, commonly on its septal tricuspid leaflet side. When viewed from the left anterior oblique view, reflecting the width of the orifice of the inferior vena cava, the catheter directs toward the septal direction. It does not show tangential straight shape, which is perfectly foreshortened, even though the ventricular

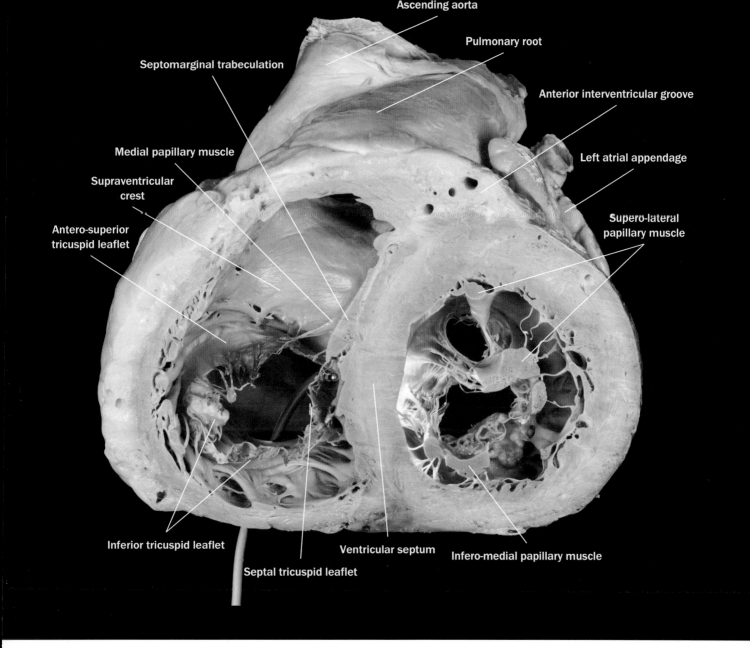

Ascending aorta

Pulmonary root

Septomarginal trabeculation

Anterior interventricular groove

Medial papillary muscle

Left atrial appendage

Supraventricular crest

Supero-lateral papillary muscle

Antero-superior tricuspid leaflet

Inferior tricuspid leaflet

Ventricular septum

Infero-medial papillary muscle

Septal tricuspid leaflet

septum is seen tangentially. If the optimal left anterior oblique angulation is defined as the view showing the ventricular septum tangentially, this indicates that setting the left anterior oblique angulation based on the shape of the His-catheter could be far left anterior oblique than the optimal angulation. Insufficient or excessive left anterior oblique angulation relative to the optimal angulation would complicate the procedure related to the ventricular septum. For example, if the left anterior oblique angulation is insufficient relative to the optimal angulation, the septal direction is readily feasible even if the catheter actually directs toward the anterior free wall. On the other hand, excessive left anterior oblique angulation could hardly allow the catheter to point the septal direction even if the catheter is actually placed on the ventricular septum.[8]

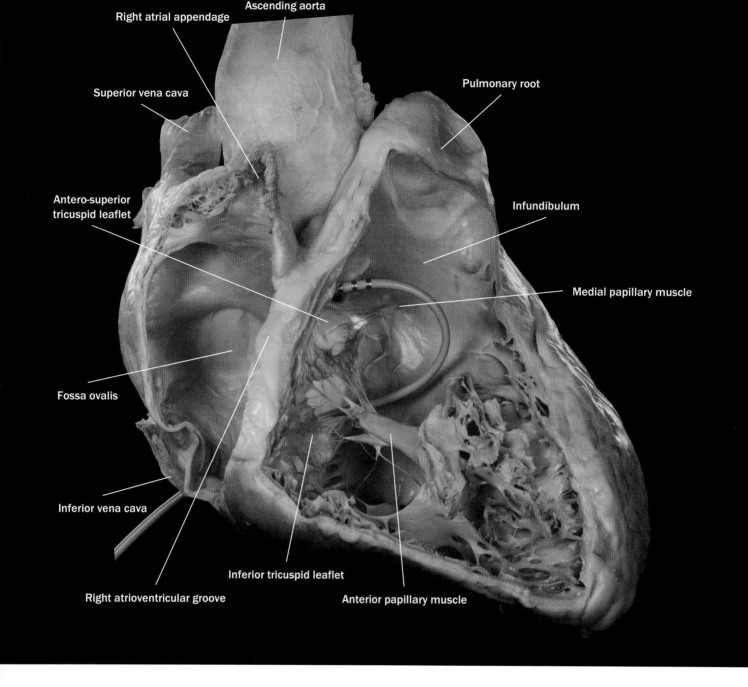

Right atrial appendage

Ascending aorta

Pulmonary root

Superior vena cava

Infundibulum

Antero-superior
tricuspid leaflet

Medial papillary muscle

Fossa ovalis

Inferior vena cava

Inferior tricuspid leaflet

Right atrioventricular groove

Anterior papillary muscle

Figure 51   The ablation catheter placed at the superior tricuspid annulus with the U-turn approach.

The left image is viewed from the right anterior oblique direction, and the right image is viewed from the left anterior oblique direction. The catheter is fixed at the superior tricuspid valve attachment. This U-turn approach can theoretically

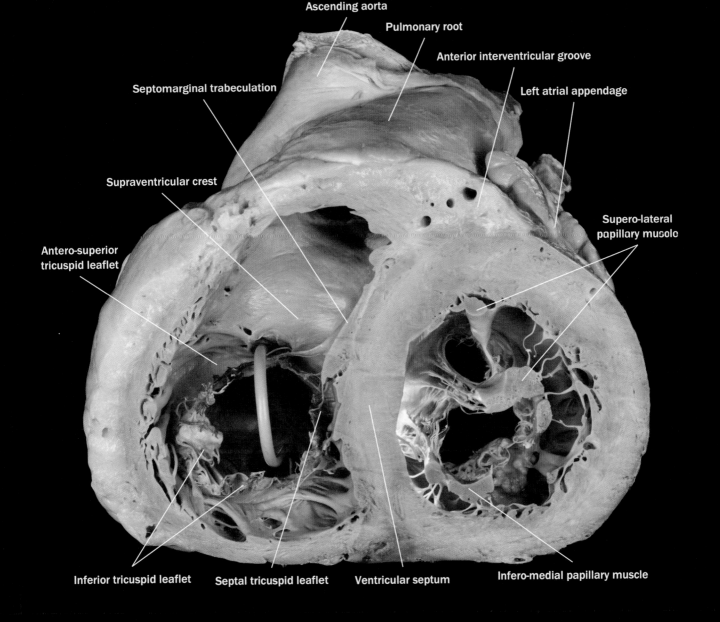

Ascending aorta

Pulmonary root

Anterior interventricular groove

Left atrial appendage

Septomarginal trabeculation

Supraventricular crest

Supero-lateral papillary muscle

Antero-superior tricuspid leaflet

Inferior tricuspid leaflet Septal tricuspid leaflet Ventricular septum Infero-medial papillary muscle

avoid direct injury to the antero-superior tricuspid leaflet,[9] compared to the conventional ablation of the tricuspid annulus, sandwiching the leaflet between the catheter tip and annulus.

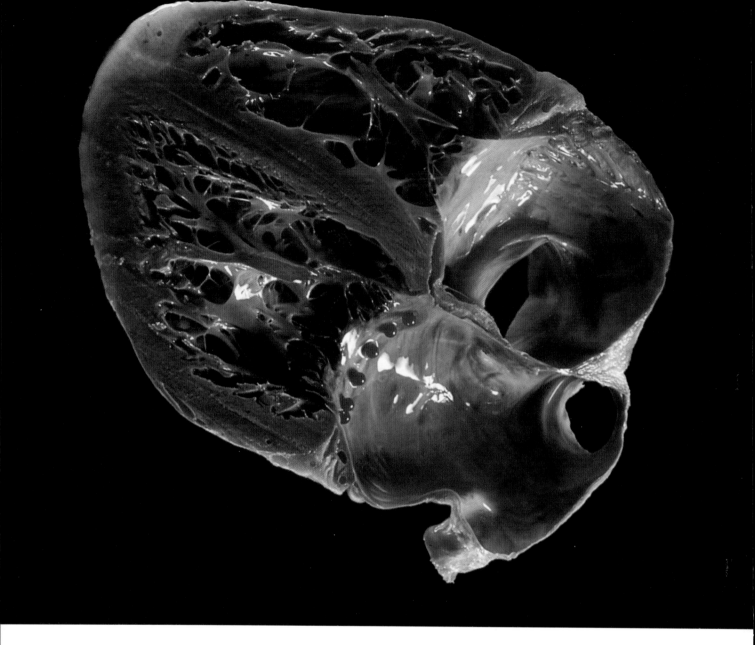

Figure 52 The horizontal section showing the four-chamber image viewed from the superior direction.[1]

The commissure between the inferior and septal tricuspid leaflets is anchored by the inferior papillary muscle. Due to deeply wedged bilateral atrioventricular groove, lateral annulus of the mitral and tricuspid valve is located medial relative to the basal-lateral free wall. Thus, the basal free wall of the right ventricle shows a right-angled bending, suggesting the need for the U-turn approach if this region is related to the accessory pathways or ventricular arrhythmias. The space between the antero-medial right atrium and the basal ventricular septum is the inferior pyramidal space. In this heart, the

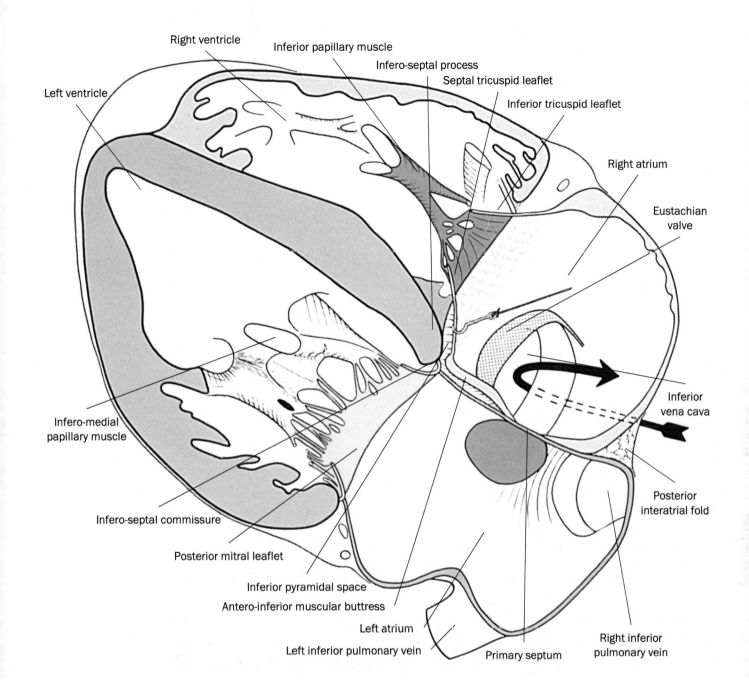

Right ventricle

Inferior papillary muscle

Infero-septal process

Septal tricuspid leaflet

Inferior tricuspid leaflet

Left ventricle

Right atrium

Eustachian valve

Infero-medial papillary muscle

Inferior vena cava

Infero-septal commissure

Posterior interatrial fold

Posterior mitral leaflet

Inferior pyramidal space

Antero-inferior muscular buttress

Left atrium

Left inferior pulmonary vein

Primary septum

Right inferior pulmonary vein

epicardial fibro-adipose tissue filling the inferior pyramidal space is removed. This basal infero-septal left ventricle found at the offset between the mitral and tricuspid annulus is referred to as the infero-septal process.[10] Refer to Figure 46. Thus, the inferior pyramidal space is sandwiched between the infero-septal process and the floor of the triangle of Koch at the antero-medial right atrium. This inferior pyramidal space allows the atrioventricular nodal artery to ascend toward the atrioventricular node located at the right-side of the central fibrous body. The paired section of this image is Figure 53.

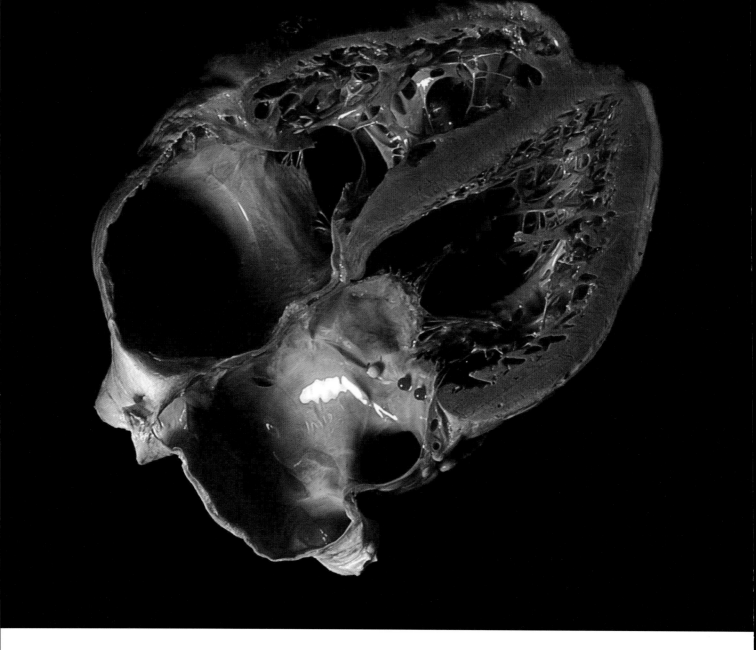

Figure 53   The horizontal section showing the four-chamber image viewed from the inferior direction.[1]

The inferior and septal tricuspid leaflet is cut on this plane. The antero-superior tricuspid leaflet is observed along the supraventricular crest away from the observer. The tricuspid annulus is located apical to the mitral annulus. The offset between the tricuspid and mitral annuli at the basal inferior ventricular septum corresponds to the region of the infero-septal process and inferior pyramidal space. Refer to Figure 46. The epicardial adipose tissue filling the inferior pyramidal

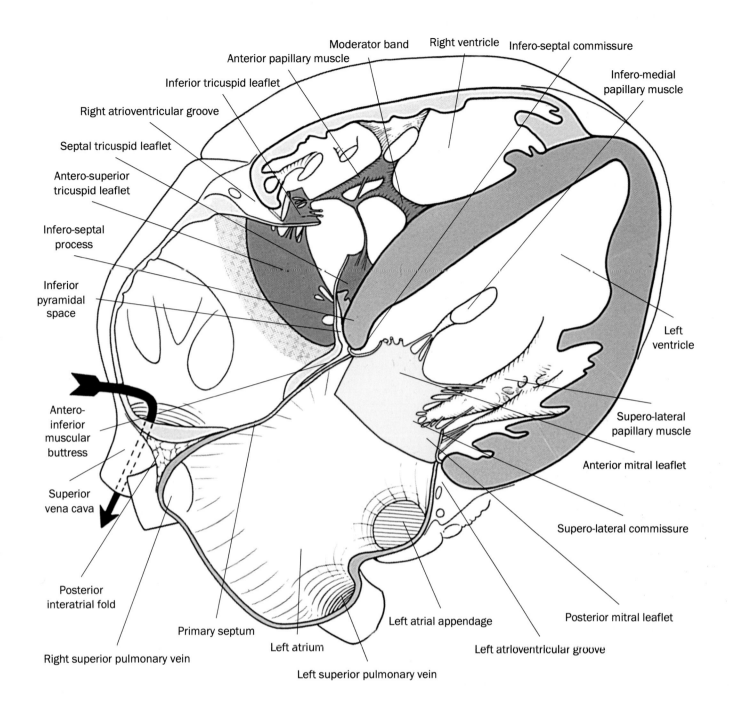

Moderator band

Right ventricle

Infero-septal commissure

Anterior papillary muscle

Infero-medial
papillary muscle

Inferior tricuspid leaflet

Right atrioventricular groove

Septal tricuspid leaflet

Antero-superior
tricuspid leaflet

Infero-septal
process

Inferior
pyramidal
space

Left
ventricle

Antero-
inferior
muscular
buttress

Supero-lateral
papillary muscle

Anterior mitral leaflet

Superior
vena cava

Supero-lateral commissure

Posterior
interatrial fold

Posterior mitral leaflet

Right superior pulmonary vein

Primary septum

Left atrial appendage

Left atrioventricular groove

Left atrium

Left superior pulmonary vein

space is removed. The antero-medial right atrium close to the septal tricuspid leaflet, corresponding to the floor of the triangle of Koch, is facing to the infero-septal process[10] intervened by the inferior pyramidal space.[11] The trabeculation is apparently coarse and extensive in the right ventricle compared to the fine trabeculation in the left ventricle. The paired section of this image is Figure 52.

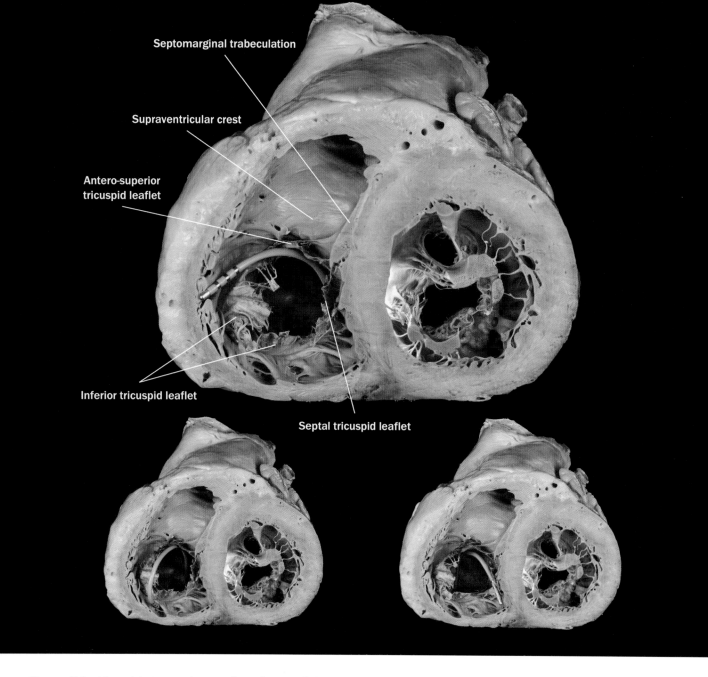

Septomarginal trabeculation

Supraventricular crest

Antero-superior tricuspid leaflet

Inferior tricuspid leaflet

Septal tricuspid leaflet

Figure 54 The ablation catheter placed around the tricuspid annulus.

The tricuspid annulus is a substrate for idiopathic ventricular arrhythmia with septal region predominance.[12] The catheter is placed at the basal-lateral right ventricle (upper), infero-lateral tricuspid annulus with the U-turn approach (lower left), and basal infero-medial right ventricle (lower right) via the inferior vena cava. The tricuspid valve is located apical relative to the mitral valve. Rich trabeculations are observed around the lateral and inferior tricuspid annulus. On the contrary, the endocardial surface is much smoother around the superior and septal tricuspid annulus.

References

1. McAlpine WA. Digitized collection of all the images created by Dr. McAlpine at UCLA. Copyright UCLA Cardiac Arrhythmia Center. Part of this collection appeared in *Heart and Coronary Arteries: An Anatomical Atlas for Clinical Diagnosis, Radiological Investigation, and Surgical Treatment*. New York: Springer-Verlag; 1975.
2. Zimmerman J, Bailey CP. The surgical significance of the fibrous skeleton of the heart. *J Thorac Cardiovasc Surg*. 1962;44:701–712.
3. Saremi F, Sánchez-Quintana D, Mori S, et al. Fibrous skeleton of the heart: Anatomic overview and evaluation of pathologic conditions with CT and MR imaging. *Radiographics*. 2017;37:1330–1351.
4. Mori S, Fukuzawa K, Takaya T, et al. Clinical structural anatomy of the inferior pyramidal space reconstructed within the cardiac contour using multidetector-row computed tomography. *J Cardiovasc Electrophysiol*. 2015;26:705–712.
5. Saremi F, Hassani C, Millan-Nunez V, et al. Imaging evaluation of tricuspid valve: Analysis of morphology and function with CT and MRI. *AJR Am J Roentgenol*. 2015;204:W531–W542.
6. Shimizu S. [Topographical anatomy of the atrioventricular node of Tawara—findings by macro-microscopic dissection under dissecting microscope] (in Japanese). *Nihon Kyobu Geka Gakkai Zasshi*. 1989;37:227–233.
7. Tretter JT, Sarwark AE, Anderson RH, et al. Assessment of the anatomical variation to be found in the normal tricuspid valve. *Clin Anat*. 2016;29:399–407.
8. Mori S, Fukuzawa K, Takaya T, et al. Optimal angulations for obtaining an *en face* view of each coronary aortic sinus and the interventricular septum: Correlative anatomy around the left ventricular outflow tract. *Clin Anat*. 2015;28:494–505.
9. Enriquez A, Tapias C, Rodriguez D, et al. Role of intracardiac echocardiography for guiding ablation of tricuspid valve arrhythmias. *Heart Rhythm Case Rep*. 2018;4:209–213.
10. Li A, Zuberi Z, Bradfield JS, et al. Endocardial ablation of ventricular ectopic beats arising from the basal inferoseptal process of the left ventricle. *Heart Rhythm*. 2018;15:1356–1362.
11. Mori S, Nishii T, Takaya T, et al. Clinical structural anatomy of the inferior pyramidal space reconstructed from the living heart: Three-dimensional visualization using multidetector-row computed tomography. *Clin Anat*. 2015;28:878–887.
12. Tada H, Tadokoro K, Ito S, et al. Idiopathic ventricular arrhythmias originating from the tricuspid annulus: Prevalence, electrocardiographic characteristics, and results of radiofrequency catheter ablation. *Heart Rhythm*. 2007;4:7–16.

10

Membranous Septum

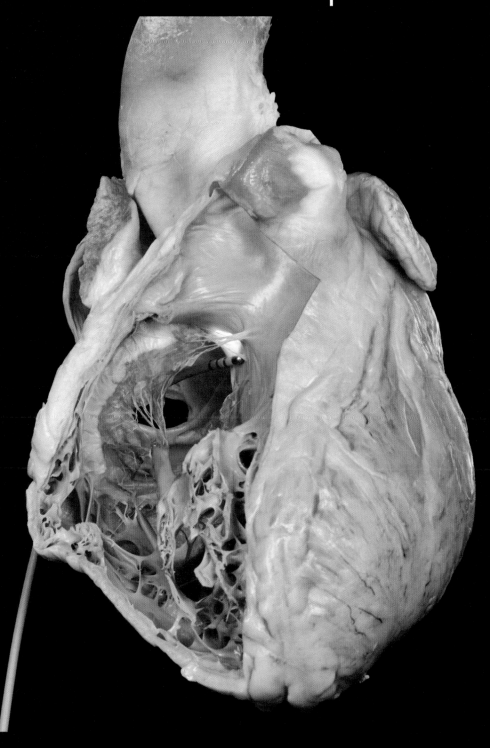

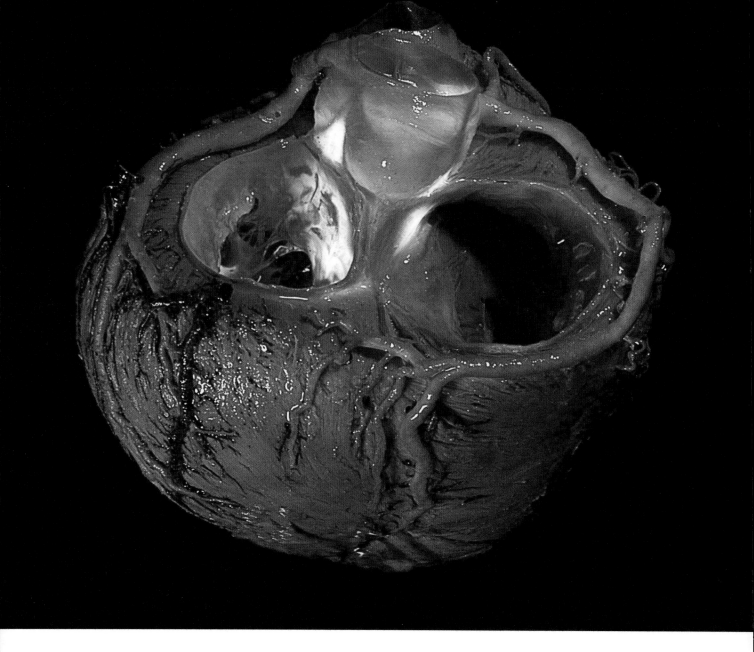

Figure 55   The atrioventricular junction viewed from the atrial side.[1]

The light source placed within the left ventricular outflow tract transilluminates the interleaflet triangles between the aortic sinuses, anterior mitral leaflet, and the atrioventricular portion of the membranous septum. The less transilluminated thick and firm fibrous tissue located at the bottom of the non-coronary aortic sinus is the right fibrous trigone, also referred to as the central fibrous body.[1] This firm, fibrous tissue connects the aortic root (non-coronary aortic sinus), anterior mitral leaflet, atrial septum (antero-inferior muscular buttress), ventricular septum, infero-septal process, the membranous septum, and the septal tricuspid leaflet. The interleaflet triangle between the non-coronary and right coronary aortic sinuses is located superior to the membranous septum. It is separated from the membranous septum by the ventriculo-infundibular

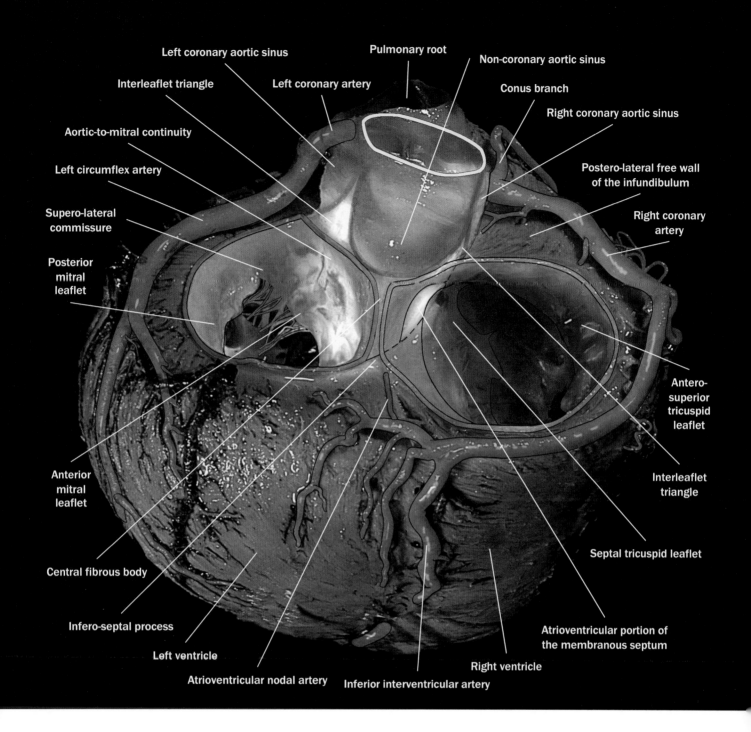

Left coronary aortic sinus

Pulmonary root

Non-coronary aortic sinus

Interleaflet triangle

Left coronary artery

Conus branch

Right coronary aortic sinus

Aortic-to-mitral continuity

Postero-lateral free wall
of the infundibulum

Left circumflex artery

Right coronary
artery

Supero-lateral
commissure

Posterior
mitral
leaflet

Antero-
superior
tricuspid
leaflet

Anterior
mitral
leaflet

Interleaflet
triangle

Central fibrous body

Septal tricuspid leaflet

Infero-septal process

Atrioventricular portion of
the membranous septum

Left ventricle

Right ventricle

Atrioventricular nodal artery

Inferior interventricular artery

fold.[2] Thus, the membranous septum is the anatomically true septum between the right atrium/ventricle and the left ventricular outflow tract. On the contrary, the interleaflet triangle above the membranous septum is not the septum, but it just separates the distal end of the left ventricular outflow tract from the right-side transverse sinus. As all of three interleaflet triangles incorporated into the aortic root are located beneath the semi-lunar hingelines of the aortic valve leaflets, they are hemodynamically the components of the left ventricular outflow tract.[3] These interleaflet triangles are structurally the components of the aortic root extending between the virtual basal ring and sinutubular junction,[4] though. The atrioventricular nodal artery ascends toward the central fibrous body, posterior to the infero-septal process. Refer to Figure 46.

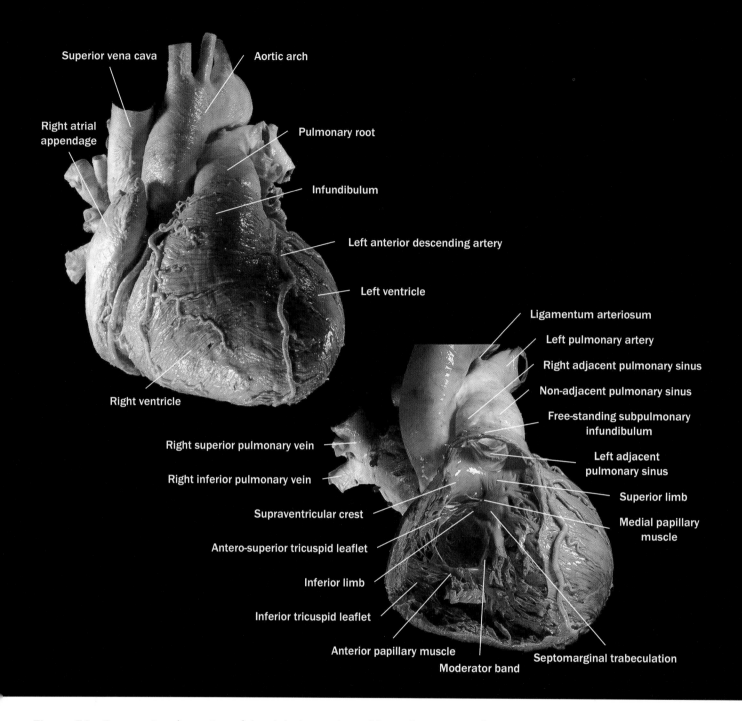

Superior vena cava

Aortic arch

Right atrial appendage

Pulmonary root

Infundibulum

Left anterior descending artery

Left ventricle

Right ventricle

Ligamentum arteriosum

Left pulmonary artery

Right adjacent pulmonary sinus

Non-adjacent pulmonary sinus

Free-standing subpulmonary infundibulum

Left adjacent pulmonary sinus

Right superior pulmonary vein

Right inferior pulmonary vein

Superior limb

Medial papillary muscle

Supraventricular crest

Antero-superior tricuspid leaflet

Inferior limb

Inferior tricuspid leaflet

Anterior papillary muscle

Septomarginal trabeculation

Moderator band

Figure 56 Progressive dissection of the right heart viewed from the anterior direction.[1]

The whole heart is viewed from the anterior direction (upper left). The progressive dissection of the right heart (lower left and right) reveals the deep and central location of the membranous septum inferior to the aortic root. The membranous septum is located on the crest of the ventricular septum, inferior to the interleaflet triangle between the non-coronary and right coronary aortic sinuses. The membranous septum composes supero-medial part of the right ventricular inflow. The black line in the image on the right page shows the postero-lateral attachment of the right ventricle, corresponding to the inferior margin of the ventriculo-infundibular fold.[1] The membranous septum is separated from the interleaflet triangle by this line. The nadir of the right coronary aortic sinus is located inferior to this line. In other words, this line is located superior to the virtual basal ring at the base of the right coronary aortic sinus. Thus, this line corresponds to the

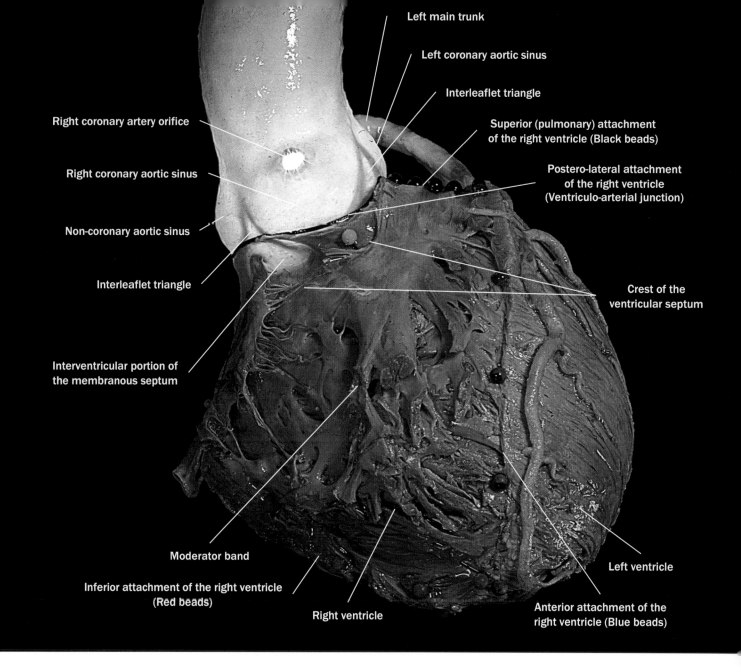

Left main trunk

Left coronary aortic sinus

Interleaflet triangle

Right coronary artery orifice

Superior (pulmonary) attachment
of the right ventricle (Black beads)

Right coronary aortic sinus

Postero-lateral attachment
of the right ventricle
(Ventriculo-arterial junction)

Non-coronary aortic sinus

Interleaflet triangle

Crest of the
ventricular septum

Interventricular portion of
the membranous septum

Moderator band

Left ventricle

Inferior attachment of the right ventricle
(Red beads)

Right ventricle

Anterior attachment of the
right ventricle (Blue beads)

ventriculo-arterial junction at this region. This means the part of the crest of the ventricular septum is incorporated at the base of the right coronary aortic sinus.[5] This structural anatomy is also referred to as the myocardial crescent supporting the right coronary aortic sinus.[5] This myocardial crescent is the potential substrate of ventricular arrhythmia ablated from the right coronary aortic sinus.[6] Left antero-superior to the membranous septum, the medial papillary muscle is located anterior to the nadir of the right coronary aortic sinus. The medial papillary muscle is generally found close to the bifurcation of the superior and inferior limbs of the septomarginal trabeculation, at its inferior limb side. The superior limb of the septo-marginal trabeculation ascends toward the left adjacent pulmonary sinus. The proximal part of the superior limb is the superior limit of the ventricular septum in the right ventricular outflow tract. Refer to Figure 81.

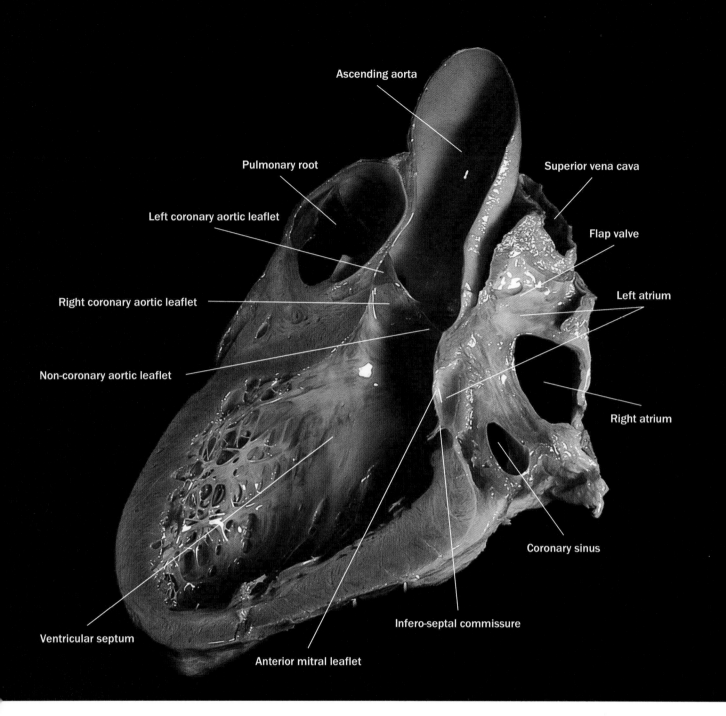

Ascending aorta

Pulmonary root

Superior vena cava

Left coronary aortic leaflet

Flap valve

Right coronary aortic leaflet

Left atrium

Non-coronary aortic leaflet

Right atrium

Coronary sinus

Ventricular septum

Infero-septal commissure

Anterior mitral leaflet

Figure 57 Left ventricular aspect of the membranous septum.[1]

The heart is viewed from the left postero-superior direction. The atrial septum is sectioned almost tangentially. Transillumination reveals the location of the membranous septum (right), infero-apical to the interleaflet triangle between the right and non-coronary aortic sinuses.[7] The crest of the ventricular septum just apical to the inferior margin of the membranous septum, corresponding to the origin of the left bundle branch, bulges toward the left ventricular outflow tract.

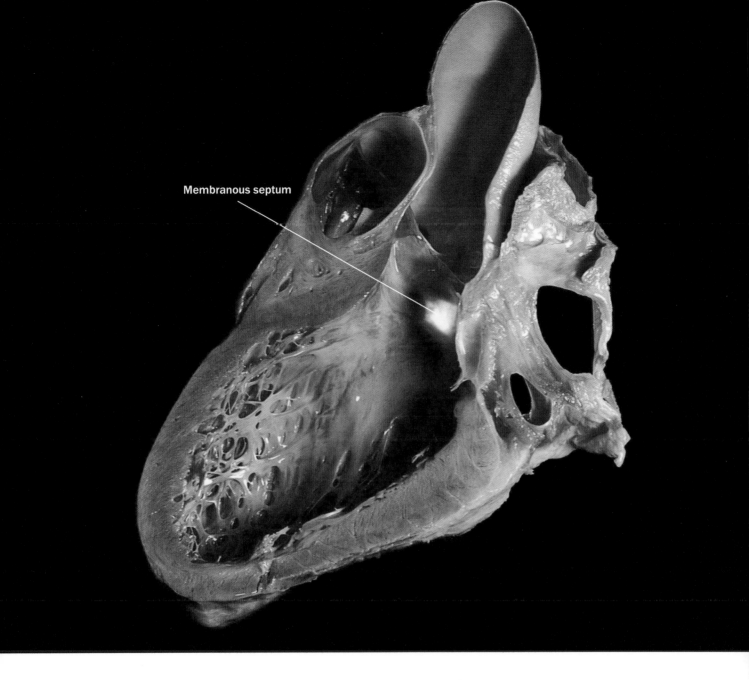

Membranous septum

The extent of this bulging varies among individuals.[8] The muscular ventricular septum shows many fine apical trabeculations without papillary muscles. The location of the membranous septum relative to the virtual basal ring plane of the aortic root is variable.[2]

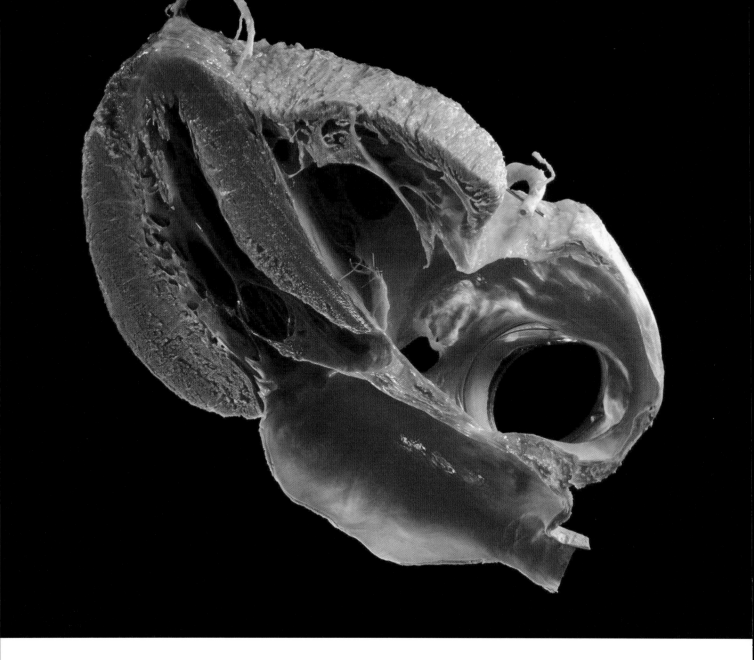

Figure 58 The horizontal section at the level of the membranous septum viewed from the superior direction.[1]

The horizontal section is made at the level of the atrioventricular portion of the membranous septum below the bottom of the non-coronary aortic sinus. The membranous septum is located between the crest of the muscular ventricular septum and the atrial septum, corresponding to the antero-inferior muscular buttress. The septal tricuspid leaflet divides the membranous septum into the atrioventricular and interventricular portions in unequal fashion. Therefore, the membranous septum separates the right atrial vestibule and right ventricular inflow from the left ventricular outflow tract. The right fibrous trigone is the triangular-shaped, firm, fibrous thickening continuing from the bottom of the non-coronary aortic sinus toward the infero-septal commissure to support the medial part of the anterior mitral leaflet.[9] The septal tricuspid leaflet, anterior mitral leaflet, and the membranous septum are connected to this thick fibrous tissue. This fibrous tissue

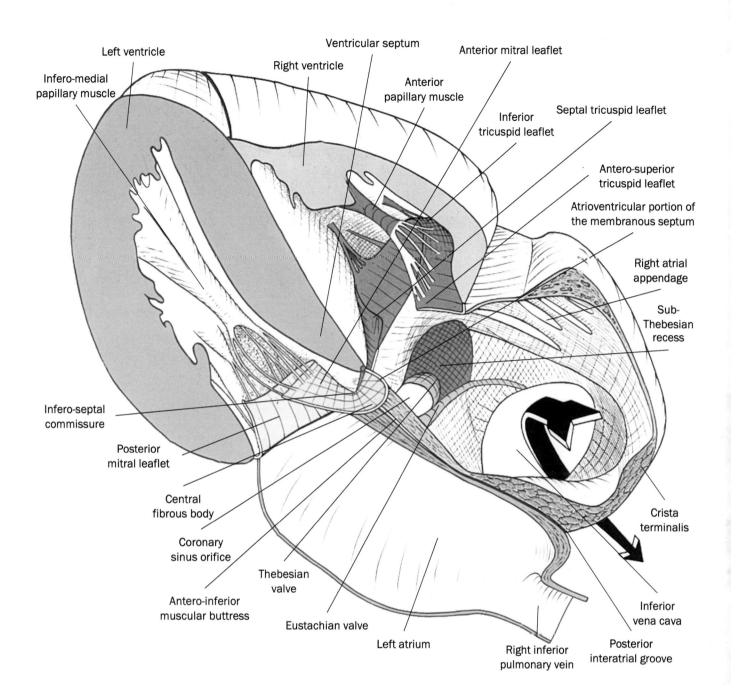

Left ventricle

Infero-medial
papillary muscle

Ventricular septum

Right ventricle

Anterior
papillary muscle

Anterior mitral leaflet

Inferior
tricuspid leaflet

Septal tricuspid leaflet

Antero-superior
tricuspid leaflet

Atrioventricular portion of
the membranous septum

Right atrial
appendage

Sub-
Thebesian
recess

Infero-septal
commissure

Posterior
mitral leaflet

Central
fibrous body

Coronary
sinus orifice

Antero-inferior
muscular buttress

Thebesian
valve

Eustachian valve

Left atrium

Right inferior
pulmonary vein

Crista
terminalis

Inferior
vena cava

Posterior
interatrial groove

also connects the aortic root (non-coronary aortic sinus), ventricular septum, atrial septum (antero-inferior buttress), and infero-septal process of the left ventricle. The right fibrous trigone is also referred to as the central fibrous body,[1,9,10] which is the keystone of the fibrous cardiac skeleton.[11] Sometimes, the central fibrous body is described as the concept involving both the right fibrous trigone and the atrioventricular portion of the membranous septum.[11] Macroscopically, even using the transillumination, clear demarcation between the right fibrous trigone and the membranous septum is difficult. The atrioventricular node is generally located on the right atrial side of the central fibrous body[9] at the apex of the inferior pyramidal space. The bundle of His penetrates the central fibrous body to emerge to the inferior rim of the atrioventricular portion of the membranous septum. The paired section of this image is Figure 59.

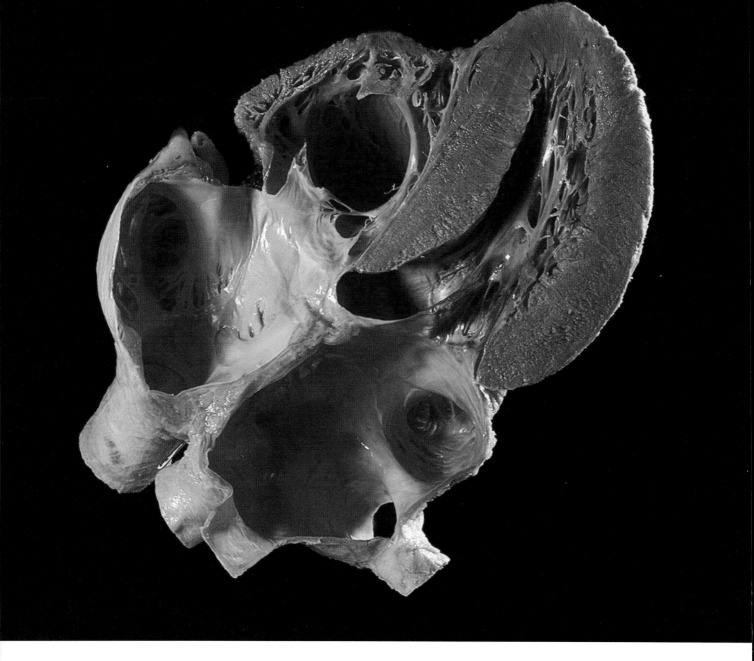

Figure 59 The horizontal section at the level of the membranous septum viewed from the inferior direction.[1]

The membranous septum is located between the crest of the muscular ventricular septum and the atrial septum (antero-inferior muscular buttress). The membranous septum is in continuity with the right fibrous trigone, which is the firm fibrous thickening extending inferiorly from the bottom of the non-coronary aortic sinus.[9] The right fibrous trigone is also referred to as the central fibrous body.[1,9,10] The central fibrous body is the keystone of the cardiac skeleton,[11] connecting the

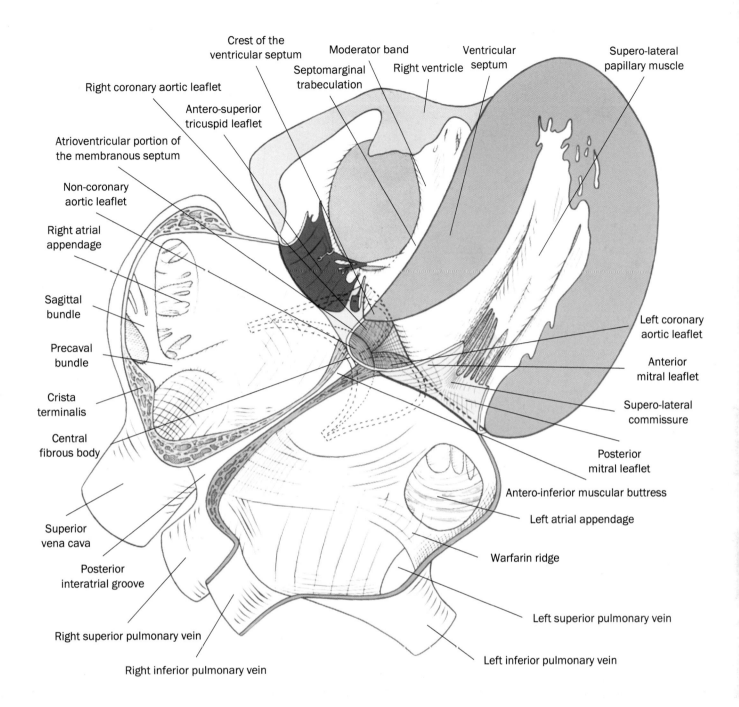

Crest of the ventricular septum

Moderator band

Right coronary aortic leaflet

Antero-superior tricuspid leaflet

Septomarginal trabeculation

Right ventricle

Ventricular septum

Supero-lateral papillary muscle

Atrioventricular portion of the membranous septum

Non-coronary aortic leaflet

Right atrial appendage

Sagittal bundle

Precaval bundle

Crista terminalis

Central fibrous body

Superior vena cava

Posterior interatrial groove

Right superior pulmonary vein

Right inferior pulmonary vein

Left coronary aortic leaflet

Anterior mitral leaflet

Supero-lateral commissure

Posterior mitral leaflet

Antero-inferior muscular buttress

Left atrial appendage

Warfarin ridge

Left superior pulmonary vein

Left inferior pulmonary vein

membranous septum, septal tricuspid leaflet, and anterior mitral leaflet. It also supports the aortic root (non-coronary aortic sinus), atrial septum (antero-inferior muscular buttress), crest of the ventricular septum, and infero-septal process of the left ventricle. The non-coronary and right coronary aortic sinuses are located superior to the membranous septum. The paired section of this image is Figure 58.

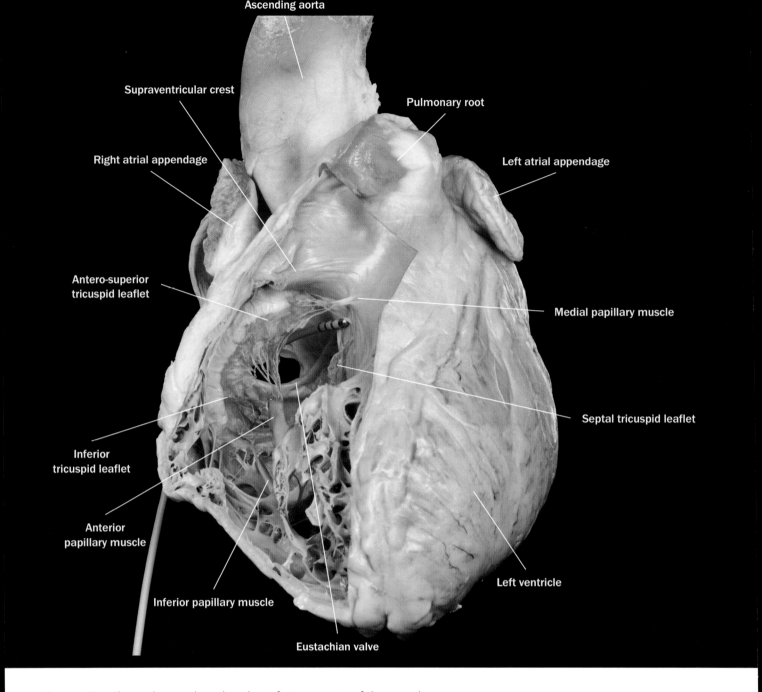

Ascending aorta

Supraventricular crest

Pulmonary root

Right atrial appendage

Left atrial appendage

Antero-superior
tricuspid leaflet

Medial papillary muscle

Inferior
tricuspid leaflet

Septal tricuspid leaflet

Anterior
papillary muscle

Inferior papillary muscle

Left ventricle

Eustachian valve

Figure 60   The catheter placed at the inferior margin of the membranous septum.

The heart is viewed from the left anterior oblique direction. The catheter is placed at the approximate location of the atrioventricular conduction axis, at the inferior margin of the membranous septum. The tip is on the superior septal attachment of the septal tricuspid leaflet. Transillumination from the left ventricular outflow tract (right) reveals the

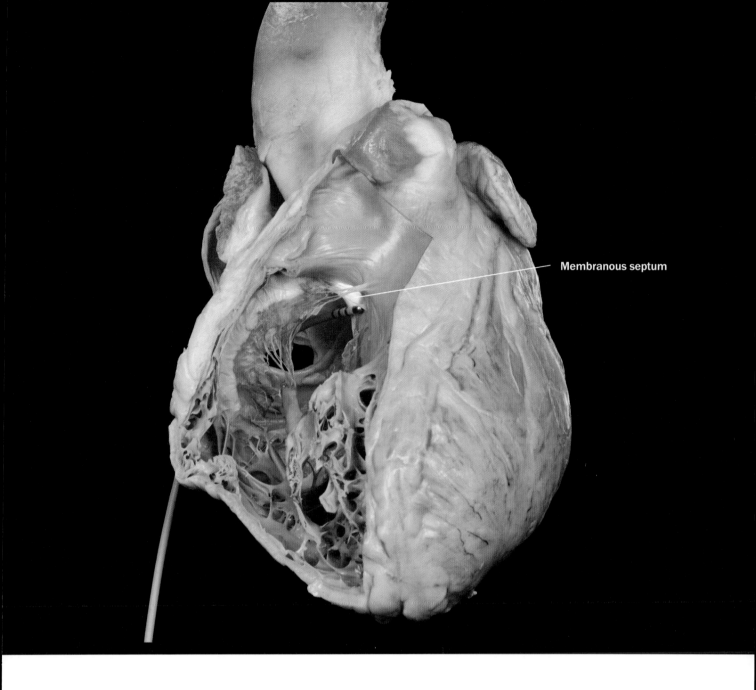

Membranous septum

membranous septum. The membranous septum tilts toward the lateral direction against the muscular ventricular septum, along with the lateral tilting of the aortic root.

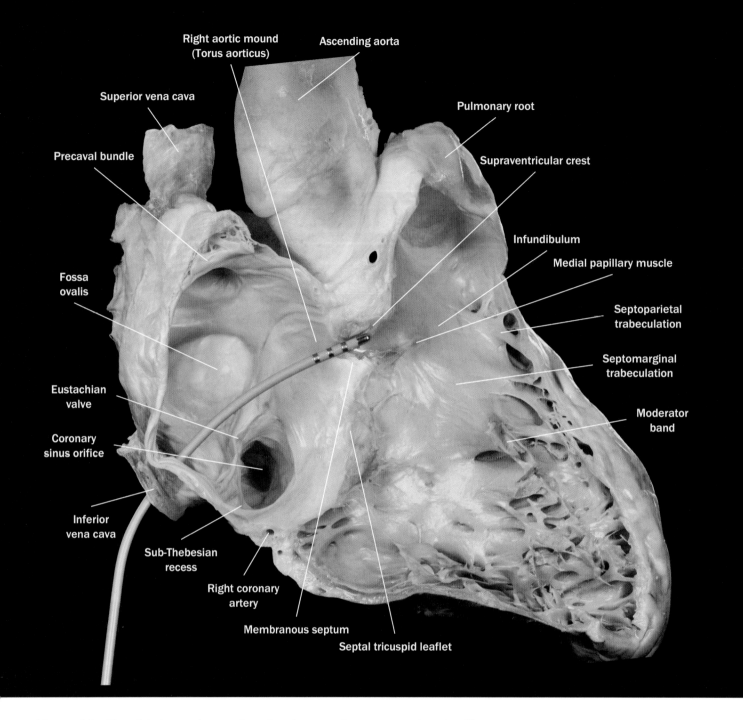

Right aortic mound (Torus aorticus)

Ascending aorta

Superior vena cava

Pulmonary root

Precaval bundle

Supraventricular crest

Infundibulum

Medial papillary muscle

Fossa ovalis

Septoparietal trabeculation

Septomarginal trabeculation

Eustachian valve

Moderator band

Coronary sinus orifice

Inferior vena cava

Sub-Thebesian recess

Right coronary artery

Membranous septum

Septal tricuspid leaflet

Figure 61 The ablation catheter placed at the superior paraseptal region.[12]

The images are viewed from the right anterior oblique (left) and left anterior oblique (right) directions. The membranous septum is transilluminated in the left image. The catheter is placed on the infero-medial part of the supraventricular crest. This region corresponds to the supero-medial tricuspid annulus. It is superior and lateral to the membranous septum. The ventricular aspect of this region is the supraventricular crest adjacent to the right coronary aortic sinus. The atrial aspect of

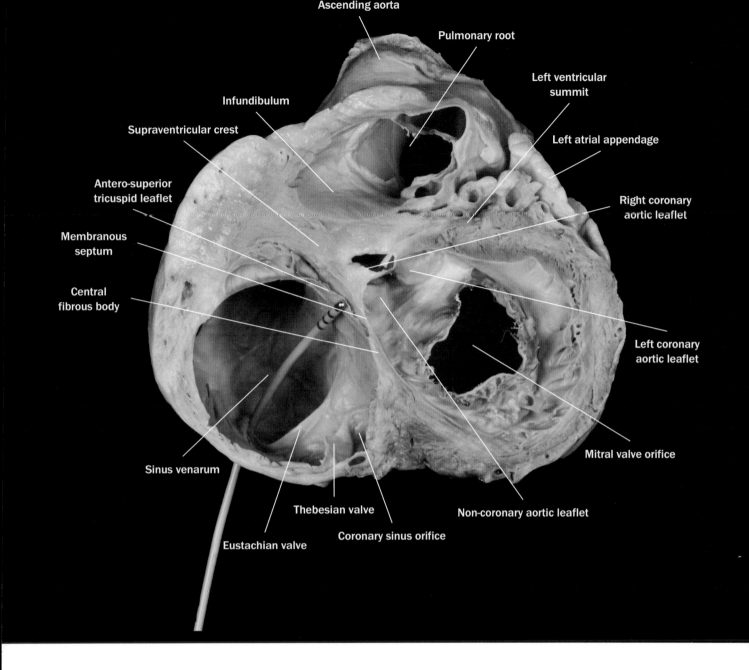

Ascending aorta

Pulmonary root

Left ventricular summit

Left atrial appendage

Infundibulum

Supraventricular crest

Right coronary aortic leaflet

Antero-superior tricuspid leaflet

Membranous septum

Central fibrous body

Left coronary aortic leaflet

Sinus venarum

Mitral valve orifice

Thebesian valve

Non-coronary aortic leaflet

Eustachian valve

Coronary sinus orifice

this region is the right atrial vestibule. If the tip is pulled back medially closer to the superior margin of the atrioventricular portion of the membranous septum, the region corresponds to the right aortic mound adjacent to the anterior half of the non-coronary aortic sinus. Refer to Figures 9 and 10. These regions are safe in terms of the injury to the atrioventricular conduction axis.

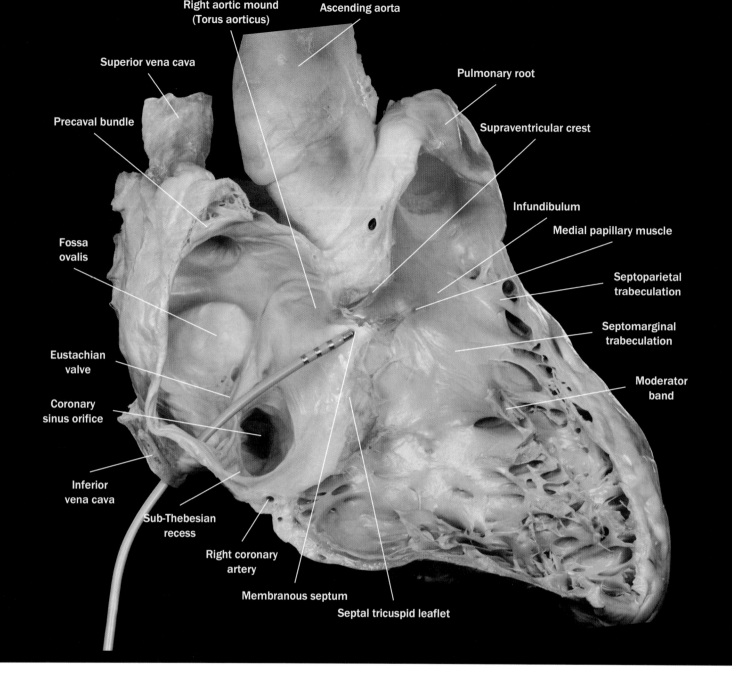

Figure 62 The ablation catheter placed at the septal region.[12]

The images are viewed from the right anterior oblique (left) and left anterior oblique (right) directions. The membranous septum is transilluminated in the left image. The catheter is placed at the membranous septum, which is the true anatomical septum between the right atrium/ventricle and left ventricular outflow tract. Thus, this approach has a potential risk

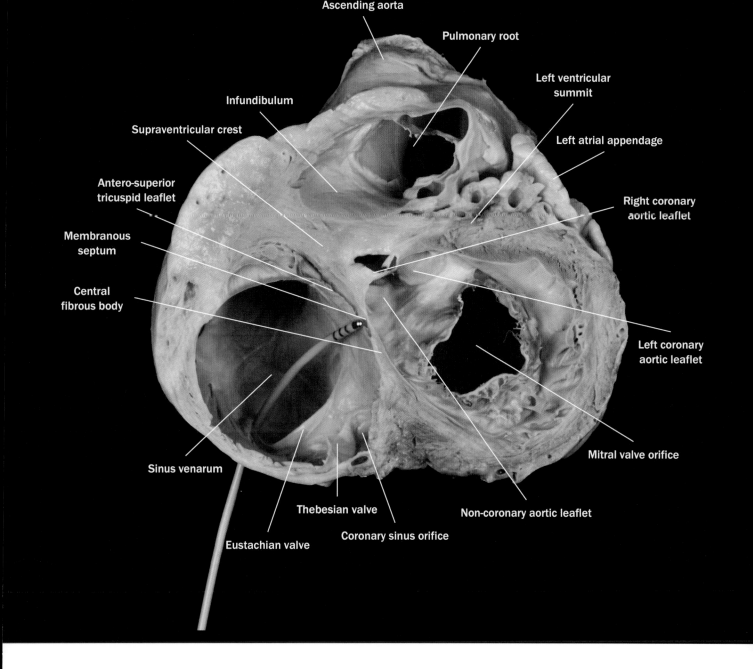

Ascending aorta

Pulmonary root

Left ventricular summit

Infundibulum

Left atrial appendage

Supraventricular crest

Right coronary aortic leaflet

Antero-superior tricuspid leaflet

Membranous septum

Central fibrous body

Left coronary aortic leaflet

Mitral valve orifice

Sinus venarum

Thebesian valve

Non-coronary aortic leaflet

Eustachian valve

Coronary sinus orifice

to create iatrogenic Gerbode-type atrioventricular shunt,[13] or interventricular shunt depending on the location of the tip relative to the attachment of the septal tricuspid leaflet.[14]

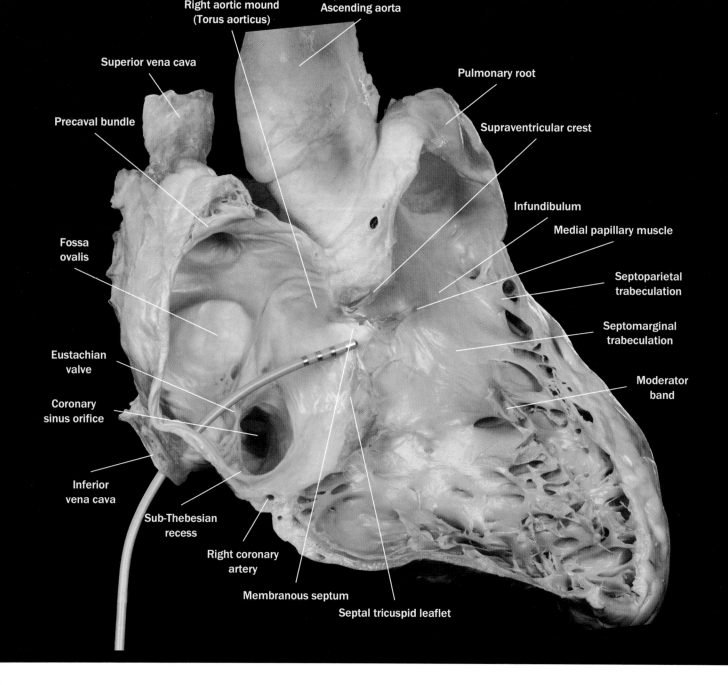

Figure 63 The ablation catheter placed at the bundle of His.[12]

The images are viewed from the right anterior oblique (left) and left anterior oblique (right) directions. The membranous septum is transilluminated in the left image. The catheter is placed at the inferior margin of the atrioventricular portion of the membranous septum. This is exact location of the penetrating bundle of the atrioventricular conduction axis, referred

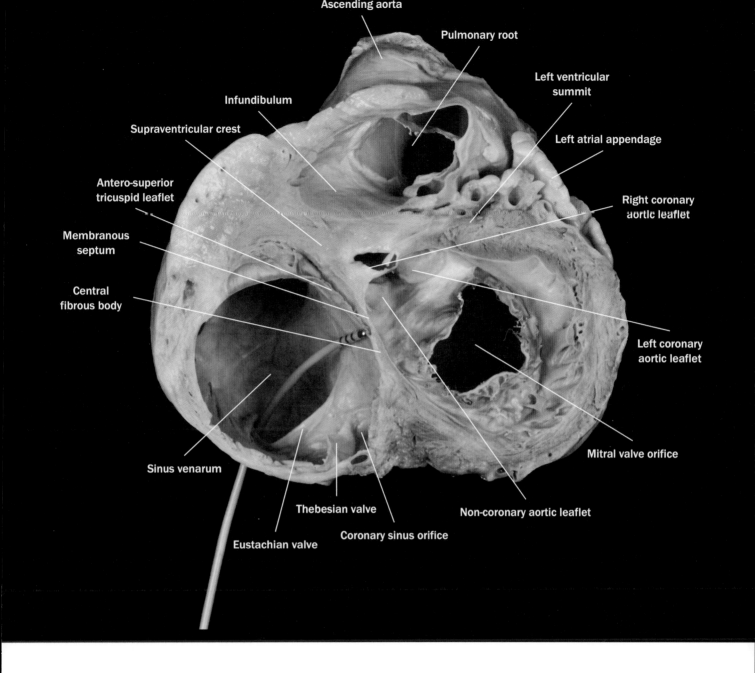

Ascending aorta

Pulmonary root

Infundibulum

Left ventricular
summit

Supraventricular crest

Left atrial appendage

Antero-superior
tricuspid leaflet

Right coronary
aortic leaflet

Membranous
septum

Central
fibrous body

Left coronary
aortic leaflet

Sinus venarum

Mitral valve orifice

Thebesian valve

Non-coronary aortic leaflet

Eustachian valve

Coronary sinus orifice

to as the bundle of His. Therefore, any invasive approach should be withheld at this region except the His-bundle pacing or intentional blockade of the atrioventricular conduction.

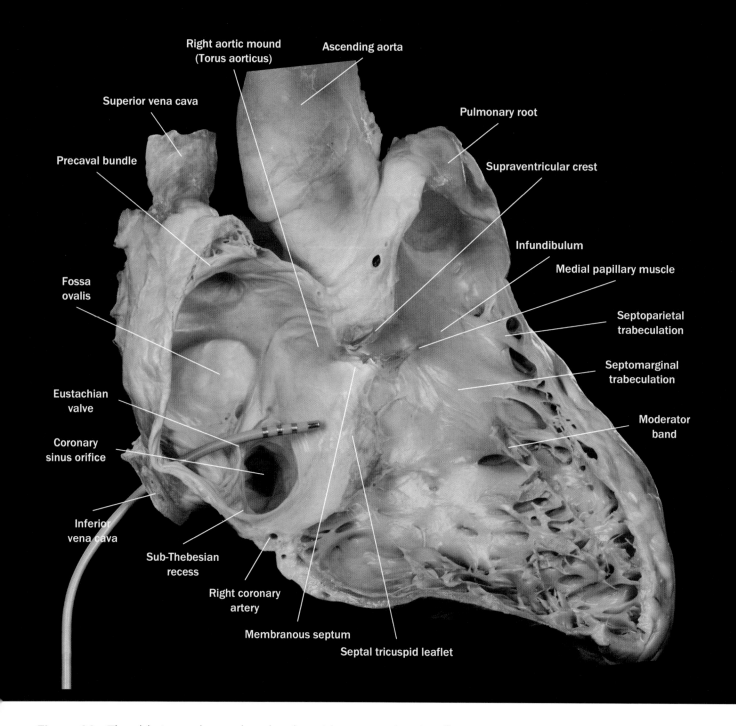

Figure 64 The ablation catheter placed at the mid-paraseptal region.[12]

The images are viewed from the right anterior oblique (left) and left anterior oblique (right) directions. The membranous septum is transilluminated in the left image. The catheter is placed at the mid-paraseptal region, the floor of the triangle of Koch between the membranous septum and the coronary sinus orifice. In the left image, the tip is located at the inferior part of the mid-paraseptal region slightly away from the main body of the atrioventricular node. The compact atrioventricular node is commonly located between this tip location and infero-posterior margin of the membranous

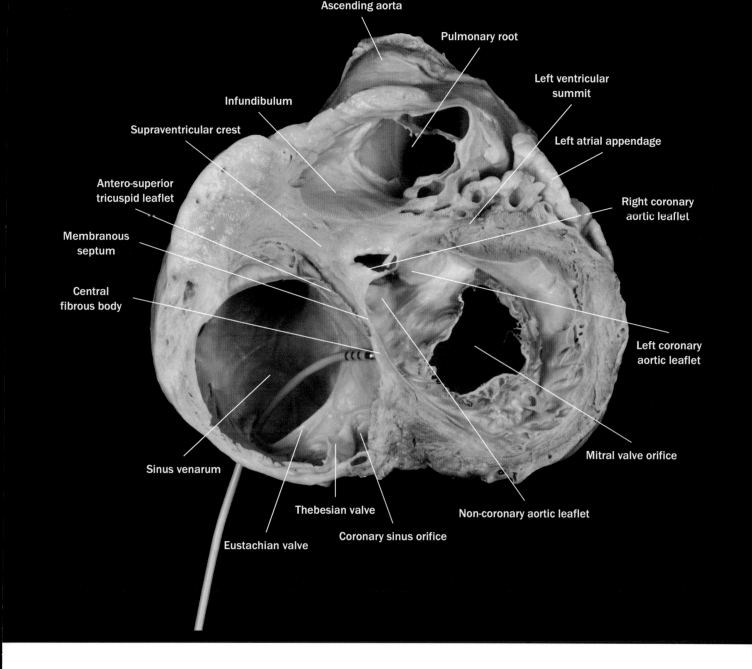

Ascending aorta

Pulmonary root

Left ventricular
summit

Infundibulum

Left atrial appendage

Supraventricular crest

Antero-superior
tricuspid leaflet

Right coronary
aortic leaflet

Membranous
septum

Central
fibrous body

Left coronary
aortic leaflet

Mitral valve orifice

Sinus venarum

Thebesian valve

Non-coronary aortic leaflet

Eustachian valve

Coronary sinus orifice

septum. Therefore, any invasive approach to the mid-paraseptal region should be withheld to protect the compact atrioventricular node. On the contrary, atrioventricular nodal ablation can be tried within this mid-paraseptal region between the membranous septum and coronary sinus orifice.[15] As estimated from the left image, the compact atrioventricular node should be located slightly to the atrial and inferior side relative to the bundle of His. Refer to Figure 67.

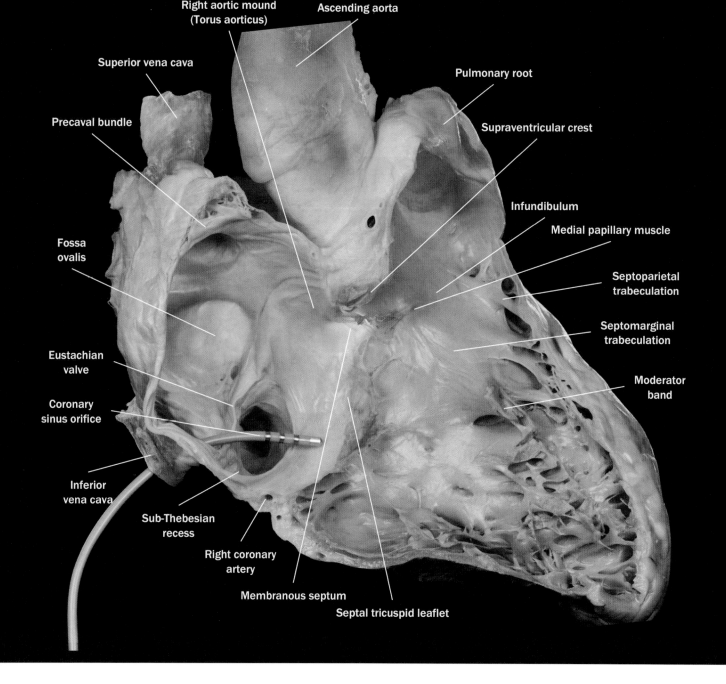

Right aortic mound
(Torus aorticus)

Ascending aorta

Superior vena cava

Pulmonary root

Precaval bundle

Supraventricular crest

Infundibulum

Medial papillary muscle

Fossa
ovalis

Septoparietal
trabeculation

Septomarginal
trabeculation

Eustachian
valve

Moderator
band

Coronary
sinus orifice

Inferior
vena cava

Sub-Thebesian
recess

Right coronary
artery

Membranous septum

Septal tricuspid leaflet

Figure 65   The ablation catheter placed at the inferior-paraseptal region.[12]

The images are viewed from the right anterior oblique (left) and left anterior oblique (right) directions. The membranous septum is transilluminated in the left image. The catheter is placed at the inferior-paraseptal region, corresponding to the septal isthmus between the septal attachment of the septal tricuspid leaflet and the coronary sinus orifice. This is the common site to modify the slow pathway that is related to the right inferior nodal extension.[16] The septal isthmus is not a simple, flat plane facing toward the observer viewing from the right anterior oblique direction. Rather, the plane involving the septal isthmus is almost perpendicular relative to the plane involving the membranous septum.[12] Therefore, the

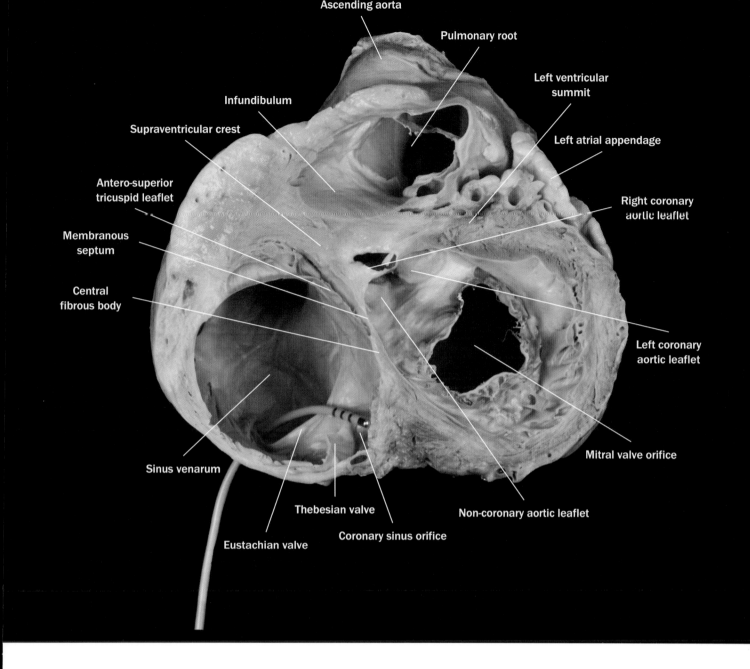

Ascending aorta

Pulmonary root

Left ventricular summit

Left atrial appendage

Infundibulum

Supraventricular crest

Right coronary aortic leaflet

Antero-superior tricuspid leaflet

Membranous septum

Central fibrous body

Left coronary aortic leaflet

Mitral valve orifice

Sinus venarum

Thebesian valve

Non-coronary aortic leaflet

Eustachian valve

Coronary sinus orifice

catheter tip has to trace this funnel-like anatomy continuing to the coronary sinus orifice to modify the slow pathway. This means that a pull-back manipulation requires concomitant clockwise torque to keep the tip attach to the region. Therefore, to successfully perform the slow pathway modification during radiofrequency catheter ablation, delicate clockwise rotation torque combined with intermittent counter torque needs to be applied referring to the left anterior oblique view, in addition to the careful pull-back manipulation referring to the right anterior oblique view.

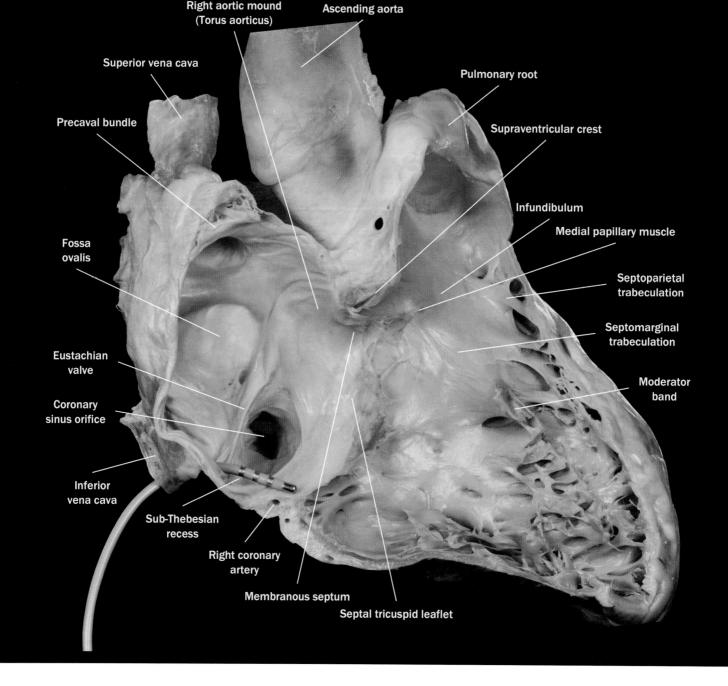

Right aortic mound (Torus aorticus)

Ascending aorta

Superior vena cava

Pulmonary root

Precaval bundle

Supraventricular crest

Infundibulum

Medial papillary muscle

Fossa ovalis

Septoparietal trabeculation

Septomarginal trabeculation

Eustachian valve

Moderator band

Coronary sinus orifice

Inferior vena cava

Sub-Thebesian recess

Right coronary artery

Membranous septum

Septal tricuspid leaflet

Figure 66   The ablation catheter placed at the cavotricuspid isthmus.[12]

The images are viewed from the right anterior oblique (left) and left anterior oblique (right) directions. The catheter is placed at the cavotricuspid isthmus between the tricuspid annulus and inferior vena cava. The pectinate muscles radiating from the crista terminalis run within this isthmus in oblique fashion. The sub-Thebesian recess,[17] also referred to as the sub-Eustachian pouch,[18] is noted infero-lateral to the coronary sinus orifice. The Eustachian valve is guarding the orifice

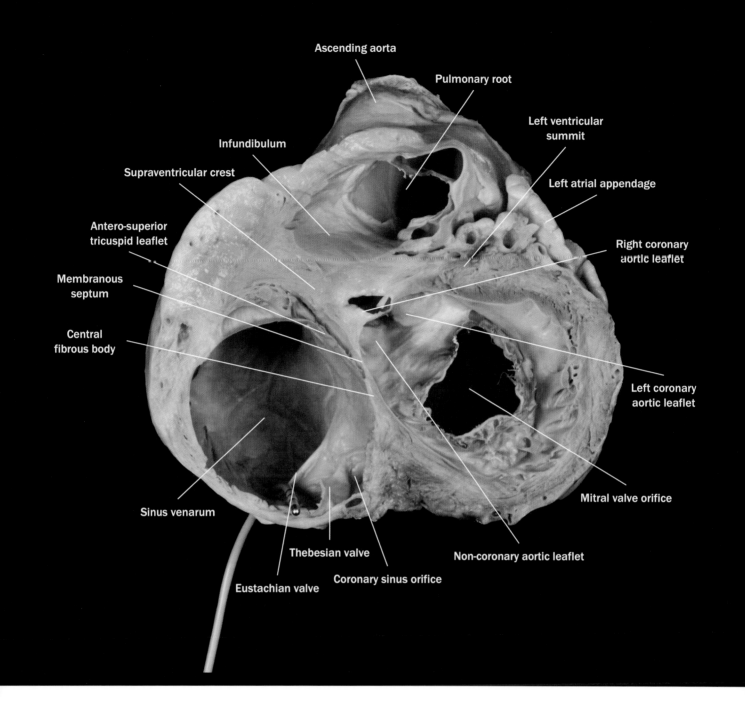

Ascending aorta

Pulmonary root

Left ventricular summit

Left atrial appendage

Infundibulum

Supraventricular crest

Right coronary aortic leaflet

Antero-superior tricuspid leaflet

Membranous septum

Central fibrous body

Left coronary aortic leaflet

Mitral valve orifice

Sinus venarum

Thebesian valve

Non-coronary aortic leaflet

Eustachian valve

Coronary sinus orifice

of the inferior vena cava. The height of the Eustachian valve is higher in medial attachment and less prominent in the lateral portion. The Eustachian valve continues to the anterior limbus of the fossa ovalis. Along the septal attachment of the Eustachian valve, the tendon of Todaro runs within the anterior limbus to the left antero-superior direction to eventually fuse with the central fibrous body. Refer to Figure 40.

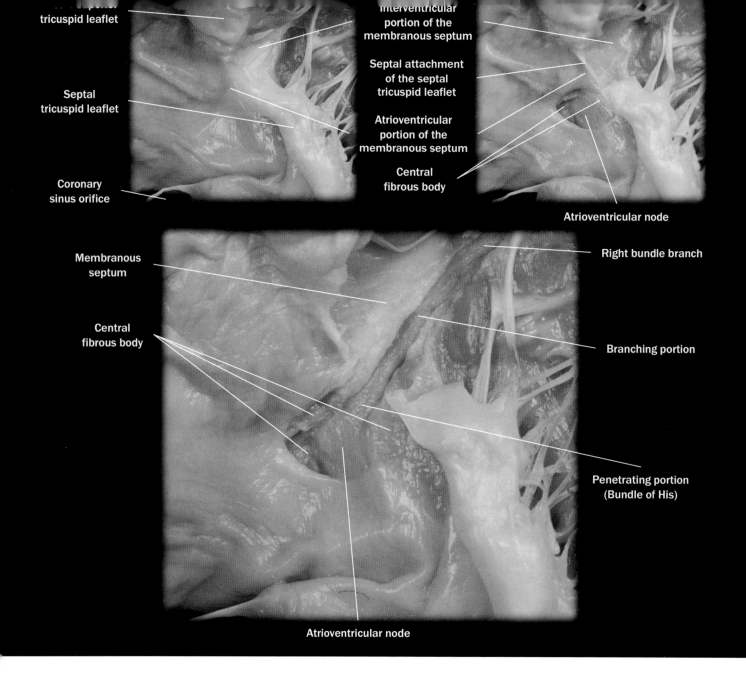

Figure 67 The macroscopic image of the atrioventricular node and conduction axis with progressive dissection.

The images are viewed from the right anterior oblique direction. The atrioventricular conduction axis is dissected using stereoscopic microscope. Transillumination of the membranous septum (upper left) reveals the predominant interventricular portion, compared to the small atrioventricular portion. The proportion of each portion is variable depending on the location of the attachment of the septal tricuspid leaflet. The small part of the septal tricuspid leaflet, as well as the right atrial myocardium at the apex of the triangle of Koch are removed (upper right). The compact atrioventricular node is found at the postero-inferior corner of the membranous septum,[19] lying on the thick central fibrous body. Beneath the right atrial myocardium, the node is covered by the thin epicardial adipose tissue of the apex of the inferior pyramidal space. The bundle of His (penetrating bundle) cannot be observed, as it is covered by the central fibrous body. The central fibrous body covering the bundle of His as well as the thin fibrous tissue at the inferior rim of the membranous septum is further carefully removed (lower) to reveal the atrioventricular conduction axis. The location of the bundle of His relative to the membranous septum[20,21] and relative to the crest of the ventricular septum[22] is variable.

References

1. McAlpine WA. Digitized collection of all the images created by Dr. McAlpine at UCLA. Copyright UCLA Cardiac Arrhythmia Center. Part of this collection appeared in *Heart and Coronary Arteries: An Anatomical Atlas for Clinical Diagnosis, Radiological Investigation, and Surgical Treatment*. New York: Springer-Verlag; 1975.
2. Mori S, Tretter JT, Toba T, et al. Relationship between the membranous septum and the virtual basal ring of the aortic root in candidates for transcatheter implantation of the aortic valve. *Clin Anat.* 2018;31:525–534.
3. Sutton JP 3rd, Ho SY, Anderson RH. The forgotten interleaflet triangles: A review of the surgical anatomy of the aortic valve. *Ann Thorac Surg.* 1995;59:419–427.
4. Tretter JT, Izawa Y, Spicer DE, et al. Understanding the aortic root using computed tomographic assessment: A potential pathway to improved customized surgical repair. *Circ Cardiovasc Imaging.* 2021;14:e013134.
5. Toh H, Mori S, Tretter JT, et al. Living anatomy of the ventricular myocardial crescents supporting the coronary aortic sinuses. *Semin Thorac Cardiovasc Surg.* 2020;32:230–241.
6. Wang Y, Liang Z, Wu S, et al. Idiopathic ventricular arrhythmias originating from the right coronary sinus: Prevalence, electrocardiographic and electrophysiological characteristics, and catheter ablation. *Heart Rhythm.* 2018;15:81–89.
7. Tretter JT, Mori S, Anderson RH, et al. Anatomical predictors of conduction damage after transcatheter implantation of the aortic valve. *Open Heart.* 2019;6:e000972.
8. Tsuda D, Mori S, Izawa Y, et al. Diversity and determinants of the sigmoid septum and its impact on morphology of the outflow tract as revealed using cardiac computed tomography. *Echocardiography.* 2022;39:248-259.
9. Zimmerman J, Bailey CP. The surgical significance of the fibrous skeleton of the heart. *J Thorac Cardiovasc Surg.* 1962;44:701–712.
10. Racker DK. The AV junction region of the heart: A comprehensive study correlating gross anatomy and direct three-dimensional analysis. Part I. Architecture and topography. *Anat Rec.* 1999;256:49–63.
11. Saremi F, Sánchez-Quintana D, Mori S, et al. Fibrous skeleton of the heart: Anatomic overview and evaluation of pathologic conditions with CT and MR imaging. *Radiographics.* 2017;37:1330–1351.
12. Mori S, Fukuzawa K, Takaya T, et al. Clinical structural anatomy of the Inferior pyramidal space reconstructed within the cardiac contour using multidetector-row computed tomography. *J Cardiovasc Electrophysiol.* 2015;26:705–712.
13. Can I, Krueger K, Chandrashekar Y, et al. Images in cardiovascular medicine. Gerbode-type defect induced by catheter ablation of the atrioventricular node. *Circulation.* 2009;119:e553–556.
14. Gerbode F, Hultgren H, Melrose D, et al. Syndrome of left ventricular-right atrial shunt: Successful surgical repair of defect in five cases, with observation of bradycardia on closure. *Ann Surg.* 1958;148:433–446.
15. Marshall HJ, Griffith MJ. Ablation of the atrioventricular junction: Technique, acute and long-term results in 115 consecutive patients. *Europace.* 1999;1:26–29.
16. Inoue S, Becker AE. Posterior extensions of the human compact atrioventricular node: A neglected anatomic feature of potential clinical significance. *Circulation.* 1998;97:188–193.
17. Mori S, Tretter JT, Spicer DE, et al. What is the real cardiac anatomy? *Clin Anat.* 2019;32:288–309.
18. Sánchez-Quintana D, Doblado-Calatrava M, Cabrera JA, et al. Anatomical basis for the cardiac interventional electrophysiologist. *Biomed Res Int.* 2015;2015:547364.
19. Shimizu S. [Topographical anatomy of the atrioventricular node of Tawara—findings by macro-microscopic dissection under dissecting microscope] (in Japanese). *Nihon Kyobu Geka Gakkai Zasshi.* 1989;37:227–233.
20. Massing GK, James TN. Anatomical configuration of the His bundle and bundle branches in the human heart. *Circulation.* 1976;53:609–621.
21. Kawashima T, Sato F. Visualizing anatomical evidences on atrioventricular conduction system for TAVI. *Int J Cardiol.* 2014;174:1–6.
22. Kawashima T, Sasaki H. A macroscopic anatomical investigation of atrioventricular bundle locational variation relative to the membranous part of the ventricular septum in elderly human hearts. *Surg Radiol Anat.* 2005;27:206–213.

11

Right Ventricular Trabeculation/ Band/Papillary Muscles, Right Ventricular Apex

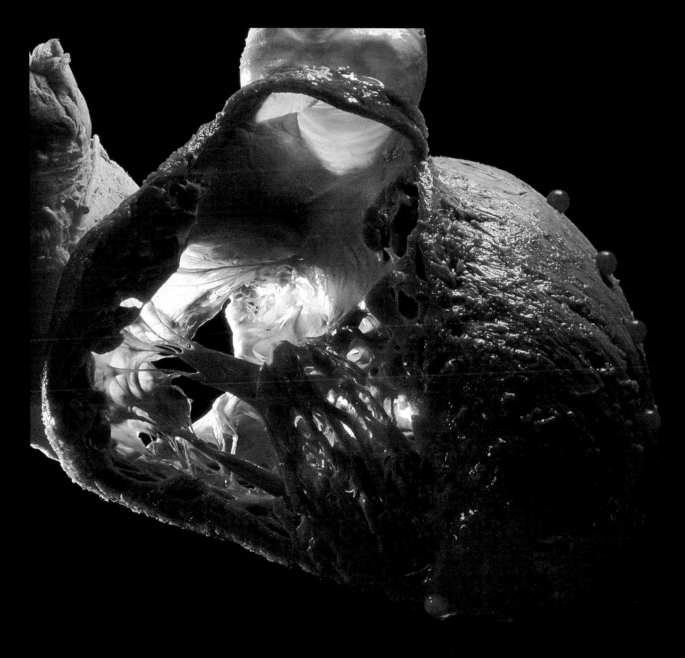

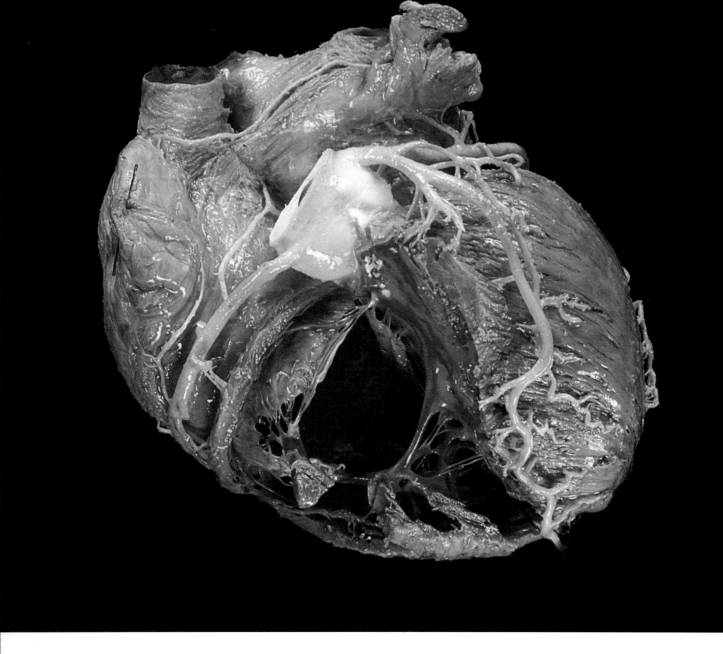

Figure 68 The inner aspect of the right ventricular inlet and apex.[1]

The heart is viewed from the antero-superior direction. The free wall of the right ventricle, the right ventricular outflow tract, and the pulmonary root are removed. The posterior attachment of the right ventricle is where the right ventricular outflow tract starts to separate from the left ventricle. Behind the posterior attachment, the major septal branch enters into the basal superior ventricular septum. The moderator band arises from the septomarginal trabeculation from the supero-septum at the mid-ventricular level. The morphology of the moderator band is variable with mean thickness and length of 4.5 mm and 16.2 mm, respectively.[2] It traverses the mid-right ventricle toward the base of the anterior papillary muscle. The medial papillary muscle is located at the base of the septomarginal trabeculation, just anterior to the right coronary aortic sinus. The medial papillary muscle anchors the medial part of the antero-superior tricuspid leaflet.[3] The

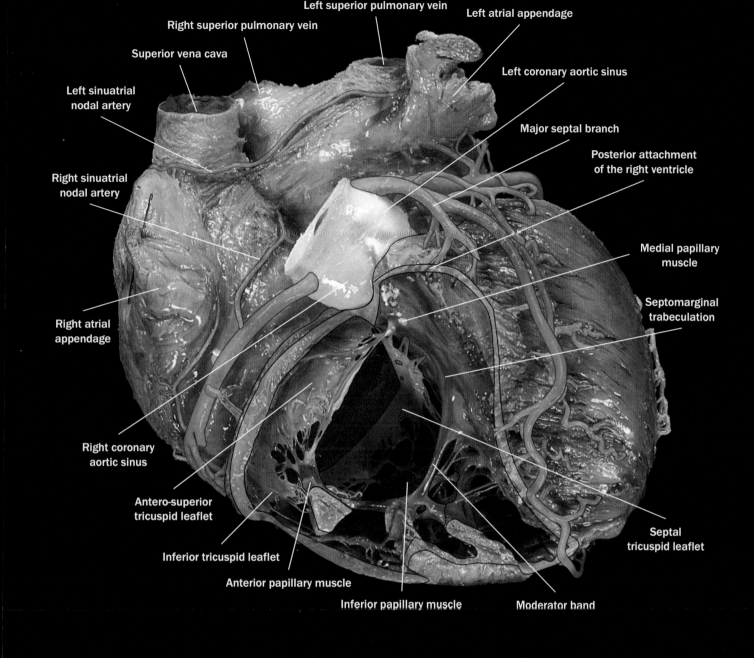

Left superior pulmonary vein

Right superior pulmonary vein

Left atrial appendage

Superior vena cava

Left coronary aortic sinus

Left sinuatrial nodal artery

Major septal branch

Posterior attachment of the right ventricle

Right sinuatrial nodal artery

Medial papillary muscle

Septomarginal trabeculation

Right atrial appendage

Right coronary aortic sinus

Antero-superior tricuspid leaflet

Inferior tricuspid leaflet

Septal tricuspid leaflet

Anterior papillary muscle

Inferior papillary muscle

Moderator band

medial papillary muscle, septomarginal trabeculation, moderator band, and the base of the anterior papillary muscle are important as they are related to the course of the right bundle branch.[4] Endocardial activation of the right ventricle starts near the insertion of the anterior papillary muscle approximately 5 to 10 ms after the onset of the left ventricular activation.[5] The moderator band is connected with multiple trabeculations. The anterior papillary muscle anchors the commissure between the antero-superior and inferior tricuspid leaflets. Septal tricuspid leaflet is anchored by the chordae tendineae attaching directly to the ventricular septum. The inferior papillary muscle anchors the commissure between the septal and inferior tricuspid leaflets.

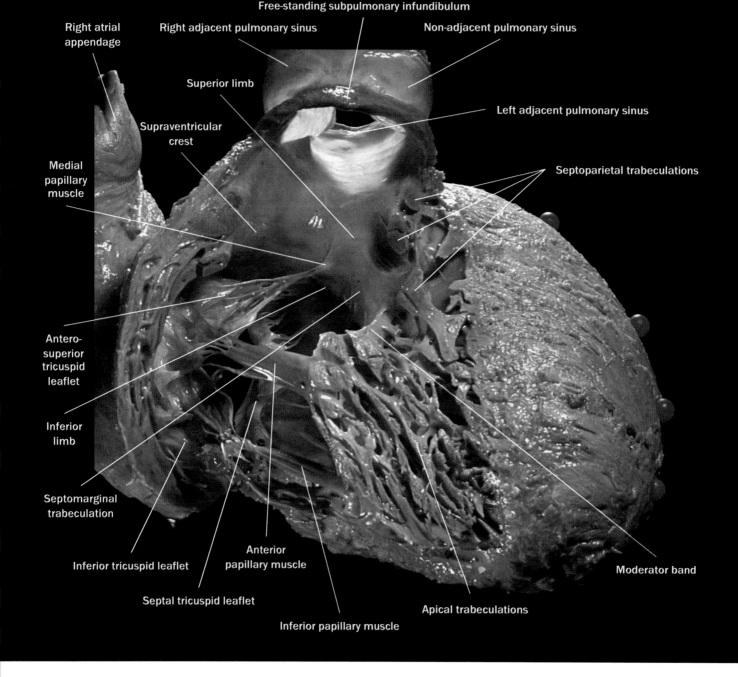

Free-standing subpulmonary infundibulum

Right atrial appendage

Right adjacent pulmonary sinus

Non-adjacent pulmonary sinus

Superior limb

Left adjacent pulmonary sinus

Supraventricular crest

Medial papillary muscle

Septoparietal trabeculations

Antero-superior tricuspid leaflet

Inferior limb

Septomarginal trabeculation

Inferior tricuspid leaflet

Anterior papillary muscle

Septal tricuspid leaflet

Inferior papillary muscle

Apical trabeculations

Moderator band

Figure 69 The right ventricular apical trabeculations.[1]

The heart is viewed from the anterior direction. The free wall of the right ventricle is removed. The medial papillary muscle is located at the base of the septomarginal trabeculation, at the bifurcation of the superior and inferior limbs of the septo-marginal trabeculation, at its inferior limb side. The medial papillary muscle anchors the medial part of the antero-superior tricuspid leaflet. The superior limb directs toward the left adjacent pulmonary sinus, and the inferior limb directs toward the membranous septum. The supraventricular crest arises from the bifurcation of the superior and inferior limbs. It runs along the superior tricuspid annulus. Thus, the supraventricular crest is in orthogonal relationship to the septomarginal trabeculation. The supraventricular crest is also referred to as the ventriculo-infundibular fold, forming the postero-lateral

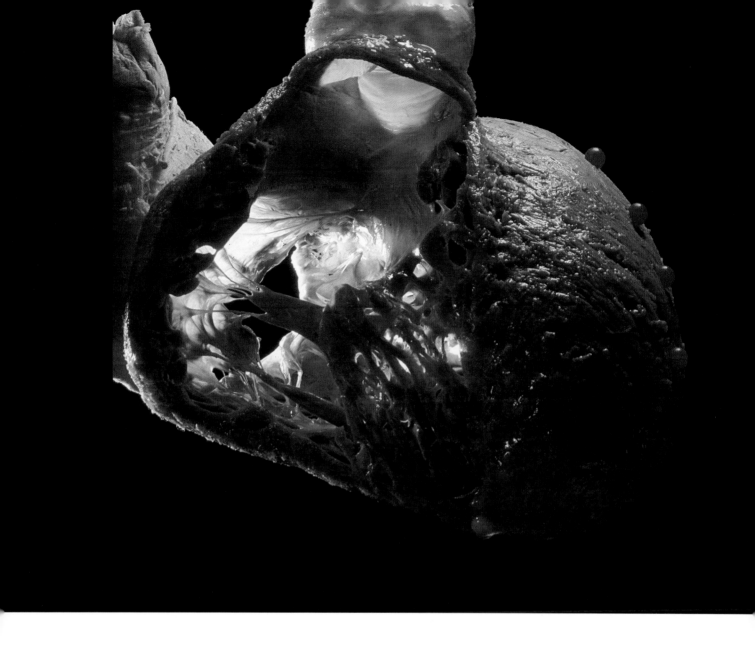

free wall of the infundibulum that lifts the pulmonary valve away from the tricuspid valve. Coarse and dense apical and basal trabeculations are noted, which actually extend over the lateral free wall. On the contrary, the subpulmonary region shows a smooth endocardial surface, except the septoparietal trabeculation, which arises from the superior limb of the septomarginal trabeculation, coursing on the medial infundibulum. The anterior papillary muscle is supported by the mid-lateral trabeculations and anchors the commissure between the antero-superior and inferior tricuspid leaflets. The inferior papillary muscle anchors the commissure between the inferior and septal tricuspid leaflets. The septal leaflet is anchored by multiple chordae tendineae attaching to the ventricular septum.

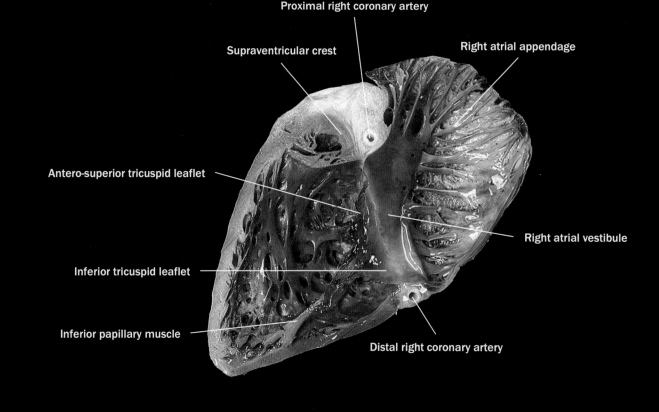

Proximal right coronary artery

Supraventricular crest

Right atrial appendage

Antero-superior tricuspid leaflet

Right atrial vestibule

Inferior tricuspid leaflet

Inferior papillary muscle

Distal right coronary artery

Figure 70   Open image of the right ventricle.[1]

The free wall of the right heart is cut and opened (left) then viewed from the left posterior oblique direction. The main specimen (right) is viewed from the right anterior oblique direction. At the right ventricular free wall, the coarse and dense trabeculations extend from apical to basal regions. Only the right atrial vestibule shows the smooth endocardial surface sandwiched between the trabeculations of the right ventricle and pectinate muscles of the right atrial appendage. The moderator band and the body of the anterior papillary muscle is left on the main specimen. The anterior papillary muscle anchors the commissure between the antero-superior and inferior tricuspid leaflets. The close proximity of the right atrial vestibule and the right coronary artery running in the right atrioventricular groove can be recognized at both superior

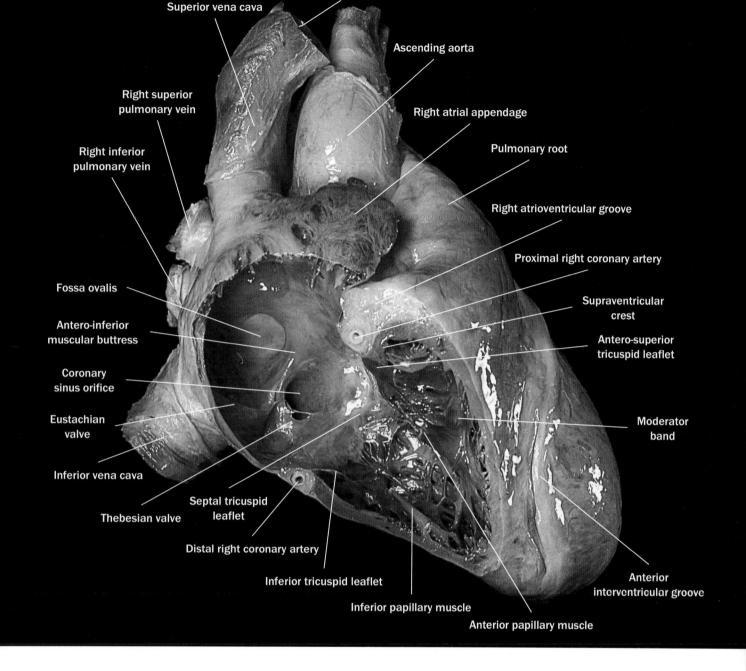

Superior vena cava

Ascending aorta

Right superior
pulmonary vein

Right atrial appendage

Right inferior
pulmonary vein

Pulmonary root

Right atrioventricular groove

Proximal right coronary artery

Fossa ovalis

Supraventricular
crest

Antero-inferior
muscular buttress

Antero-superior
tricuspid leaflet

Coronary
sinus orifice

Eustachian
valve

Moderator
band

Inferior vena cava

Thebesian valve

Septal tricuspid
leaflet

Distal right coronary artery

Anterior
interventricular groove

Inferior tricuspid leaflet

Inferior papillary muscle

Anterior papillary muscle

and inferior tricuspid annulus. The average minimum distance between the endocardium at the inferior right atrial vestibule to the distal right coronary artery is 3 mm,[6] which suggests the potential risk of inadvertent injury to the right coronary artery during catheter ablation of the cavotricuspid isthmus.[7] The supraventricular crest extends superior to the tricuspid annulus to lift up the pulmonary valve. In other words, this structural anatomy renders the superior atrioventricular groove as deeply wedged between the right atrial appendage and supraventricular crest. This peculiar shape suggests the need for the U-turn approach if the superior tricuspid annulus is related to the accessory pathways or ventricular arrhythmias. Refer to Figure 51.

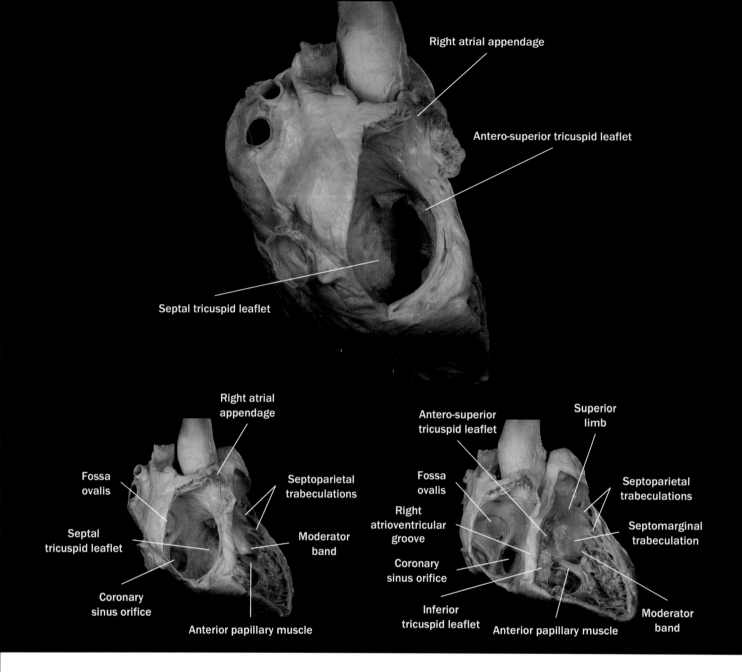

Figure 71   Rotational observation of the right ventricle. 🔲🔲 Anaglyph 14.

The free wall of the right heart is removed, except for the right atrioventricular groove. The heart is viewed from the right posterior oblique 105-degree (upper image on the left page), right anterior oblique 75-degree (lower left image on the left page), 45-degree (lower right image on the left page), 15-degree (upper left image on the right page) directions, and left anterior oblique 15-degree (upper right image on the right page), 45-degree (lower image on the right page) directions. The moderator band traverses the middle part of the right ventricle. Dense and coarse apical trabeculations are left by only removing the thin right ventricular free wall. The endocardial surface of the basal-mid septum and right ventricular outflow tract is smooth, except for the septoparietal trabeculations originating from the superior limb of the septomarginal trabeculation. The septoparietal trabeculations on the medial infundibulum directs toward the anterior free wall of the right ventricular outflow tract. The septomarginal trabeculation is less prominent in this heart. *En face* and tangential views of the atrial and ventricular septum are obtained at right anterior oblique 45-degree view (lower right image on the left

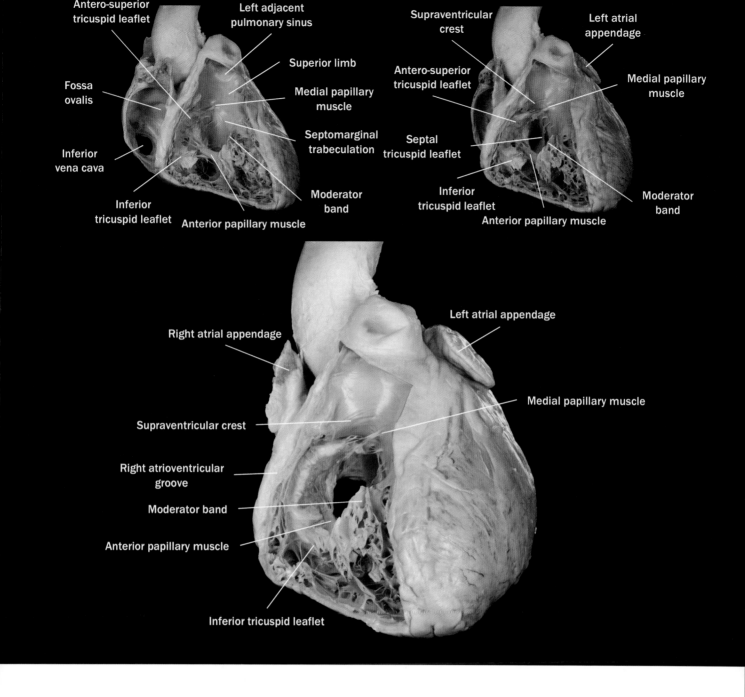

Antero-superior tricuspid leaflet

Left adjacent pulmonary sinus

Superior limb

Medial papillary muscle

Fossa ovalis

Septomarginal trabeculation

Inferior vena cava

Inferior tricuspid leaflet

Anterior papillary muscle

Moderator band

Supraventricular crest

Left atrial appendage

Antero-superior tricuspid leaflet

Medial papillary muscle

Septal tricuspid leaflet

Inferior tricuspid leaflet

Anterior papillary muscle

Moderator band

Right atrial appendage

Left atrial appendage

Medial papillary muscle

Supraventricular crest

Right atrioventricular groove

Moderator band

Anterior papillary muscle

Inferior tricuspid leaflet

page), and left anterior oblique 45-degree view (lower image on the right page), respectively.[8] Therefore, in this heart, a right anterior oblique 45-degree view provides optimal separation of the structures on the atrial or ventricular septa. On the contrary, every structural relationship on the atrial and ventricular septa are foreshortened in the left anterior oblique 45-degree view. Therefore, the left anterior oblique view cannot secure the precise septal approach.[9] If the right anterior oblique angulation is shallower, it is insufficient for optimal separation of the septal structures.[10] Less right anterior oblique angulation, relative to the *en face* view of the ventricular septum, makes the right-hand margin of the cardiac silhouette increasingly occupied by the left ventricle (upper left image on the right page). X-shaped crisscrossing of the right and left ventricular outflow tracts between the both atrial appendages are best shown in the left anterior oblique 45-degree view (lower image on the right page), as the optimal separation of the left and right ventricles is achieved. The supraventricular crest, also referred to as the ventriculo-infundibular fold composing the postero-lateral free wall of the right ventricular outflow tract covers the aortic root at its crossing point.

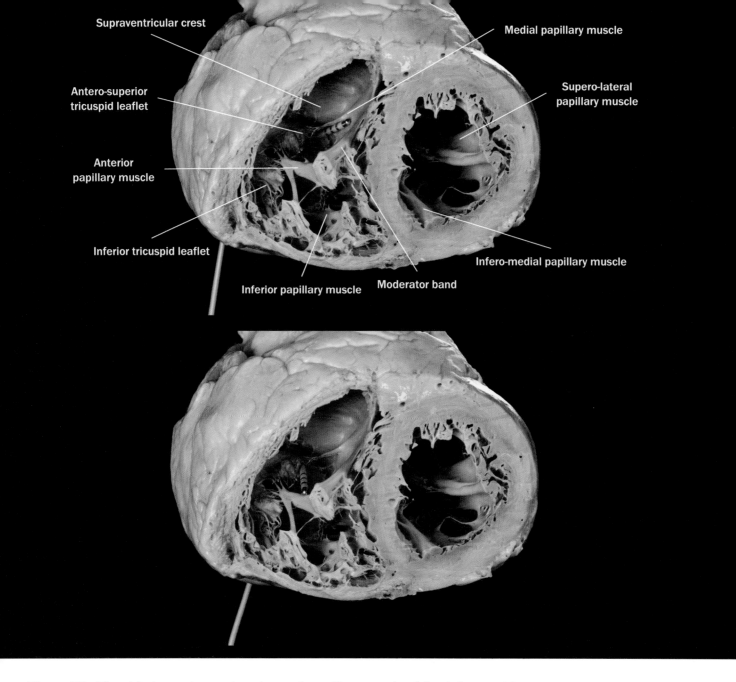

Figure 72 The ablation catheter placed at each papillary muscle of the right ventricle.

The images are viewed from the left anterior oblique direction. Right ventricular trabeculations[11] and papillary muscles[12] can be the substrate for idiopathic ventricular arrhythmia. The catheter is placed on the medial papillary muscle (upper image on the left page), moderator band (upper image on the right page), anterior papillary muscle (lower image on the left

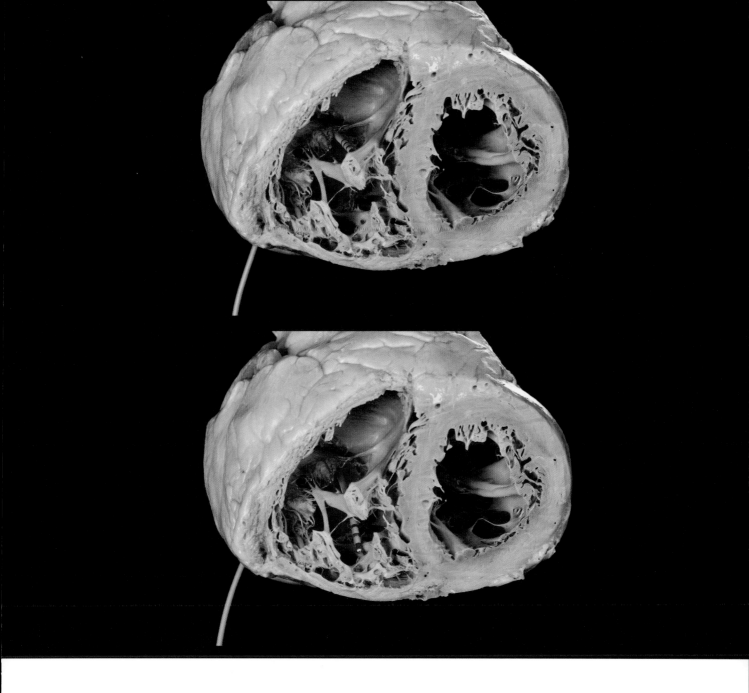

page), and inferior papillary muscle (lower image on the right page). Any injury to the moderator band and these papillary muscles, except the inferior papillary muscle, has a potential risk to damage the right bundle branch.

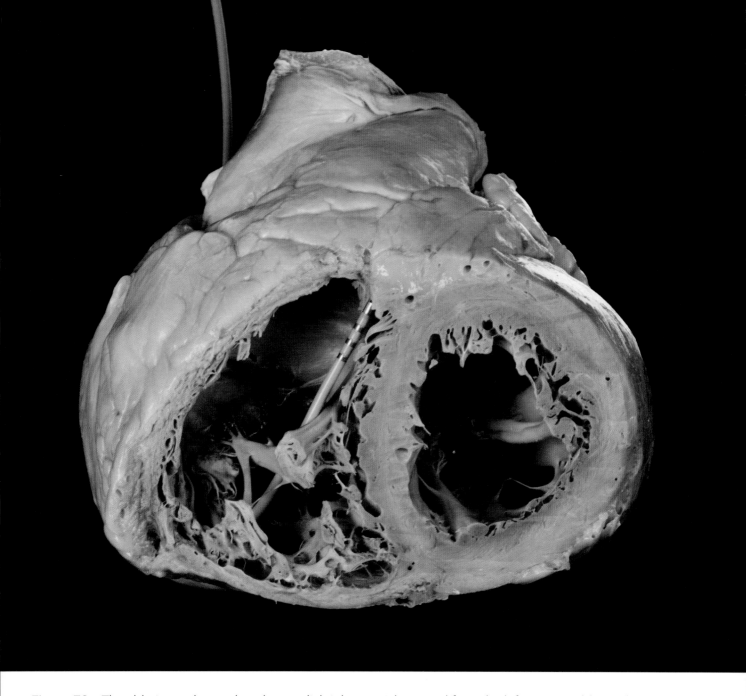

Figure 73 The ablation catheter placed at medial right ventricle viewed from the left anterior oblique direction.

The catheter is placed on the medial free wall of the right ventricular outflow tract superior to the moderator band and septomarginal trabeculation (left) using superior approach. Even though this region looks like septal direction, it is actually not the muscular ventricular septum but the medial free wall of the right ventricular outflow tract (infundibulum) superior to the anterior attachment of the right ventricle. Thus, it has a potential risk of cardiac perforation toward the anterior interventricular groove. On the contrary, the catheter is placed on the middle ventricular septum inferior to the moderator band and septomarginal trabeculation (right). This region is the true muscular ventricular septum, and it has

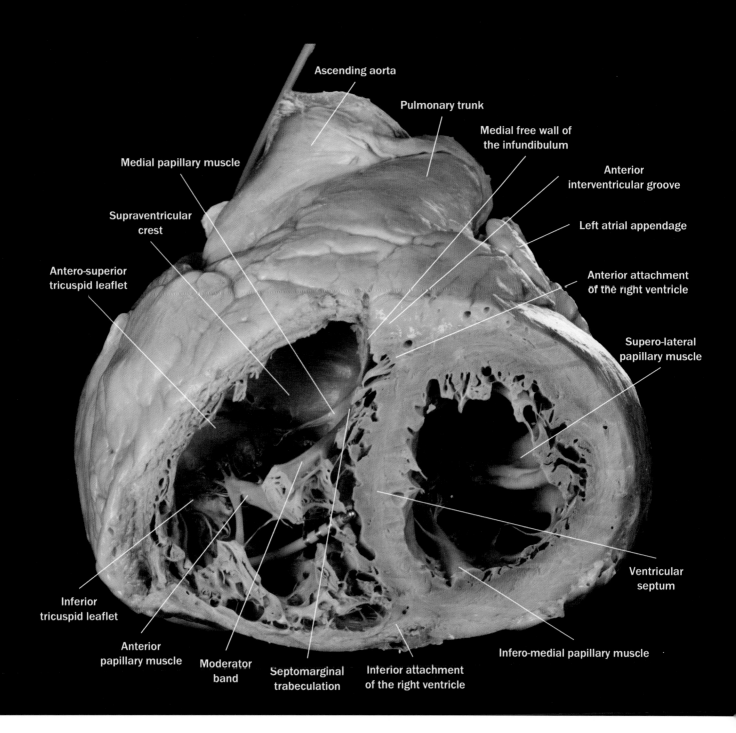

Ascending aorta

Pulmonary trunk

Medial free wall of
the infundibulum

Anterior
interventricular groove

Medial papillary muscle

Left atrial appendage

Supraventricular
crest

Anterior attachment
of the right ventricle

Antero-superior
tricuspid leaflet

Supero-lateral
papillary muscle

Inferior
tricuspid leaflet

Ventricular
septum

Anterior
papillary muscle

Infero-medial papillary muscle

Moderator
band

Septomarginal
trabeculation

Inferior attachment
of the right ventricle

much less risk of cardiac perforation and inadvertent injuries to the right bundle branch, septal tricuspid leaflet, and its chordae tendineae. Therefore, endomyocardial biopsy for diffuse myocardial disease[13] is recommended from this region, the mid-septum of the mid-right ventricle inferior to the septomarginal trabeculation. The right anterior oblique view is useful to confirm the safe region.[14] During the endomyocardial biopsy, general risk of perforation is less than 1% by the skilled hand.[15]

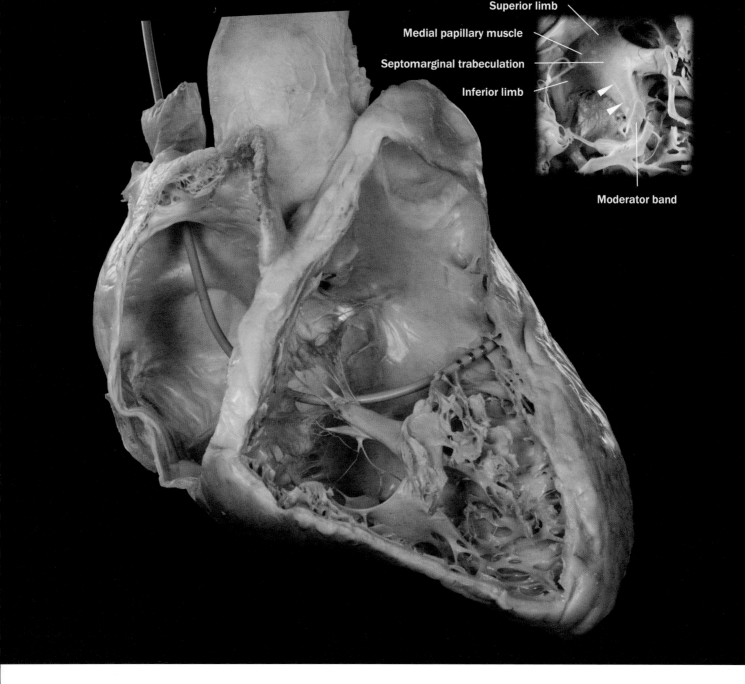

Superior limb

Medial papillary muscle

Septomarginal trabeculation

Inferior limb

Moderator band

Figure 74 The ablation catheter placed at the right ventricular outflow tract viewed from the right anterior oblique direction.

The images are viewed from the right anterior oblique 30-degree direction. The membranous septum is transilluminated. The catheter is placed on the antero-medial free wall of the low right ventricular outflow tract at the anterior attachment of the right ventricle (left). The tip of the catheter is located at the base of the septoparietal trabeculation originating from the superior limb of the septomarginal trabeculation. Although the distance from the tip to the cardiac contour is secured, this region is not the ventricular septum but the medial free wall adjacent to the anterior interventricular groove. Therefore, catheter ablation or misplacement of the septal pacing lead into this region has the potential risk of cardiac perforation,[16] unexpected anterior free wall pacing,[9] and injury to the left anterior descending artery, including occlusion[17] or extravasation.[18] If the catheter tip is bent back on the septomarginal trabeculation (right), this region is the superior ventricular

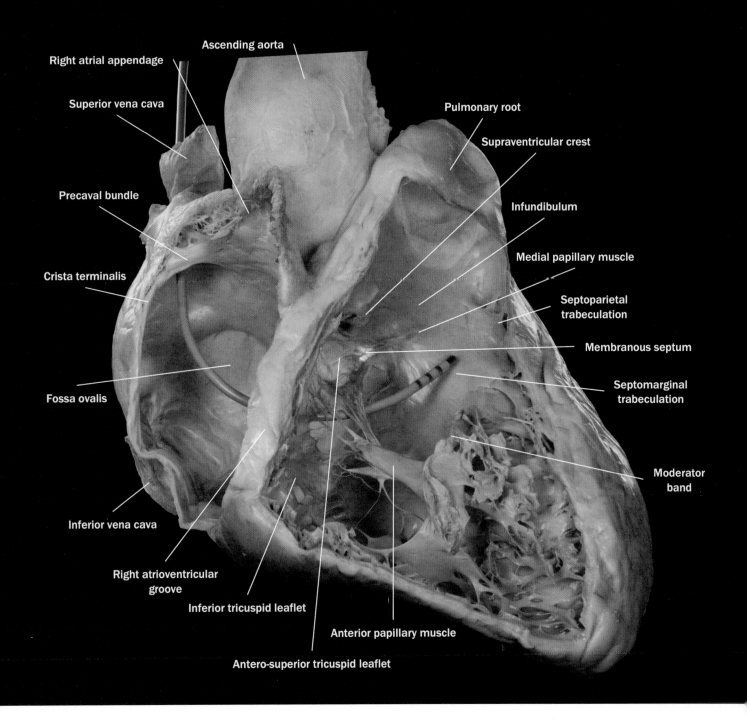

Right atrial appendage

Ascending aorta

Superior vena cava

Pulmonary root

Supraventricular crest

Precaval bundle

Infundibulum

Medial papillary muscle

Crista terminalis

Septoparietal
trabeculation

Membranous septum

Fossa ovalis

Septomarginal
trabeculation

Inferior vena cava

Moderator
band

Right atrioventricular
groove

Inferior tricuspid leaflet

Anterior papillary muscle

Antero-superior tricuspid leaflet

septum. The septomarginal trabeculation itself is not prominent in this heart. Smooth endocardial surface is recognized, indicating the technical difficulty to keep this position. While the cardiac perforation is less likely at this region as this is the true ventricular septum, procedure on the septomarginal trabeculation has a potential risk of injury to the right bundle branch. The right bundle branch generally passes just inferior to the base of the medial papillary muscle, then runs within the septomarginal trabeculation, and travels through the moderator band to reach the base of the anterior papillary muscle.[19] The depth of the right bundle branch measured from the endocardial surface is variable.[19] In some cases, the right bundle branch can be observed macroscopically on the endocardial surface (arrowheads on the inset image on the left page recorded from another heart with the prominent septomarginal trabeculation).

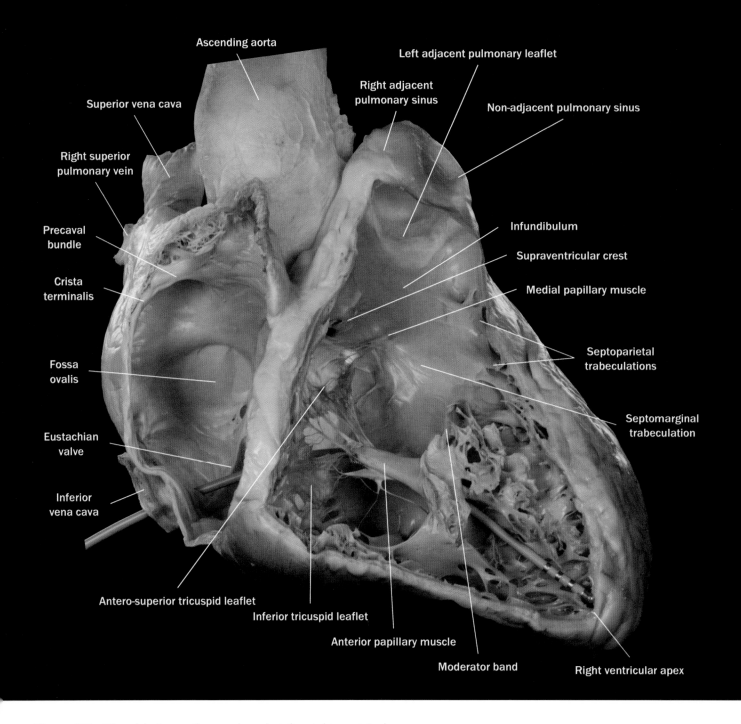

Ascending aorta

Left adjacent pulmonary leaflet

Right adjacent pulmonary sinus

Non-adjacent pulmonary sinus

Superior vena cava

Right superior pulmonary vein

Infundibulum

Supraventricular crest

Precaval bundle

Medial papillary muscle

Crista terminalis

Septoparietal trabeculations

Fossa ovalis

Septomarginal trabeculation

Eustachian valve

Inferior vena cava

Antero-superior tricuspid leaflet

Inferior tricuspid leaflet

Anterior papillary muscle

Moderator band

Right ventricular apex

Figure 75 The ablation catheter placed at the right ventricular apex.

The images are viewed from the right anterior oblique direction, corresponding roughly 30 degrees. Even though the apical trabeculation is dense, the myocardial wall thickness of the right ventricle is thin. This increases the risk of perforation during invasive procedures within the right ventricle, including catheter ablation and implantation of cardiac rhythm management device.[20] From this view, the tip of the catheter placed at the very apical region is still distant from the right-hand margin of the apical cardiac contour. This is simply because the right ventricle does not represent the cardiac contour. The left ventricular anterior wall and apex, as well as epicardial adipose tissue, composes the right-hand apical cardiac contour in shallow right anterior oblique view. Thus, when using shallow right anterior oblique view, the finding that the tip of the catheter or lead is within the cardiac silhouette does not exclude the perforation of the right ventricular anterior wall or apex. In other words, it is not a safe approach to use the cardiac contour to estimate the right ventricular apical orientation. It is also true for frontal[21] and left anterior oblique views. The tip within the cardiac silhouette does not secure the intracardiac location, even if the image indicates no extensive displacement of the catheter or lead. In this regard, deeper right anterior oblique view (45 degrees to 50 degrees), combined with optimal angiography,[22] should be most useful as it shows the *en face* view of the atrial and ventricular septa.[8] Using this approach, frequent sites of the perforation involving cardiac apex[21] and right ventricular outflow tract[16] are placed close to the margin of the contour, which makes minor displacement of the tip of the device or extravasation much easier to recognize. Furthermore, as the direction of the ventricular septum shows a wide individual variation,[8] optimal angulation to obtain the *en face* view of the ventricular septum should be customized according to each patients' anatomy.

References

1. McAlpine WA. Digitized collection of all the images created by Dr. McAlpine at UCLA. Copyright UCLA Cardiac Arrhythmia Center. Part of this collection appeared in *Heart and Coronary Arteries: An Anatomical Atlas for Clinical Diagnosis, Radiological Investigation, and Surgical Treatment*. New York: Springer-Verlag; 1975.
2. Loukas M, Klaassen Z, Tubbs RS, et al. Anatomical observations of the moderator band. *Clin Anat*. 2010;23:443–450.
3. Muresian H. The clinical anatomy of the right ventricle. *Clin Anat*. 2016;29:380–398.
4. Widran J, Lev M. The dissection of the atrioventricular node, bundle and bundle branches in the human heart. *Circulation*. 1951;4:863–867.
5. Durrer D, van Dam RT, Freud GE, et al. Total excitation of the isolated human heart. *Circulation*. 1970;41:899–912.
6. Al Aloul B, Sigurdsson G, Can I, et al. Proximity of right coronary artery to cavotricuspid isthmus as determined by computed tomography. *Pacing Clin Electrophysiol*. 2010;33:1319–1323.
7. Funayama N, Konishi T, Yamamoto T, et al. Acute right coronary artery occlusion after radiofrequency catheter ablation of cavotricuspid isthmus: Vascular response assessed by optical frequency domain imaging. *Heart Rhythm Case Rep*. 2017;3:496–498.
8. Mori S, Fukuzawa K, Takaya T, et al. Optimal angulations for obtaining an *en face* view of each coronary aortic sinus and the interventricular septum: Correlative anatomy around the left ventricular outflow tract. *Clin Anat*. 2015;28:494–505.
9. Burri H, Domenichini G, Sunthorn H, et al. Comparison of tools and techniques for implanting pacemaker leads on the ventricular mid-septum. *Europace*. 2012;14:847–852.
10. Osmancik P, Stros P, Herman D, et al. The insufficiency of left anterior oblique and the usefulness of right anterior oblique projection for correct localization of a computed tomography-verified right ventricular lead into the mid-septum. *Circ Arrhythm Electrophysiol*. 2013;6:719–725.
11. Sadek MM, Benhayon D, Sureddi R, et al. Idiopathic ventricular arrhythmias originating from the moderator band: Electrocardiographic characteristics and treatment by catheter ablation. *Heart Rhythm*. 2015;12:67–75.
12. Crawford T, Mueller G, Good E, et al. Ventricular arrhythmias originating from papillary muscles in the right ventricle. *Heart Rhythm*. 2010;7:725–730.
13. Konno S, Sakakibara S. Endo-myocardial biopsy. *Dis Chest*. 1963;44:345–350.
14. Burri H, Domenichini G, Sunthorn H, et al. Comparison of tools and techniques for implanting pacemaker leads on the ventricular mid-septum. *Europace*. 2012;14:847–852.
15. Hiramitsu S, Hiroe M, Uemura A, et al. National survey of the use of endomyocardial biopsy in Japan. *Jpn Circ J*. 1998 Dec;62:909–912.
16. Tokuda M, Kojodjojo P, Epstein LM, et al. Outcomes of cardiac perforation complicating catheter ablation of ventricular arrhythmias. *Circ Arrhythm Electrophysiol*. 2011;4:660–666.
17. Parwani AS, Rolf S, Haverkamp W. Coronary artery occlusion due to lead insertion into the right ventricular outflow tract. *Eur Heart J*. 2009;30:425.
18. Hayase J, Shapiro H, Bae D, et al. Dual chamber pacemaker implantation complicated by left anterior ascending coronary artery injury. *JACC Case Rep*. 2019;1:633–637.
19. Shimizu S. [Topographical anatomy of the atrioventricular node of Tawara—findings by macro-microscopic dissection under dissecting microscope] (in Japanese). *Nihon Kyobu Geka Gakkai Zasshi*. 1989;37:227–233.
20. Cano Ó, Andrés A, Alonso P, et al. Incidence and predictors of clinically relevant cardiac perforation associated with systematic implantation of active-fixation pacing and defibrillation leads: A single-centre experience with over 3800 implanted leads. *Europace*. 2017;19:96–102.
21. Zhang X, Zheng C, Wang P, et al. Assessment of cardiac lead perforation: Comparison among chest radiography, transthoracic echocardiography and electrocardiography-gated contrast-enhanced cardiac CT. *Eur Radiol*. 2019;29:963–974.
22. Shenthar J, Singh B, Banavalikar B, et al. Cardiac perforation complicating cardiac electrophysiology procedures: Value of angiography and use of a closure device to avoid cardiac surgery. *J Interv Card Electrophysiol*. 2020;58:193–201.

12

Right Ventricular Outflow Tract

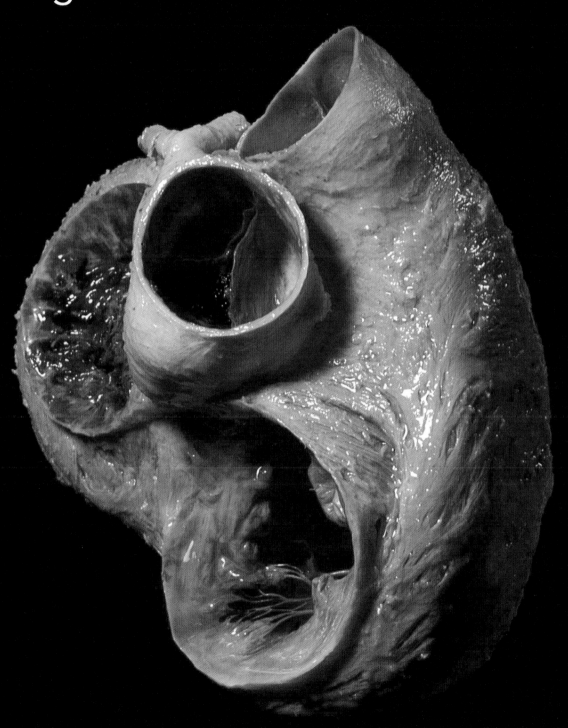

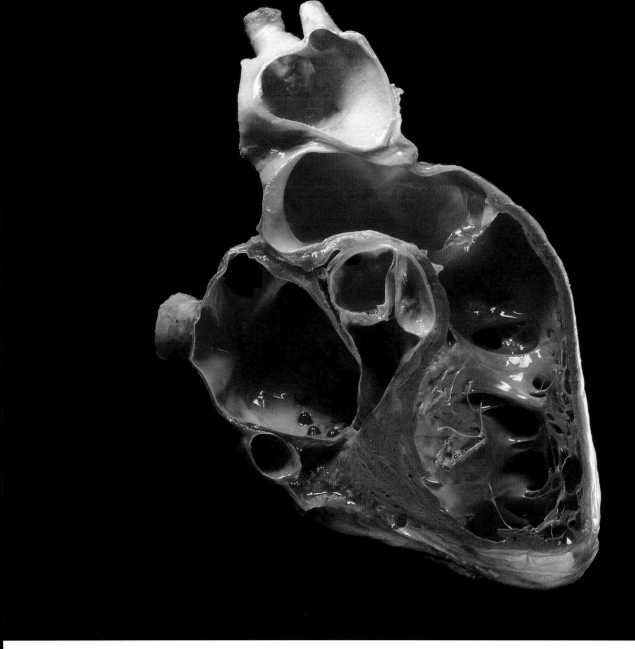

Figure 76 Sagittal section of the right ventricle viewed from the right direction.[1]

The septomarginal trabeculation and moderator band demarcate the boundary between the right ventricular outflow tract (infundibulum) and the rest of the right ventricle, involving the inflow and apical components. The small medial papillary muscle is located at the base of the septomarginal trabeculation, anterior to the right coronary aortic sinus, commonly anchoring the antero-superior tricuspid leaflet. The right bundle branch runs just inferior to this medial papillary muscle coursing within the septomarginal trabeculation and moderator band.[2] The pulmonary valve is lifted up over the aortic valve by the right ventricular outflow tract. Thus, the postero-lateral free wall of the infundibulum covers the substantial part of the right coronary aortic sinus anteriorly. The pulmonary root directs toward the postero-superior direction. In

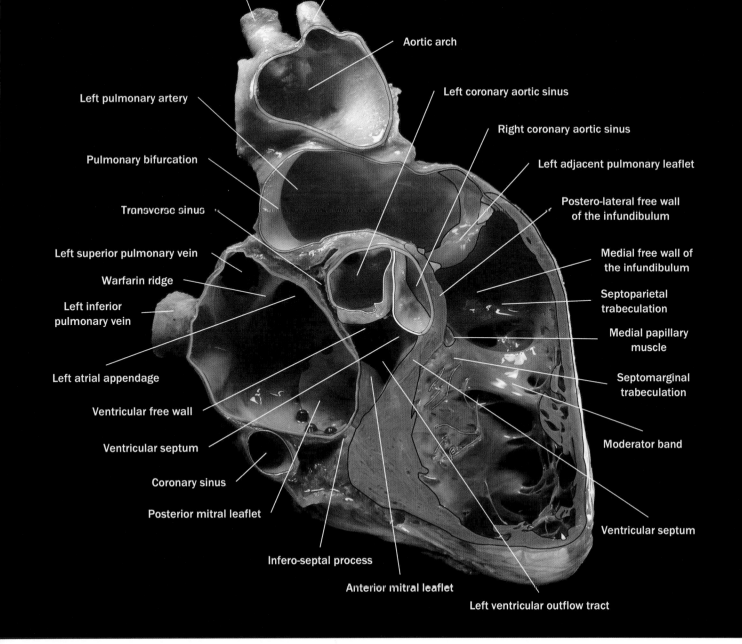

Aortic arch

Left pulmonary artery

Pulmonary bifurcation

Transverse sinus

Left superior pulmonary vein

Warfarin ridge

Left inferior pulmonary vein

Left atrial appendage

Ventricular free wall

Ventricular septum

Coronary sinus

Posterior mitral leaflet

Infero-septal process

Anterior mitral leaflet

Left coronary aortic sinus

Right coronary aortic sinus

Left adjacent pulmonary leaflet

Postero-lateral free wall of the infundibulum

Medial free wall of the infundibulum

Septoparietal trabeculation

Medial papillary muscle

Septomarginal trabeculation

Moderator band

Ventricular septum

Left ventricular outflow tract

contrast to the aortic root, the base of the pulmonary root has encircling muscular support by free-standing subpulmonary infundibulum.[3] Although the coarse trabeculations are found in the right ventricular apical and lateral walls, the endocardial surface of the right ventricular outflow tract and inflow septum is relatively smooth, except for the septoparietal trabeculation located medial within the outflow tract. This medial wall of the right ventricular outflow tract facing toward the observer is not the septum but the free wall. The anterior wall of the right ventricle faces to the chest wall along the left sternal boarder. The superior part of the basal muscular ventricular septum separates the right ventricular inflow from the left ventricular outflow.[4] The paired section of this image is Figure 128.

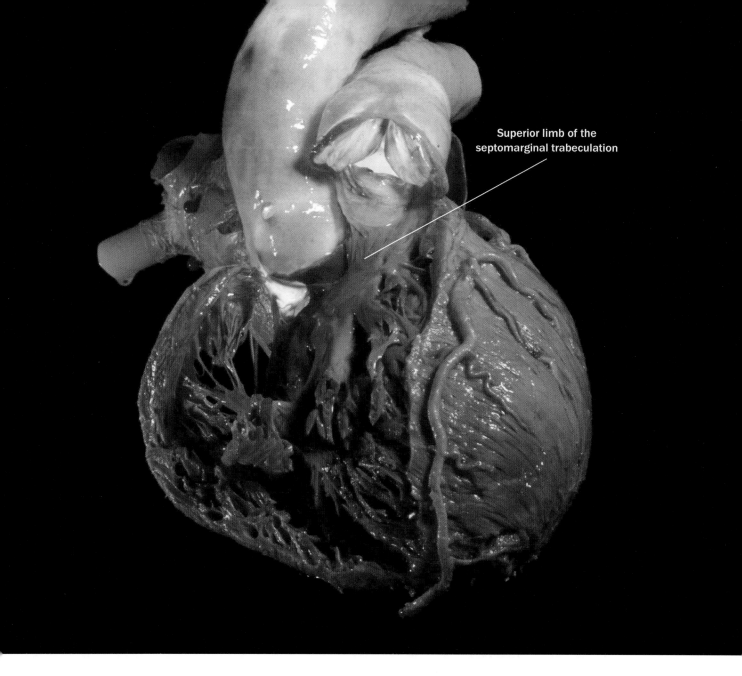

Superior limb of the
septomarginal trabeculation

Figure 77 The inner aspect of the right ventricle viewed from the left anterior oblique direction.[1]

The right ventricular free wall is removed, except for the inferior wall. The membranous septum is transilluminated. The postero-lateral free wall of the right ventricular outflow tract is also removed, which covers substantial part of the right coronary aortic sinus. Although the aortic root is adjacent to the right ventricular outflow tract and pulmonary root, they are separated each other by the thin fibrous tissue plane.[5] Within such tissue plane, the so-called tendon of the infundibulum or conus tendon[6] is generally illustrated in the figures showing fibrous skeleton of the heart[7,8] as the firm, fibrous structure connecting the aortic and pulmonary roots. However, this structure is rarely found consistently.[6] The base of the right coronary aortic sinus is directly supported by the crest of the ventricular septum,[9] referred to as the myocardial crescent.[10] The superior margin of this myocardial crescent corresponds to the ventriculo-arterial junction,[11] identical to the postero-lateral attachment of the right ventricle at the inferior margin of the ventriculo-infundibular fold. Until reaching this ventriculo-arterial junction, the dissector can easily divide the right ventricular outflow tract from the right coronary aortic sinus. Due to this close anatomical relationship between the postero-lateral free wall of the right ventricular outflow tract and the right coronary aortic sinus, ventricular arrhythmias showing earliest activation at the right coronary aortic sinus[12] also requires detailed mapping from the

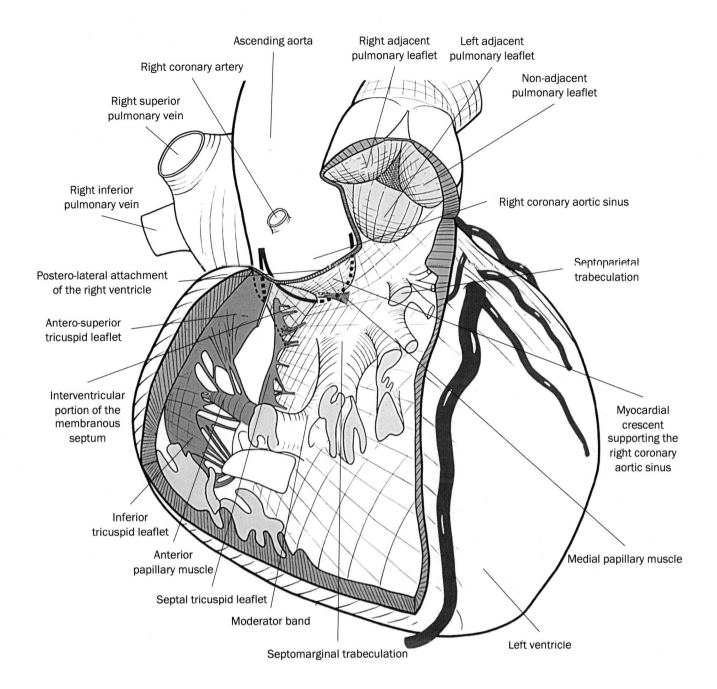

Ascending aorta

Right coronary artery

Right superior
pulmonary vein

Right adjacent
pulmonary leaflet

Left adjacent
pulmonary leaflet

Non-adjacent
pulmonary leaflet

Right inferior
pulmonary vein

Right coronary aortic sinus

Septoparietal
trabeculation

Postero-lateral attachment
of the right ventricle

Antero-superior
tricuspid leaflet

Interventricular
portion of the
membranous
septum

Myocardial
crescent
supporting the
right coronary
aortic sinus

Inferior
tricuspid leaflet

Anterior
papillary muscle

Medial papillary muscle

Septal tricuspid leaflet

Moderator band

Left ventricle

Septomarginal trabeculation

adjacent right ventricular outflow tract at its postero-lateral part, corresponding to the medial part of the supraventricular crest. The insulated preferential conductions connecting the right/left coronary aortic sinuses and right ventricular outflow tract/para-Hisian region have been reported in the setting of the ventricular arrhythmias ablated from the aortic sinuses. Those reports reveal the remote exit at the right ventricular outflow tract,[13] or connection to the His-Purkinje system[14,15] that can be ablated from the right or left coronary aortic sinuses. The substrate of this insulated preferential conduction is considered to be the dead-end tract.[16] The dead-end tract is the remnant of the aortic ring,[17,18] which is the conducting tissues initially encircling the developing interventricular communication and eventually surrounding the aortic root.[19] The superior limb of the septo-marginal trabeculation directs toward the left adjacent pulmonary sinus, which is located the most postero-inferior among the three pulmonary sinuses. From the superior limb, several septoparietal trabeculations originate running toward the left anterior direction at the medial infundibulum. The proximal part of this superior limb is the superior limit of the ventricular septum in the right ventricular outflow tract. At the bifurcation of the superior and inferior limbs of the septoparietal trabeculation, medial papillary muscle is located at its inferior limb side, anchoring the medial part of the antero-superior tricuspid leaflet.

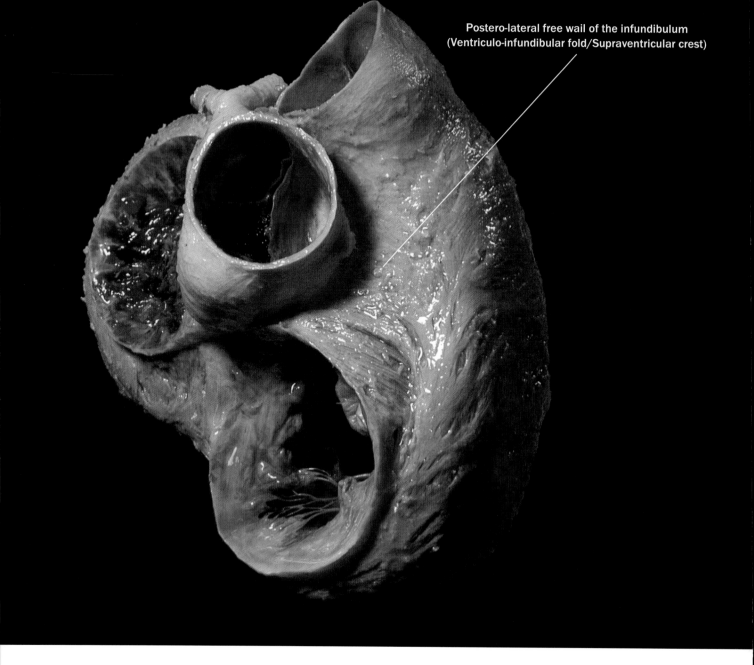

Figure 78   The crisscross relationship between the right ventricular outflow tract and the aortic root.[1]

The pulmonary valve is lifted up from the tricuspid valve by the right ventricular outflow tract. The right ventricular outflow tract and the aortic root show crisscross relationship each other. The postero-lateral free wall of the right ventricular outflow tract and pulmonary root override the right and left coronary aortic sinuses. The left main trunk of the left coronary artery is located distal to the sinutubular junction of the pulmonary root. Thus, it is the pulmonary trunk that overrides the left main trunk. The encircling myocardium of the free-standing subpulmonary infundibulum supports the base of the all three pulmonary sinuses. Therefore, ventriculo-arterial junction is located above the virtual basal ring in constant fashion in the pulmonary root. In contrast, the ventriculo-arterial junction is only seen at the base of the right and left coronary aortic sinuses in the aortic root,[3] as the rest of the aortic root is supported by the fibrous tissue, including right and left fibrous trigones, aortic-to-mitral (aortomitral) continuity, and membranous septum. The apex of the

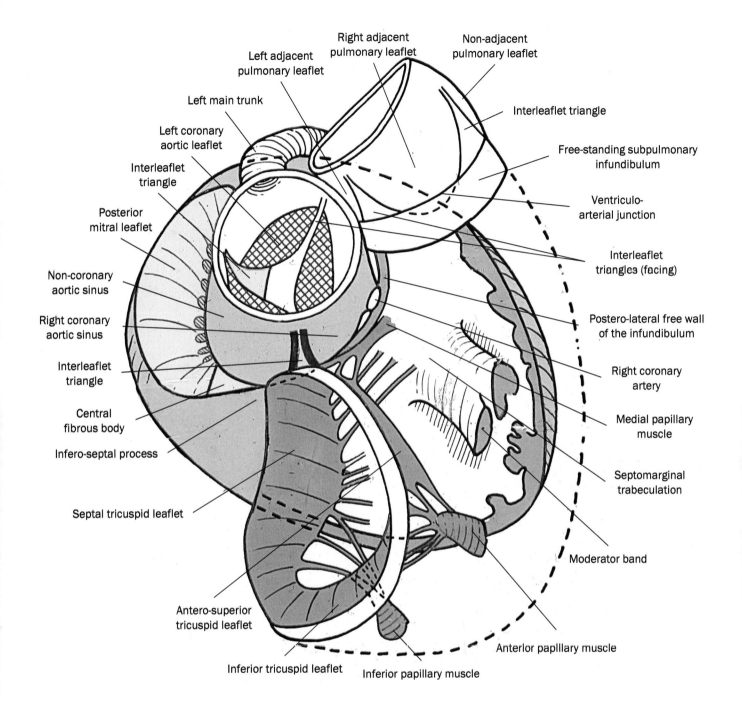

Right adjacent
pulmonary leaflet

Left adjacent
pulmonary leaflet

Non-adjacent
pulmonary leaflet

Left main trunk

Interleaflet triangle

Left coronary
aortic leaflet

Free-standing subpulmonary
infundibulum

Interleaflet
triangle

Ventriculo-
arterial junction

Posterior
mitral leaflet

Interleaflet
triangles (facing)

Non-coronary
aortic sinus

Postero-lateral free wall
of the infundibulum

Right coronary
aortic sinus

Right coronary
artery

Interleaflet
triangle

Medial papillary
muscle

Central
fibrous body

Septomarginal
trabeculation

Infero-septal process

Septal tricuspid leaflet

Moderator band

Antero-superior
tricuspid leaflet

Anterior papillary muscle

Inferior tricuspid leaflet

Inferior papillary muscle

interleaflet triangle between the right and left coronary aortic sinuses is close to the apex of the interleaflet triangle between the right and left adjacent pulmonary sinuses. The close anatomical relationship between the postero-lateral free wall of the right ventricular outflow tract and the right coronary aortic sinus suggests the necessity of thorough mapping of the right ventricular outflow tract and pulmonary root in the setting of ventricular arrhythmias seemingly originating from the right coronary aortic sinus or the interleaflet triangle between the right and left coronary aortic sinuses. The region of the interleaflet triangle between the right and left coronary aortic sinuses is also referred to as the *junction* of both sinuses.[20] As both facing interleaflet triangles are located proximal to the semilunar attachment of arterial leaflets, both facing *junctions* are hemodynamically outflow tracts facing to the thin fibro-adipose tissue plane between both arterial roots. Refer to Figure 79.

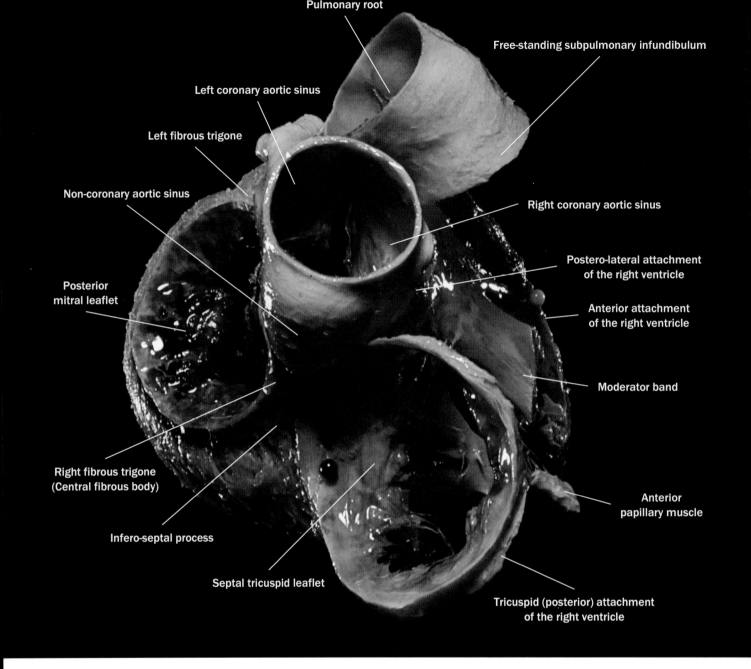

Pulmonary root

Free-standing subpulmonary infundibulum

Left coronary aortic sinus

Left fibrous trigone

Non-coronary aortic sinus

Right coronary aortic sinus

Posterior mitral leaflet

Postero-lateral attachment of the right ventricle

Anterior attachment of the right ventricle

Moderator band

Right fibrous trigone (Central fibrous body)

Anterior papillary muscle

Infero-septal process

Septal tricuspid leaflet

Tricuspid (posterior) attachment of the right ventricle

Figure 79   Removal of the free wall of the right ventricle.[1]

The free-wall components of the right ventricle are removed, except the encircling free-standing subpulmonary infundibulum supporting the pulmonary root. The two images on the right page show a part removed from the left iamge. In contrast to the left heart, the atrioventricular and arterial valves are distant separated by the postero-lateral free wall of the right ventricular outflow tract (infundibulum). This curved part is also referred to as the ventriculo-infundibular fold. The endocardial side of this ventriculo-infundibular fold corresponds to the supraventricular crest. This postero-lateral free wall

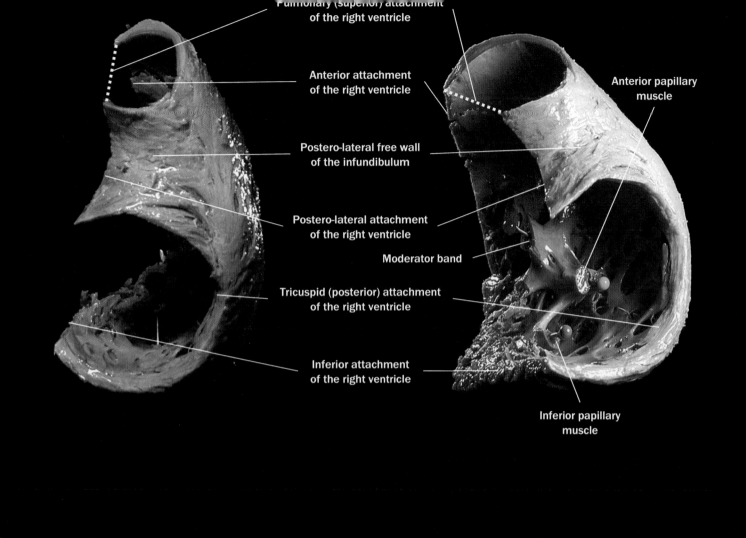

Pulmonary (superior) attachment
of the right ventricle

Anterior attachment
of the right ventricle

Postero-lateral free wall
of the infundibulum

Postero-lateral attachment
of the right ventricle

Moderator band

Tricuspid (posterior) attachment
of the right ventricle

Inferior attachment
of the right ventricle

Anterior papillary
muscle

Inferior papillary
muscle

is adjacent to the right coronary aortic sinus separated by the thin fibrous tissue plane.[21] In the image on the left page, the moderator band is sectioned. In the left image on the right page, the *en face* view of the postero-lateral free wall of the right ventricular outflow tract is shown. In the right image on the right page, the red, yellow, and blue beads indicate the moderator band, anterior papillary muscle, and inferior papillary muscle, respectively. Refer to Figure 78.

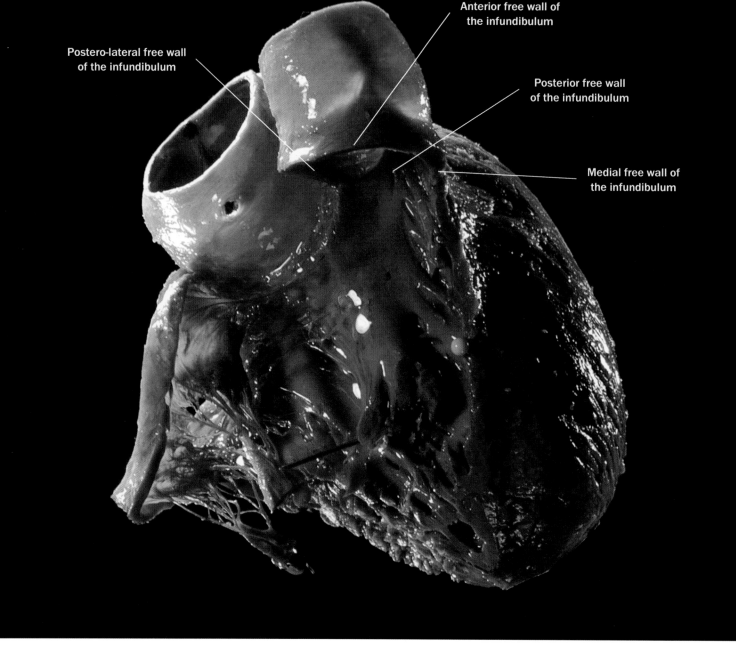

Figure 80 Removal of the free wall of the right ventricle viewed from the anterior direction.[1]

The free wall component of the right ventricle is removed, except the encircling free-standing subpulmonary infundibulum. It is the presence of this encircling free-standing subpulmonary infundibulum that permits the entirety of the pulmonary root to be removed and used as an aortic autograft in the Ross procedure.[22] Only the superior attachment (white dotted lines) is left connected in this specimen to leave the pulmonary root *in situ*. The postero-lateral free wall of the right ventricular outflow tract covering the right coronary aortic sinus is removed. The posterior free wall of the right ventricular outflow tract beneath the pulmonary valve is left intact, covered by the superior limb of the septomarginal trabeculation directing toward the left adjacent pulmonary sinus. The free wall of the right ventricle has five attachments: anterior, postero-lateral, inferior, tricuspid (posterior), and pulmonary (superior). They correspond to the anterior interventricular groove, inferior border of the ventriculo-infundibular fold (ventriculo-arterial junction), inferior interventricular groove, right atrioventricular groove, and posterior border of the free-standing subpulmonary infundibulum, respectively. Within the right ventricular outflow tract, the anterior, postero-lateral, and pulmonary attachments are related to medial, postero-lateral, and posterior free wall

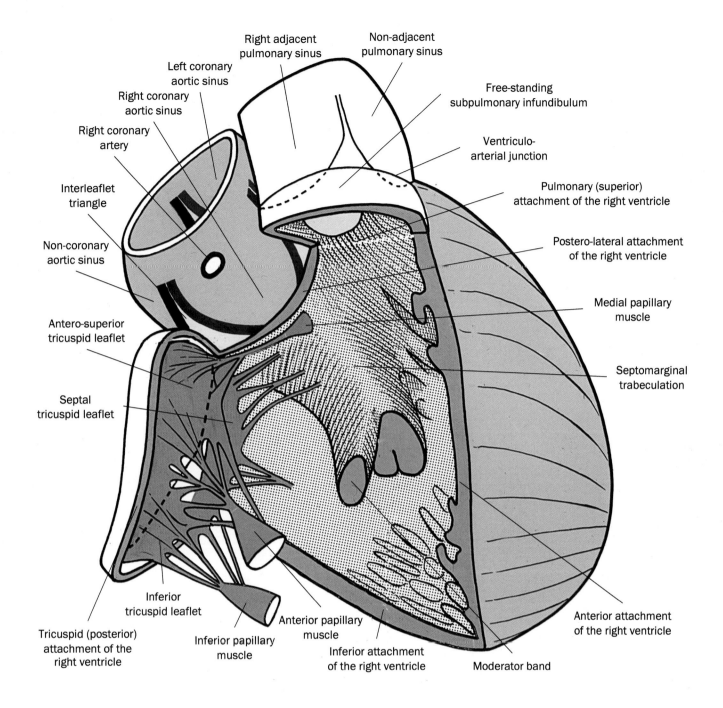

Right adjacent
pulmonary sinus

Non-adjacent
pulmonary sinus

Left coronary
aortic sinus

Right coronary
aortic sinus

Free-standing
subpulmonary infundibulum

Right coronary
artery

Ventriculo-
arterial junction

Interleaflet
triangle

Pulmonary (superior)
attachment of the right ventricle

Non-coronary
aortic sinus

Postero-lateral attachment
of the right ventricle

Antero-superior
tricuspid leaflet

Medial papillary
muscle

Septomarginal
trabeculation

Septal
tricuspid leaflet

Inferior
tricuspid leaflet

Anterior attachment
of the right ventricle

Tricuspid (posterior)
attachment of the
right ventricle

Inferior papillary
muscle

Anterior papillary
muscle

Inferior attachment
of the right ventricle

Moderator band

of the infundibulum, respectively. The medial free wall of the infundibulum is close to the proximal-mid left anterior descending artery. The postero-lateral free wall of the infundibulum is adjacent to the right coronary aortic sinus. The posterior free wall of the infundibulum is related to the left coronary aortic sinus and left ventricular summit. A substantial part of the right coronary aortic sinus is covered by the postero-lateral free wall of the right ventricular outflow tract, intervened by the thin fibrous tissue plane. The cutting line at the postero-lateral attachment demarcates the ventriculo-arterial junction at the base of the aortic root. By the crest of the ventricular septum at this region, the bottom of the right coronary aortic sinus is firmly supported. The ventriculo-arterial junction of the aortic root is only found at the base of the right and left coronary aortic sinuses, whereas it is found at every sinus of the pulmonary root.[3] In these regions, the ventriculo-arterial junction located superior to the virtual basal ring of the arterial roots is a normal structural anatomy. Therefore, it should not be deemed as the myocardial sleeve or extensions.[23] Similarly, the postero-lateral free wall of the right ventricular outflow tract covering the right coronary aortic sinus should not be deemed as the myocardial sleeve or extensions of the aortic root.

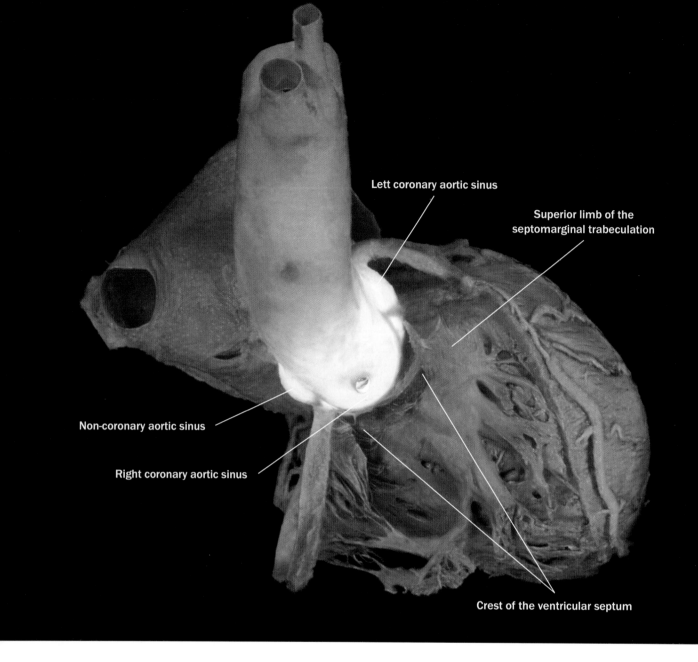

Left coronary aortic sinus

Superior limb of the
septomarginal trabeculation

Non-coronary aortic sinus

Right coronary aortic sinus

Crest of the ventricular septum

Figure 81   Five attachments of the right ventricle viewed from the right antero-superior direction.[1]

The five attachments of the right ventricle are shown. At the pulmonary (superior) attachment of the right ventricle, the posterior free wall of the right ventricular outflow tract detaches from the ventricular mass to elevate the pulmonary valve. At this elevated posterior free wall, the right ventricular outflow tract starts to override the left coronary aortic sinus and left coronary artery. Refer to Figure 135. Therefore, the superior attachment demarcates the margin between the ventricular septum of the right ventricular outflow tract and the basal superior left ventricular free wall, referred to as the left ventricular summit.[24] Thus, the septal region of the right ventricular outflow tract is located antero-inferior relative to the posterior free wall of the right ventricular outflow tract, and it is located medial relative to the postero-lateral free wall of the right ventricular outflow tract covering the right coronary aortic sinus. In the context of the entire right ventricular outflow tract, this septal region is located postero-inferior.[4] The interleaflet triangle between the right and left coronary aortic sinuses is located close to the junction between the pulmonary and postero-lateral attachments. The postero-lateral attachment corresponds to the ventriculo-arterial junction, that is, the superior margin of the crest of the ventricular septum. Thus, the base of the right coronary aortic sinus is related to the crest of the ventricular septum, and the base of the anterior half of

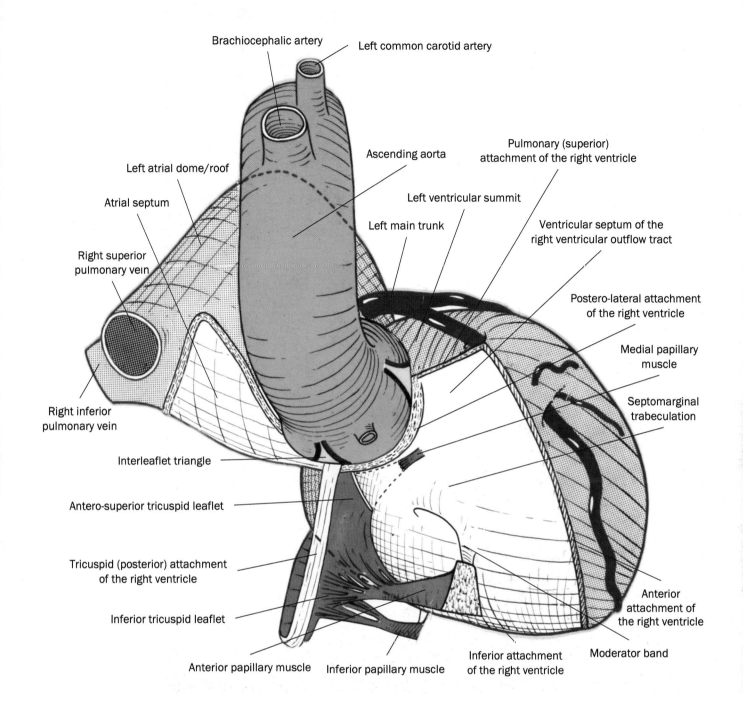

Brachiocephalic artery

Left common carotid artery

Ascending aorta

Pulmonary (superior) attachment of the right ventricle

Left atrial dome/roof

Left ventricular summit

Atrial septum

Left main trunk

Ventricular septum of the right ventricular outflow tract

Right superior pulmonary vein

Postero-lateral attachment of the right ventricle

Medial papillary muscle

Right inferior pulmonary vein

Septomarginal trabeculation

Interleaflet triangle

Antero-superior tricuspid leaflet

Tricuspid (posterior) attachment of the right ventricle

Anterior attachment of the right ventricle

Inferior tricuspid leaflet

Anterior papillary muscle

Inferior papillary muscle

Inferior attachment of the right ventricle

Moderator band

the left coronary aortic sinus is related to the left ventricular free wall.[10] In addition, the right coronary aortic sinus and the interleaflet triangle between the right and left coronary aortic sinuses are, in part, covered by the postero-lateral free wall of the right ventricular outflow tract, separated by the thin fibro-adipose tissue plane. Considering these structural relationships, the crest of the ventricular septum supporting the right coronary aortic sinus, the basal superior left ventricular free wall at the left ventricular summit supporting the left coronary aortic sinus, and the postero-lateral free wall of the right ventricular outflow tract covering the right coronary aortic sinus can all be substrates of the ventricular arrhythmias ablated from the right or left coronary aortic sinuses or their so-called *junction*, corresponding to the interleaflet triangle.[20] In this situation, these ventricular arrhythmias do not actually originate from the sinuses of Valsalva, *junction*, or something like myocardial sleeve or extensions,[23] but they should be deemed as originating from ventricular myocardium of each location. Thus, detailed and thorough mapping of the adjacent ventricular myocardium based on the structural anatomy shown in Figure 81 is required when treating the ventricular arrhythmia seemingly originated from the right and left coronary aortic sinuses or their *junction*.

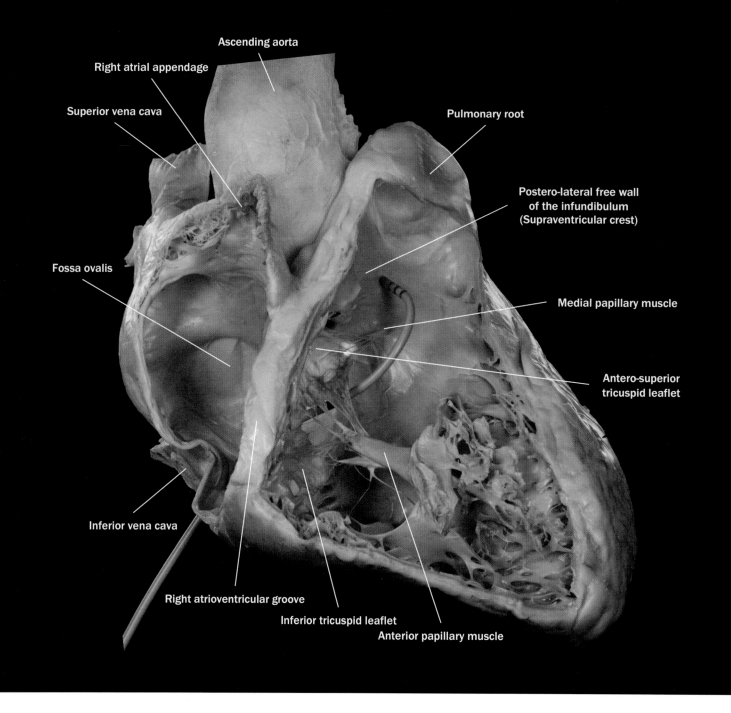

Figure 82 The ablation catheter placed at the right postero-lateral wall of the right ventricular outflow tract (supraventricular crest).

The images are viewed from the right anterior oblique (left) and left anterior oblique (right) directions. The catheter is placed at the right postero-lateral free wall of the right ventricular outflow tract, located anterior to the right coronary aortic sinus. This region is also referred to as the supraventricular crest or ventriculo-infundibular fold. At the medial part of the

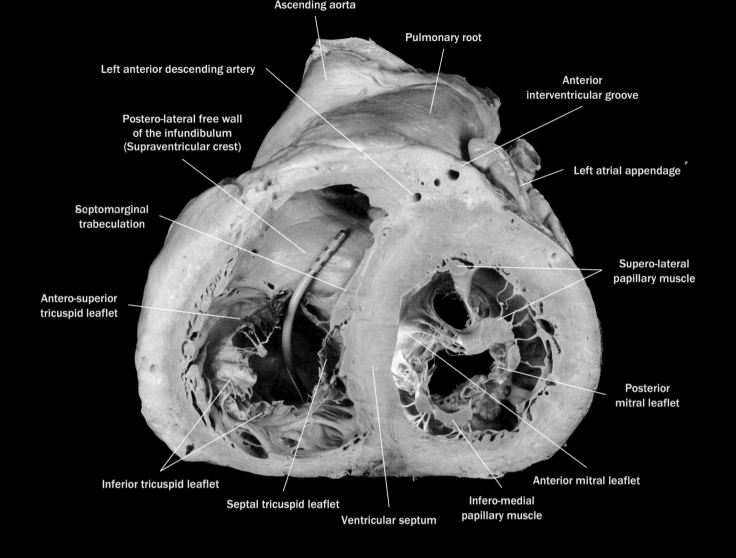

Ascending aorta

Pulmonary root

Left anterior descending artery

Anterior interventricular groove

Postero-lateral free wall of the infundibulum (Supraventricular crest)

Left atrial appendage

Septomarginal trabeculation

Supero-lateral papillary muscle

Antero-superior tricuspid leaflet

Posterior mitral leaflet

Inferior tricuspid leaflet

Anterior mitral leaflet

Septal tricuspid leaflet

Infero-medial papillary muscle

Ventricular septum

supraventricular crest, the thin fibrous tissue plane intervenes between the aortic root (right coronary aortic sinus) and right ventricular outflow tract. The endocardial surface of this region is smooth.

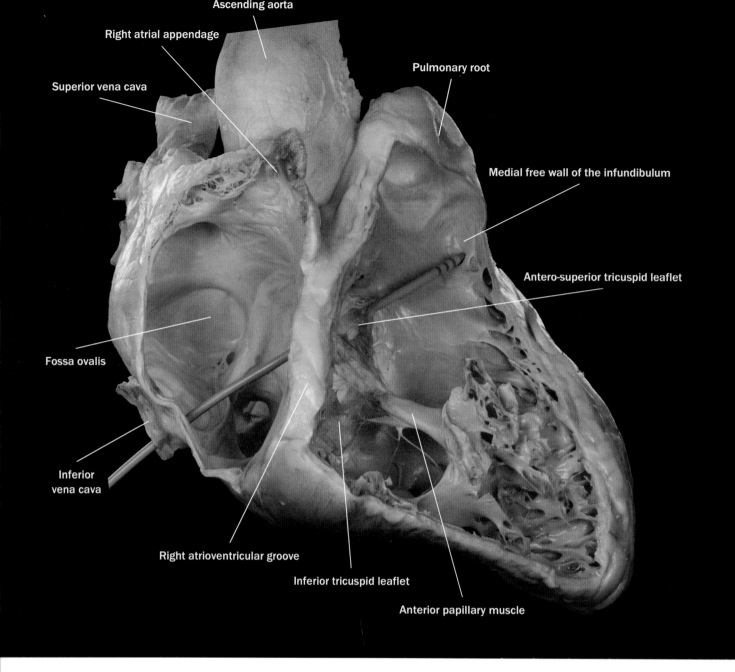

Ascending aorta

Right atrial appendage

Superior vena cava

Pulmonary root

Medial free wall of the infundibulum

Antero-superior tricuspid leaflet

Fossa ovalis

Inferior
vena cava

Right atrioventricular groove

Inferior tricuspid leaflet

Anterior papillary muscle

Figure 83   The ablation catheter placed at the medial free wall of the right ventricular outflow tract. ▭▬ Anaglyph 15.

The images are viewed from the right anterior oblique (left) and left anterior oblique (right) directions. The catheter is placed at the medial free wall of the right ventricular outflow tract, close to the base of the septoparietal trabeculation. This region, often referred to as the anterior attachment or antero-septal attachment, is a common substrate of idiopathic ventricular tachyarrhythmia originating from the right ventricular outflow tract.[25] Although the catheter appears to be directed

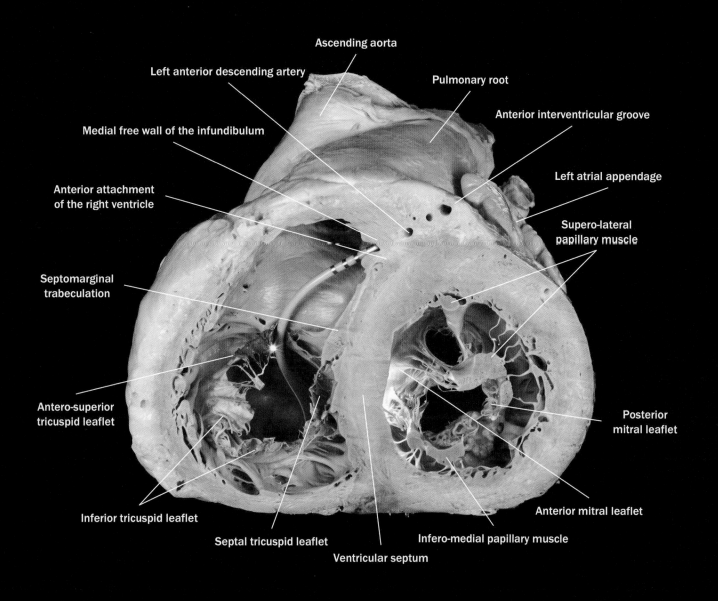

Ascending aorta

Left anterior descending artery

Pulmonary root

Medial free wall of the infundibulum

Anterior interventricular groove

Left atrial appendage

Anterior attachment of the right ventricle

Supero-lateral papillary muscle

Septomarginal trabeculation

Antero-superior tricuspid leaflet

Posterior mitral leaflet

Inferior tricuspid leaflet

Anterior mitral leaflet

Septal tricuspid leaflet

Infero-medial papillary muscle

Ventricular septum

toward the septal direction when viewed from the left anterior oblique direction (right), it is above the anterior attachment of the right ventricle to the ventricular septum. Therefore, this region is not the ventricular septum, but a thin medial free wall of the right ventricular outflow tract facing to the anterior interventricular groove. This indicates the potential risk of perforation[26] and damage to the left anterior descending artery.

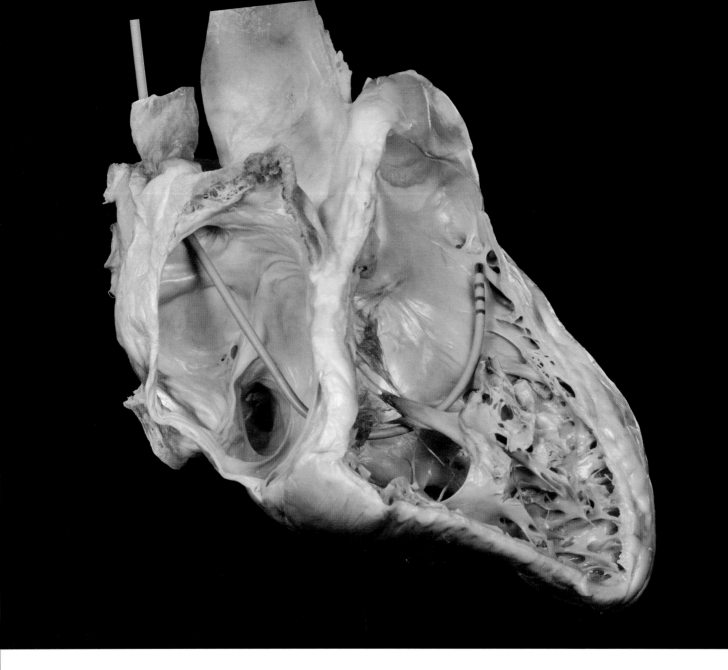

Figure 84 The superior approach to the right ventricular outflow tract using a large, U-turn curve catheter.

The images are viewed from the right anterior oblique direction. The superior approach using a large, U-turn curve is demonstrated.[27] The light source in the aortic root transilluminates the postero-lateral free wall of the right ventricular outflow tract via the right coronary aortic sinus posterior to it. The catheters are placed below the level of the pulmonary (superior) attachment of the right ventricle. In the left image, the tip is located at the medial free wall of the right ventricular outflow tract at the base of the septoparietal trabeculation. In the right image, the tip is located at the crest of the ventricular septum supporting the right coronary aortic sinus. It is just beneath the ventriculo-arterial junction of the right coronary aortic sinus, corresponding to the postero-lateral attachment of the right ventricle, which can be determined as

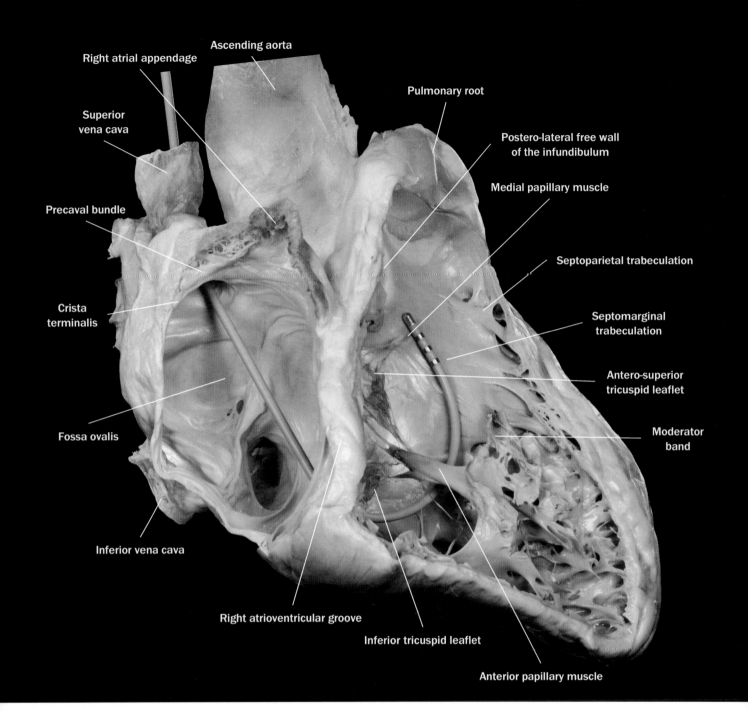

Right atrial appendage

Ascending aorta

Pulmonary root

Superior
vena cava

Postero-lateral free wall
of the infundibulum

Medial papillary muscle

Precaval bundle

Septoparietal trabeculation

Crista
terminalis

Septomarginal
trabeculation

Antero-superior
tricuspid leaflet

Moderator
band

Fossa ovalis

Inferior vena cava

Right atrioventricular groove

Inferior tricuspid leaflet

Anterior papillary muscle

the inferior margin of the transillumination. The tip is also close to the base of the medial papillary muscle. Compared to the inferior approach, which generally needs to apply double directional (sigmoid) curve on the catheter, superior approach requires single directional curve. Therefore, manipulation of the catheter is straightforward. Also, the tip can be placed less perpendicular to the medial free wall to achieve *touch ablation* rather than *push ablation*. Refer to Figure 83. Changing the bend of the catheter enables to scan left anterior (left image) and right posterior (right image) directions. Counterclockwise and clockwise rotation enables mapping to the medical and lateral directions respectively.

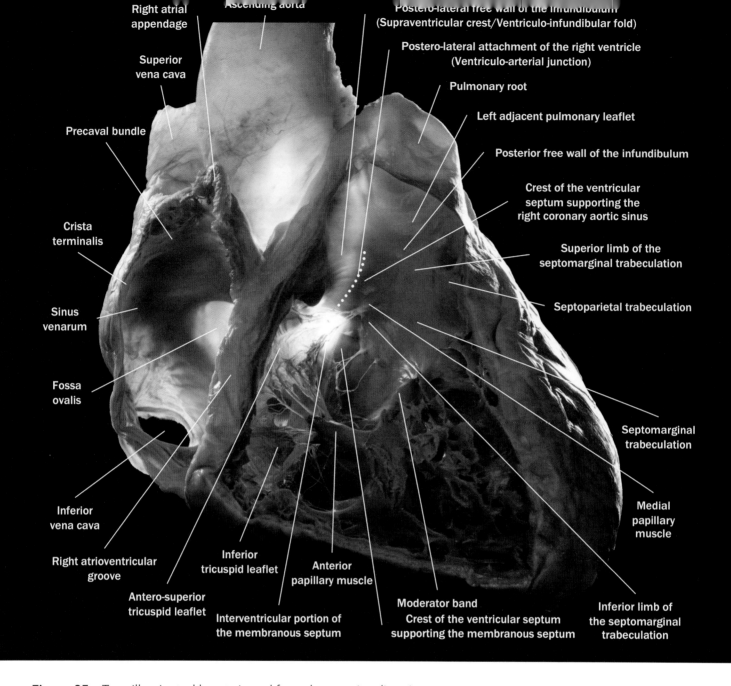

Right atrial appendage

Ascending aorta

Postero-lateral free wall of the infundibulum (Supraventricular crest/Ventriculo-infundibular fold)

Superior vena cava

Postero-lateral attachment of the right ventricle (Ventriculo-arterial junction)

Pulmonary root

Precaval bundle

Left adjacent pulmonary leaflet

Posterior free wall of the infundibulum

Crest of the ventricular septum supporting the right coronary aortic sinus

Crista terminalis

Superior limb of the septomarginal trabeculation

Septoparietal trabeculation

Sinus venarum

Fossa ovalis

Septomarginal trabeculation

Inferior vena cava

Medial papillary muscle

Right atrioventricular groove

Inferior tricuspid leaflet

Anterior papillary muscle

Antero-superior tricuspid leaflet

Interventricular portion of the membranous septum

Moderator band Crest of the ventricular septum supporting the membranous septum

Inferior limb of the septomarginal trabeculation

Figure 85   Transilluminated heart viewed from the anterior direction.

The postero-lateral free wall of the right ventricular outflow tract is transilluminated through the aortic root (right coronary aortic sinus). The posterior free wall of the right ventricular outflow tract and the crest of the muscular ventricular septum are not transilluminated. The inferior margin of the transillumination corresponds to the postero-lateral attachment of the right ventricle (white dotted line). This line also corresponds to the ventriculo-arterial junction supporting the right coronary aortic sinus, and the basal limit of the crest of the ventricular septum at the right coronary aortic sinus. The incorporated myocardium supporting the arterial root is also called as the myocardial crescent.[10] The membranous septum, fossa ovalis, and inferior sinus venarum are also transilluminated.

References

1. McAlpine WA. Digitized collection of all the images created by Dr. McAlpine at UCLA. Copyright UCLA Cardiac Arrhythmia Center. Part of this collection appeared in *Heart and Coronary Arteries: An Anatomical Atlas for Clinical Diagnosis, Radiological Investigation, and Surgical Treatment*. New York: Springer-Verlag; 1975.

2. Shimizu S. [Topographical anatomy of the atrioventricular node of Tawara—findings by macro-microscopic dissection under dissecting microscope] (in Japanese). *Nihon Kyobu Geka Gakkai Zasshi*. 1989;37 :227–233.

3. Mori S, Tretter JT, Spicer DE, et al. What is the real cardiac anatomy? *Clin Anat*. 2019;32:288–309.

4. Mori S, Fukuzawa K, Takaya T, et al. Clinical cardiac structural anatomy reconstructed within the cardiac contour using multi-detector-row computed tomography: Atrial septum and ventricular septum. *Clin Anat*. 2016;29:342–352.

5. Loukas M, Bilinsky E, Bilinsky S, et al. The anatomy of the aortic root. *Clin Anat*. 2014;27:748–756.

6. Lal M, Ho SY, Anderson RH. Is there such a thing as the "tendon of the infundibulum" in the heart? *Clin Anat*. 1997;10:307–312.

7. Zimmerman J, Bailey CP. The surgical significance of the fibrous skeleton of the heart. *J Thorac Cardiovasc Surg*. 1962;44:701–712.

8. Saremi F, Sánchez-Quintana D, Mori S, et al. Fibrous skeleton of the heart: Anatomic overview and evaluation of pathologic conditions with CT and MR imaging. *Radiographics*. 2017;37:1330–1351.

9. Mori S, Fukuzawa K, Takaya T, et al. Clinical cardiac structural anatomy reconstructed within the cardiac contour using multi-detector-row computed tomography: Left ventricular outflow tract. *Clin Anat*. 2016;29:353–363.

10. Toh H, Mori S, Tretter JT, et al. Living anatomy of the ventricular myocardial crescents supporting the coronary aortic sinuses. *Semin Thorac Cardiovasc Surg*. 2020;32:230–241.

11. Anderson RH, Mohun TJ, Sánchez-Quintana D, et al. The anatomic substrates for outflow tract arrhythmias. *Heart Rhythm*. 2019;16:290–297.

12. Wang Y, Liang Z, Wu S, et al. Idiopathic ventricular arrhythmias originating from the right coronary sinus: Prevalence, electrocardiographic and electrophysiological characteristics, and catheter ablation. *Heart Rhythm*. 2018;15:81–89.

13. Yamada T, Murakami Y, Yoshida N, et al. Preferential conduction across the ventricular outflow septum in ventricular arrhythmias originating from the aortic sinus cusp. *J Am Coll Cardiol*. 2007;50:884–891.

14. Sato E, Yagi T, Namekawa A, et al. His-Purkinje system-related incessant ventricular tachycardia arising from the left coronary cusp. *J Arrhythm*. 2014;30:323–326.

15. Han B, Li XJ, Hsia HH. Catheter ablation of arrhythmia from the aortic sinus cusp: the presence of a dead-end tract of the conduction system. *Europace*. 2013;15:1515.

16. Kurosawa H, Becker AE. Dead-end tract of the conduction axis. *Int J Cardiol*. 1985;7:13–20.

17. Anderson RH, Spicer DE, Mori S. Of tracts, rings, nodes, cusps, sinuses, and arrhythmias-A comment on Szili-Torok et al.'s paper entitled "The 'Dead-End Tract' and its role in arrhythmogenesis". J Cardiovasc. Dev. Dis. 2016, 3, 11. *J Cardiovasc Dev Dis*. 2016;3:17.

18. Anderson RH, Sánchez-Quintana D, Mori S, et al. Unusual variants of pre-excitation: From anatomy to ablation: Part I-Understanding the anatomy of the variants of ventricular pre-excitation. *J Cardiovasc Electrophysiol*. 2019;30:2170–2180.

19. Bohora S, Lokhandwala Y, Sternick EB, et al. Reappraisal and new observations on atrial tachycardia ablated from the non-coronary aortic sinus of Valsalva. *Europace*. 2018;20:124–133.

20. Yamada T, Yoshida N, Murakami Y, et al. Electrocardiographic characteristics of ventricular arrhythmias originating from the junction of the left and right coronary sinuses of Valsalva in the aorta: The activation pattern as a rationale for the electrocardiographic characteristics. *Heart Rhythm*. 2008;5:184–192.

21. Mori S, Fukuzawa K, Takaya T, et al. Optimal angulations for obtaining an *en face* view of each coronary aortic sinus and the interventricular septum: Correlative anatomy around the left ventricular outflow tract. *Clin Anat*. 2015;28:494–505.

22. Merrick AF, Yacoub MH, Ho SY, et al. Anatomy of the muscular subpulmonary infundibulum with regard to the Ross procedure. *Ann Thorac Surg*. 2000;69:556–561.

23. Hasdemir C, Aktas S, Govsa F, et al. Demonstration of ventricular myocardial extensions into the pulmonary artery and aorta beyond the ventriculo-arterial junction. *Pacing Clin Electrophysiol*. 2007; 30:534–549.

24. Yamada T, McElderry HT, Doppalapudi H, et al. Idiopathic ventricular arrhythmias originating from the left ventricular summit: Anatomic concepts relevant to ablation. *Circ Arrhythm Electrophysiol*. 2010;3:616–623.

25. Kamakura S, Shimizu W, Matsuo K, et al. Localization of optimal ablation site of idiopathic ventricular tachycardia from right and left ventricular outflow tract by body surface ECG. *Circulation*. 1998;98:1525–1533.

26. Tokuda M, Kojodjojo P, Epstein LM, et al. Outcomes of cardiac perforation complicating catheter ablation of ventricular arrhythmias. *Circ Arrhythm Electrophysiol*. 2011;4:660–666.

27. Mori S, Otomo K, Yagi T, et al. Catheter ablation for idiopathic right ventricular outflow tract premature ventricular contraction via the single right transjugular approach. *J Cardiovasc Electrophysiol*. 2013;24:229–230.

13

Pulmonary Valve

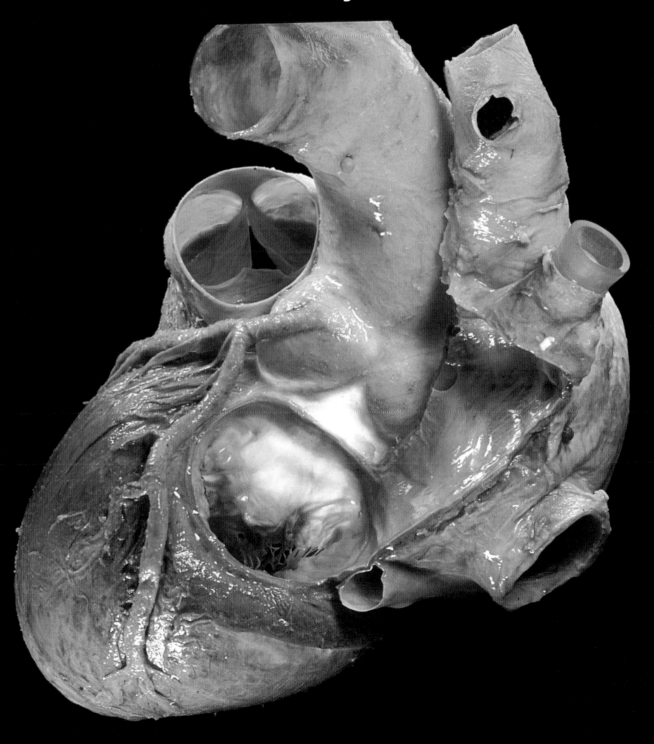

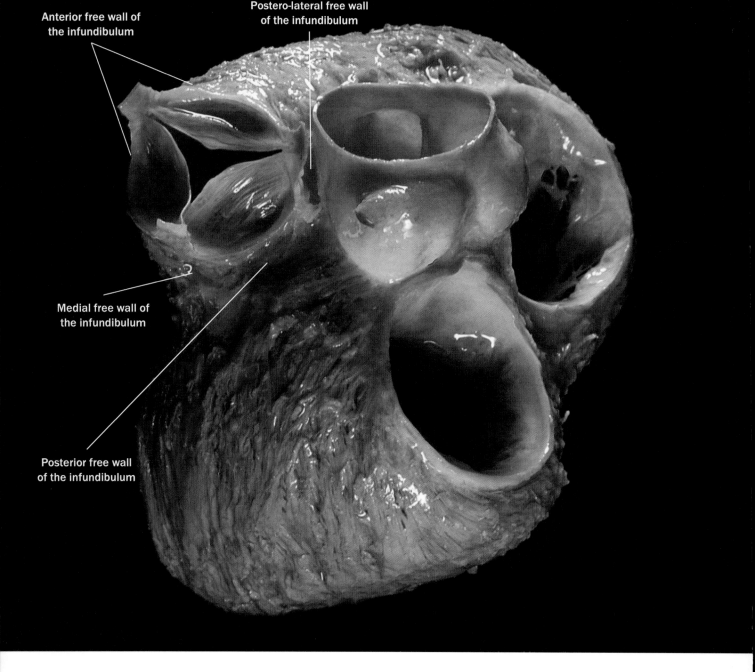

Anterior free wall of the infundibulum

Postero-lateral free wall of the infundibulum

Medial free wall of the infundibulum

Posterior free wall of the infundibulum

Figure 86   Relationship between the pulmonary valve and the aortic root.[1]

The heart is viewed from the left postero-superior direction. The four cardiac valves are not all located on a single flat plane.[2] The pulmonary valve is located at left antero-superior relative to the aortic valve.[3] The pulmonary root and the aortic root are in a crisscross relationship. The apex of the interleaflet triangle between the right and left coronary aortic sinuses is adjacent to the apex of the interleaflet triangle between the right and left adjacent pulmonary sinuses, reflecting the development of the arterial valves within the myocardial turret.[4] In the context of the correct anatomical coordinates,[5] the right adjacent and non-adjacent pulmonary sinuses are located right antero-superior and left antero-superior,

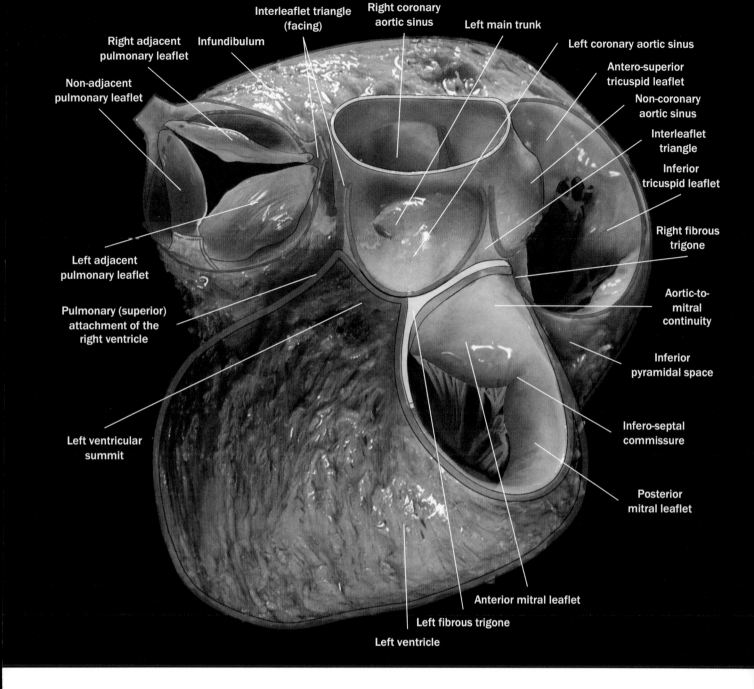

Right coronary
aortic sinus

Interleaflet triangle
(facing)

Left main trunk

Right adjacent
pulmonary leaflet

Infundibulum

Left coronary aortic sinus

Non-adjacent
pulmonary leaflet

Antero-superior
tricuspid leaflet

Non-coronary
aortic sinus

Interleaflet
triangle

Inferior
tricuspid leaflet

Right fibrous
trigone

Left adjacent
pulmonary leaflet

Aortic-to-
mitral
continuity

Pulmonary (superior)
attachment of the
right ventricle

Inferior
pyramidal space

Infero-septal
commissure

Left ventricular
summit

Posterior
mitral leaflet

Anterior mitral leaflet

Left fibrous trigone

Left ventricle

respectively, whereas the left adjacent pulmonary sinus is located most postero-inferior among the three pulmonary sinuses.[6] Therefore, the left adjacent pulmonary sinus is the closest to the left ventricular summit, where the left ventricular free wall is supporting the anterior half of the base of the left coronary aortic sinus.[7] Encircling myocardium of the right ventricular outflow tract, referred to as the free-standing subpulmonary infundibulum, supports the bases of the three pulmonary sinuses.[8]

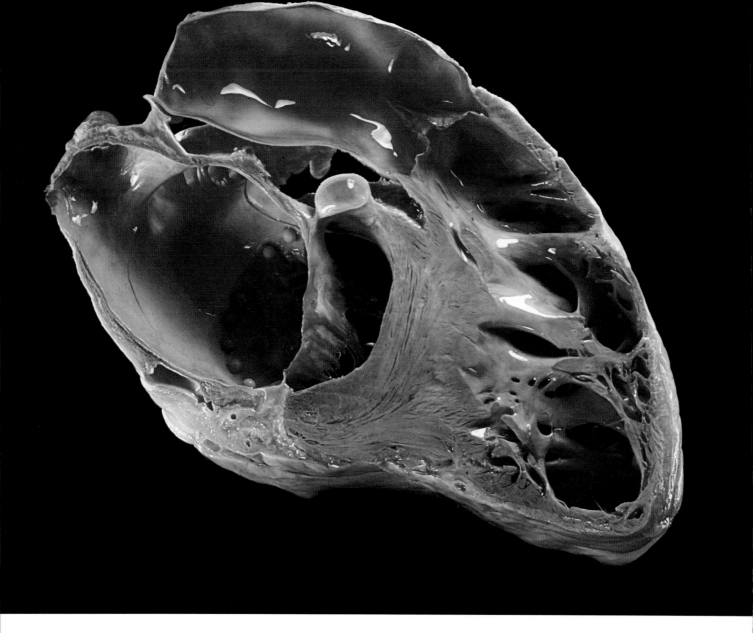

Figure 87 The sagittal section of the heart viewed from the right lateral direction.[1]

The posterior free wall of the right ventricular outflow tract is located anterior to the lateral left coronary aortic sinus. At this region, the right ventricular outflow tract separates from the ventricular mass.[9] This site corresponds to the pulmonary (superior) attachment of the right ventricle. The posterior free wall of the right ventricular outflow tract is apart from the left ventricular free wall muscle, corresponding to the left ventricular summit. The epicardial adipose tissue on the left ventricular summit, which is removed in this specimen, intervenes the space between the left coronary aortic sinus, left ventricular summit, and posterior free wall of the right ventricular outflow tract. The basal limit of this left ventricular free wall muscle, which is beak-shaped and thin (black arrow), supports the anterior half of the left coronary aortic sinus.[10] The

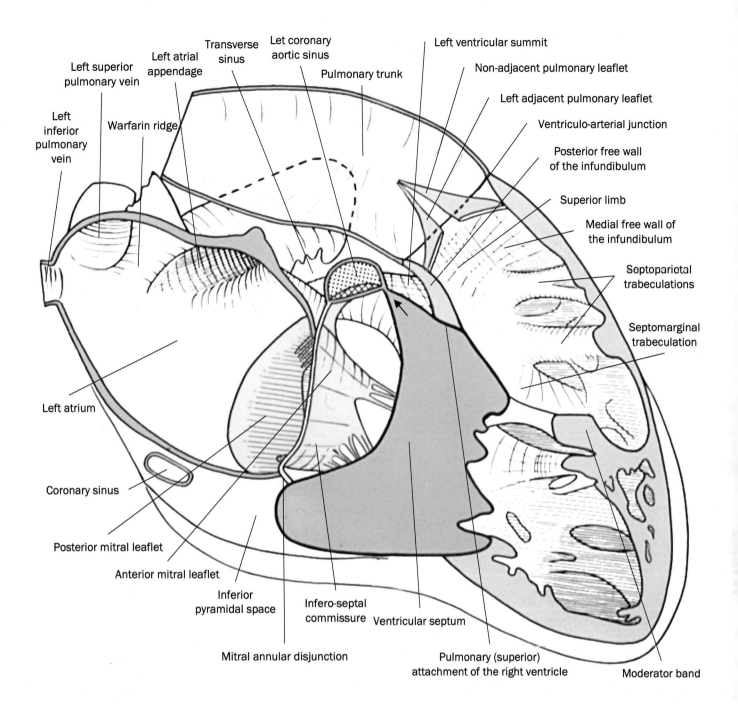

Left superior pulmonary vein

Left inferior pulmonary vein

Warfarin ridge

Left atrial appendage

Transverse sinus

Let coronary aortic sinus

Pulmonary trunk

Left ventricular summit

Non-adjacent pulmonary leaflet

Left adjacent pulmonary leaflet

Ventriculo-arterial junction

Posterior free wall of the infundibulum

Superior limb

Medial free wall of the infundibulum

Soptopariotal trabeculations

Septomarginal trabeculation

Left atrium

Coronary sinus

Posterior mitral leaflet

Anterior mitral leaflet

Inferior pyramidal space

Infero-septal commissure

Ventricular septum

Mitral annular disjunction

Pulmonary (superior) attachment of the right ventricle

Moderator band

pulmonary root and pulmonary trunk override the left coronary aortic sinus and left coronary artery. The left adjacent pulmonary sinus is located right postero-inferior to the non-adjacent pulmonary sinus, and left antero-superior to the left coronary aortic sinus. In the medial free wall of the right ventricular outflow tract, multiple septoparietal trabeculations arise from the superior limb of the septomarginal trabeculation. The superior limb of the septomarginal trabeculation directs toward the left adjacent pulmonary sinus. This section also shows how the left atrial appendage guards the left side entrance/exit of the transverse sinus. Refer to Figure 81. The paired section of this image is Figure 100.

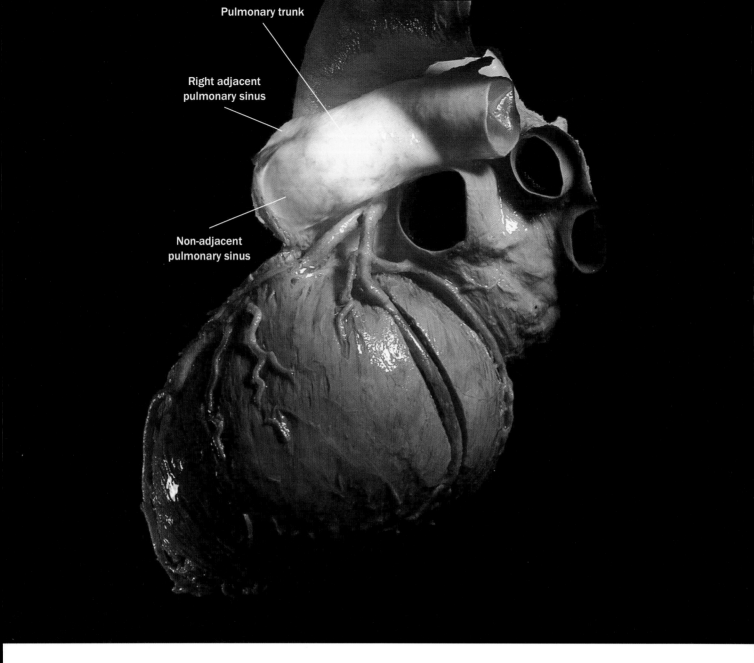

Pulmonary trunk

Right adjacent pulmonary sinus

Non-adjacent pulmonary sinus

Figure 88 Relationship between the pulmonary trunk and the left coronary artery viewed from the left lateral direction.[1]

In the right image, the pulmonary root and pulmonary trunk are removed from the left image, except the semilunar attachments of the pulmonary leaflets. The proximal left main trunk of the left coronary artery is located just beneath the proximal pulmonary trunk, which is distal to the sinutubular junction of the pulmonary root, corresponding to the plane involving

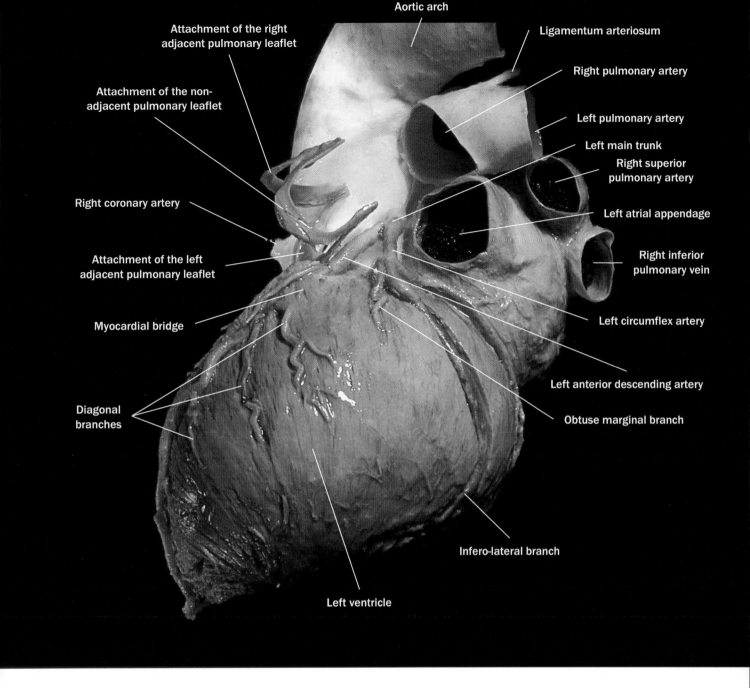

Aortic arch

Attachment of the right adjacent pulmonary leaflet

Ligamentum arteriosum

Right pulmonary artery

Attachment of the non-adjacent pulmonary leaflet

Left pulmonary artery

Left main trunk

Right superior pulmonary artery

Right coronary artery

Left atrial appendage

Attachment of the left adjacent pulmonary leaflet

Right inferior pulmonary vein

Myocardial bridge

Left circumflex artery

Left anterior descending artery

Diagonal branches

Obtuse marginal branch

Infero-lateral branch

Left ventricle

three commissures of the pulmonary leaflets. The relationship between the pulmonary root and left coronary artery shows the individual variation.[1,11] The proximal left anterior descending artery skirts the left and non-adjacent pulmonary sinuses postero-infero-laterally to them toward the anterior interventricular groove.

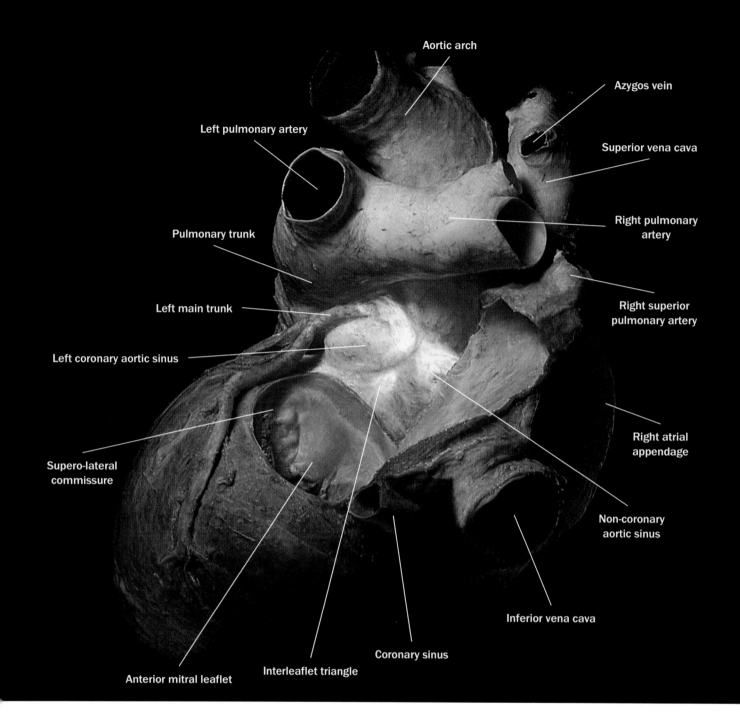

Aortic arch

Azygos vein

Left pulmonary artery

Superior vena cava

Right pulmonary artery

Pulmonary trunk

Left main trunk

Right superior pulmonary artery

Left coronary aortic sinus

Supero-lateral commissure

Right atrial appendage

Non-coronary aortic sinus

Inferior vena cava

Coronary sinus

Anterior mitral leaflet

Interleaflet triangle

Figure 89   Relationship between the pulmonary trunk and the left coronary artery viewed from the posterior direction.[1]

In the right image, the pulmonary arteries and pulmonary trunk are removed from the left image. The right pulmonary artery runs inferior to the aortic arch from the left to right direction just above the roof of the left atrium (left). The proximal left coronary artery is located just beneath the proximal pulmonary trunk. The proximal left anterior descending artery runs

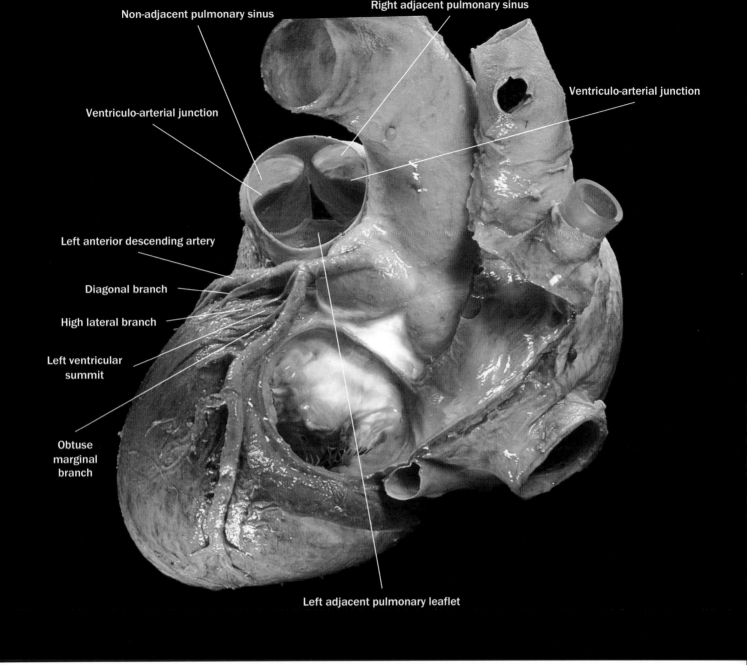

Non-adjacent pulmonary sinus

Right adjacent pulmonary sinus

Ventriculo-arterial junction

Ventriculo-arterial junction

Left anterior descending artery

Diagonal branch

High lateral branch

Left ventricular summit

Obtuse marginal branch

Left adjacent pulmonary leaflet

postero-infero-laterally to the left adjacent pulmonary sinus, skirting the sinus toward the anterior interventricular groove (right). Small diagonal, high-lateral, and obtuse marginal branches are observed on the left ventricular summit (right). Refer to Figure 92.

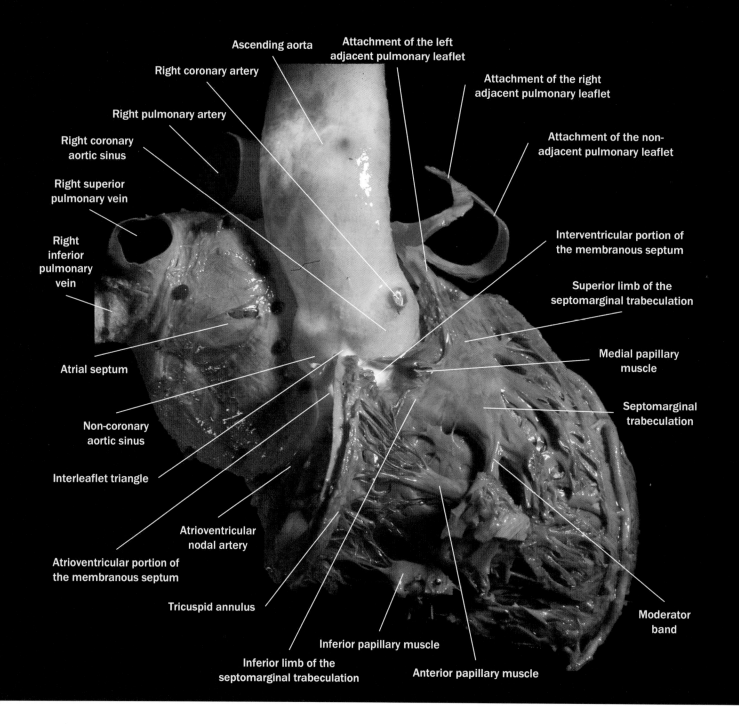

Figure 90 Relationship between the pulmonary trunk and the aortic root viewed from the right and left anterior oblique directions.[1]

When viewed from the right anterior oblique direction (left), the pulmonary valve is located left antero-superior to the aortic valve. The pulmonary root directs to the supero-posterior direction. The right and non-adjacent pulmonary sinuses are located superior to the proximal left anterior descending artery when viewed from this direction. When viewed from the left anterior oblique direction (right), the pulmonary valve is overlapped with the proximal aorta located behind. Although the aortic root commonly directs toward the right antero-superior direction, the pulmonary root directs toward the postero-superior direction. The proximal left anterior descending artery runs on the left ventricular summit behind

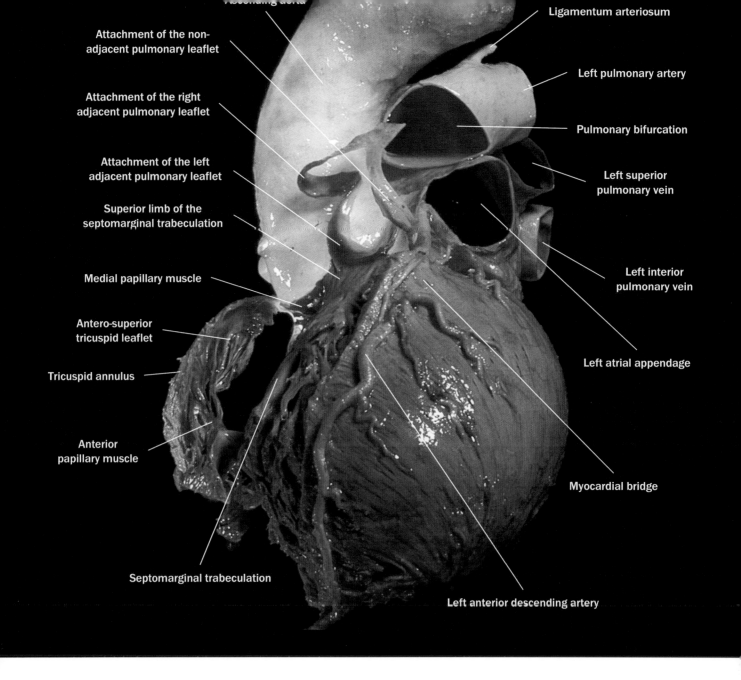

Ascending aorta

Attachment of the non-adjacent pulmonary leaflet

Attachment of the right adjacent pulmonary leaflet

Attachment of the left adjacent pulmonary leaflet

Superior limb of the septomarginal trabeculation

Medial papillary muscle

Antero-superior tricuspid leaflet

Tricuspid annulus

Anterior papillary muscle

Septomarginal trabeculation

Ligamentum arteriosum

Left pulmonary artery

Pulmonary bifurcation

Left superior pulmonary vein

Left interior pulmonary vein

Left atrial appendage

Myocardial bridge

Left anterior descending artery

the left adjacent pulmonary sinus. After it skirts the pulmonary root, it changes course along the anterior interventricular groove toward the cardiac apex. Thus, the proximal left anterior descending artery and its bending portion are the useful markers to locate the pulmonary root. The proximal-mid left anterior descending artery shows the myocardial bridge. The orifice of the left atrial appendage is located infero-lateral to the distal pulmonary trunk. This proximity between the pulmonary trunk and the left atrial appendage is important to estimate potential risk of injury to the pulmonary trunk during implantation of a left atrial appendage closure device.[12]

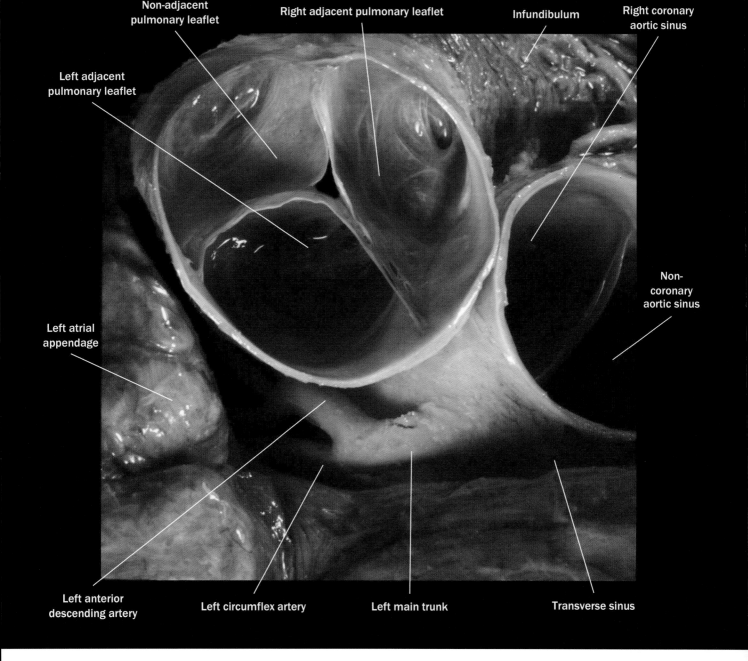

Figure 91 The pulmonary valves.[1]

The relationship between the pulmonary root, left atrial appendage, left coronary artery, and the aortic root is shown in the left image. The left adjacent pulmonary aortic sinus faces to the proximal left coronary artery. The left atrial appendage covers the left and non-adjacent pulmonary sinuses. Encircling myocardium of the right ventricular outflow tract supports the bases of the three pulmonary sinuses (right images). When viewed from the pulmonary trunk, these myocardial supports are observed as the crescent of the myocardium incorporated at the base of each sinus.[7] The distal margin of this myocardial crescent corresponds to the ventriculo-arterial junction. In the pulmonary root, the ventriculo-arterial junction

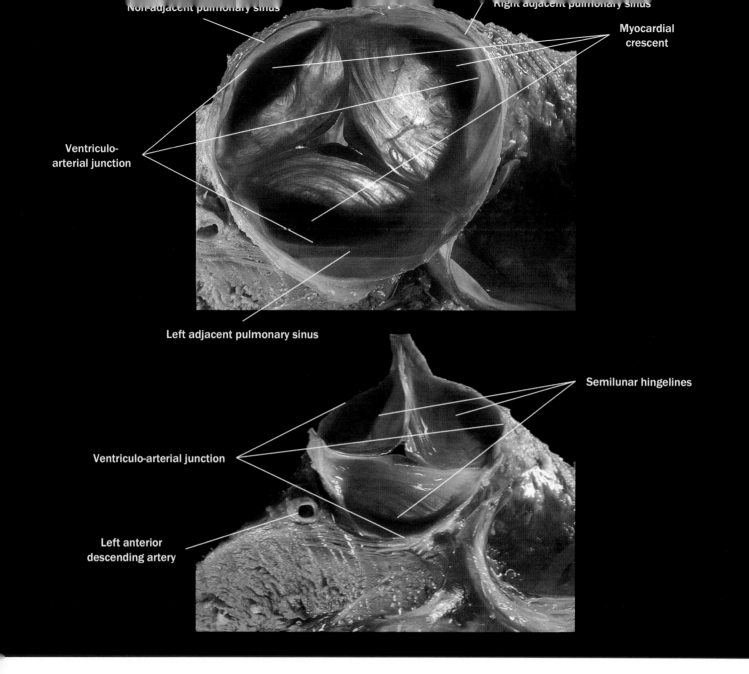

Non-adjacent pulmonary sinus

Right adjacent pulmonary sinus

Myocardial crescent

Ventriculo-arterial junction

Left adjacent pulmonary sinus

Semilunar hingelines

Ventriculo-arterial junction

Left anterior descending artery

is consistently located distal to the virtual basal ring. These myocardial crescents can be the substrate of the ventricular arrhythmia ablated from the pulmonary sinuses. The U-turn approach is an alternative option to map and ablate these myocardial crescents.[13] The fibrous wall of the pulmonary sinuses of Valsalva is removed, while the semilunar attachments of the pulmonary leaflet and myocardial crescents remain, as shown in the lower image on the right page. The proximal left anterior descending artery skirting the pulmonary root is observed adjacent to the interleaflet triangle between the left and non-adjacent pulmonary sinuses.

References

1. McAlpine WA. Digitized collection of all the images created by Dr. McAlpine at UCLA. Copyright UCLA Cardiac Arrhythmia Center. Part of this collection appeared in *Heart and Coronary Arteries: An Anatomical Atlas for Clinical Diagnosis, Radiological Investigation, and Surgical Treatment.* New York: Springer-Verlag; 1975.

2. Anderson RH, Razavi R, Taylor AM. Cardiac anatomy revisited. *J Anat.* 2004;205:159–177.

3. Mori S, Tretter JT, Spicer DE, et al. What is the real cardiac anatomy? *Clin Anat.* 2019;32:288–309.

4. Lin CJ, Lin CY, Chen CH, et al. Partitioning the heart: Mechanisms of cardiac septation and valve development. *Development.* 2012;139:3277–3299.

5. Cosío FG, Anderson RH, Kuck KH, et al. Living anatomy of the atrioventricular junctions. A guide to electrophysiologic mapping. A Consensus Statement from the Cardiac Nomenclature Study Group, Working Group of Arrhythmias, European Society of Cardiology, and the Task Force on Cardiac Nomenclature from NASPE. *Circulation.* 1999;100:e31–e37.

6. Mori S, Fukuzawa K, Takaya T, et al. Clinical cardiac structural anatomy reconstructed within the cardiac contour using multi-detector-row computed tomography: The arrangement and location of the cardiac valves. *Clin Anat.* 2016;29:364–370.

7. Anderson RH, Mohun TJ, Sánchez-Quintana D, et al. The anatomic substrates for outflow tract arrhythmias. *Heart Rhythm.* 2019;16:290–297.

8. Anderson RH, Mori S, Spicer DE, et al. Living anatomy of the pulmonary root. *J Cardiovasc Electrophysiol.* 2018;29:1238–1240.

9. Mori S, Fukuzawa K, Takaya T, et al. Clinical cardiac structural anatomy reconstructed within the cardiac contour using multi-detector-row computed tomography: Left ventricular outflow tract. *Clin Anat.* 2016;29:353–363.

10. Toh H, Mori S, Tretter JT, et al. Living anatomy of the ventricular myocardial crescents supporting the coronary aortic sinuses. *Semin Thorac Cardiovasc Surg.* 2020;32:230–241.

11. Dong X, Tang M, Sun Q, et al. Anatomical relevance of ablation to the pulmonary artery root: Clinical implications for characterizing the pulmonary sinus of Valsalva and coronary artery. *J Cardiovasc Electrophysiol.* 2018;29:1230–1237.

12. Halkin A, Cohen C, Rosso R, et al. Left atrial appendage and pulmonary artery anatomic relationship by cardiac-gated computed tomography: Implications for late pulmonary artery perforation by left atrial appendage closure devices. *Heart Rhythm.* 2016;13:2064–2069.

13. Zhang J, Tang C, Zhang Y, et al. Pulmonary sinus cusp mapping and ablation: A new concept and approach for idiopathic right ventricular outflow tract arrhythmias. *Heart Rhythm.* 2018;15:38–45.

14

Pulmonary Veins

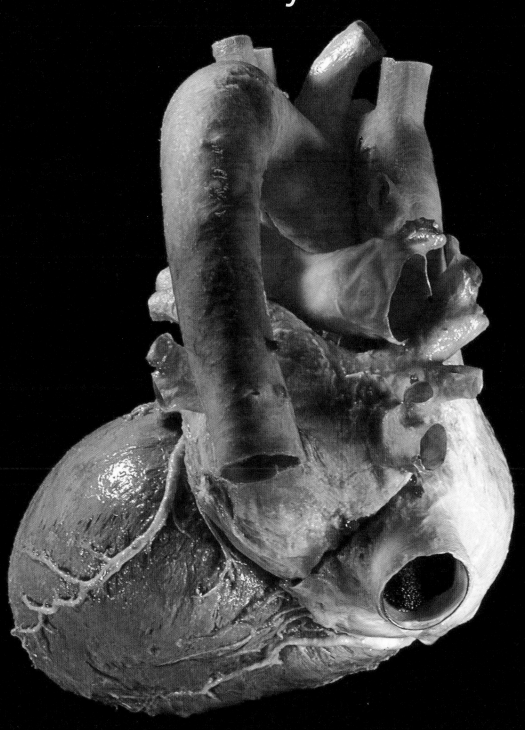

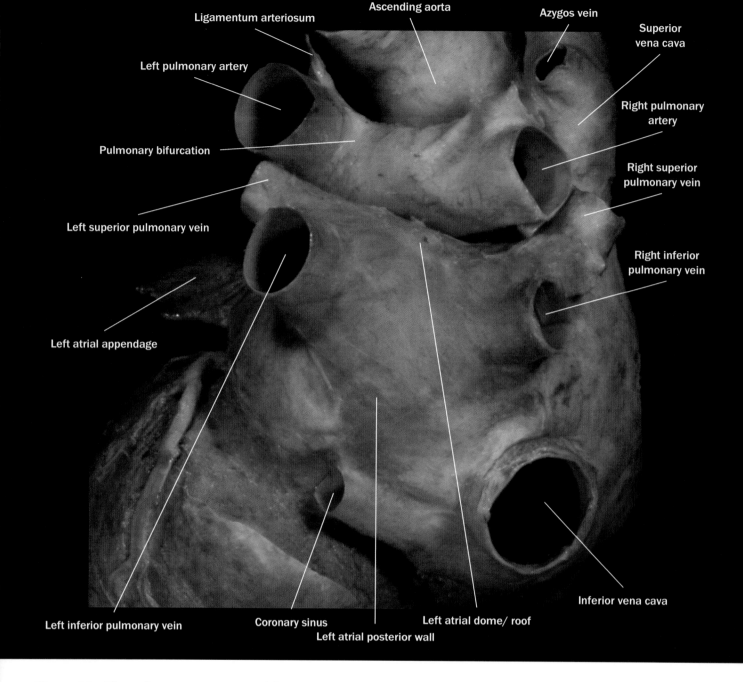

Ligamentum arteriosum

Ascending aorta

Azygos vein

Superior vena cava

Left pulmonary artery

Right pulmonary artery

Pulmonary bifurcation

Right superior pulmonary vein

Left superior pulmonary vein

Right inferior pulmonary vein

Left atrial appendage

Inferior vena cava

Left inferior pulmonary vein

Coronary sinus

Left atrial dome/ roof

Left atrial posterior wall

Figure 92   The pulmonary veins viewed from the posterior direction.[1]

The pulmonary venous component lies superior relative to the posterior wall of the left atrium, creating the dome or roof of the left atrium.[2] The left atrial dome/roof, posterior wall, and inferior pulmonary veins in the left image are removed in the right image. The pulmonary bifurcation lies on the left atrial dome/roof above the orifice of the left superior pulmonary vein. The pulmonary venous component tilts anterior. Thus, compared to the orifices of the superior pulmonary veins, the orifices of the inferior pulmonary veins are located posterior, which is commonly prominent feature in the right pulmonary veins. Therefore, the inferior half of the pulmonary venous component and the posterior wall of the left atrium are commonly closer to the structures at the posterior mediastinum, including the esophagus, descending aorta, and the vertebral column.[3] The anterior antrum of the right pulmonary veins is adjacent to the posterior interatrial groove, also referred to as the Waterston's groove or Sondergaard's groove.[4] On the other hand, the anterior antrum of the left pulmonary veins is

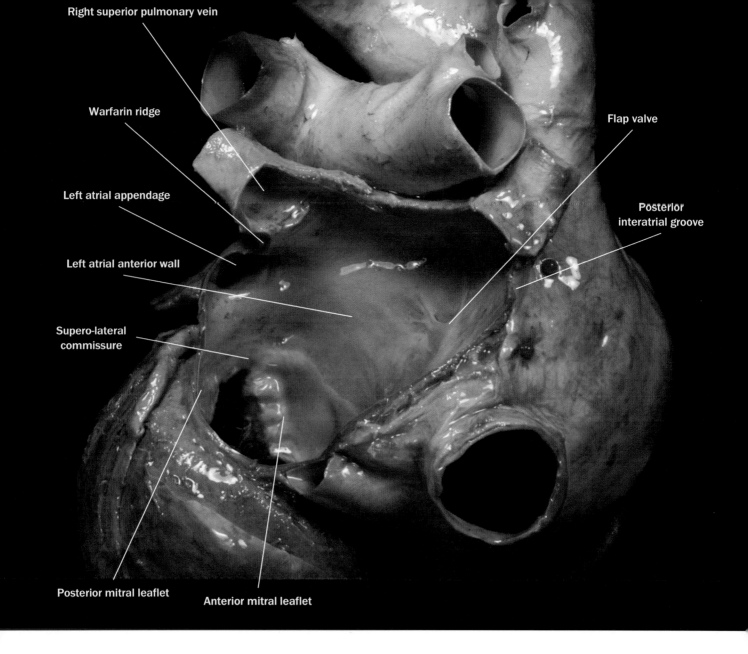

Right superior pulmonary vein

Warfarin ridge

Left atrial appendage

Left atrial anterior wall

Supero-lateral commissure

Posterior mitral leaflet

Anterior mitral leaflet

Flap valve

Posterior interatrial groove

adjacent to the fold created between the left atrial appendage and the left pulmonary veins, corresponding to the left atrial ridge or warfarin (Coumadin) ridge.[5] The mitral orifice, when compared to the plane involving four pulmonary veins, is located left antero-inferior. The orifice tilts left antero-inferior to face the cardiac apex. Because of this tilting, the distance between the pulmonary veins and the mitral annulus is significantly shorter at the left (lateral) side than the right (septal) side. Furthermore, the orifice of the left atrial appendage is located closer the orifice of the left superior pulmonary vein than the orifice of the left inferior pulmonary vein. Reflecting these anatomical relationships, the mitral isthmus, or the left atrial isthmus, is the narrowest between the left inferior pulmonary vein and the lateral mitral annulus.[6] The azygos vein is located superior to the right pulmonary artery. Refer to Figure 89.

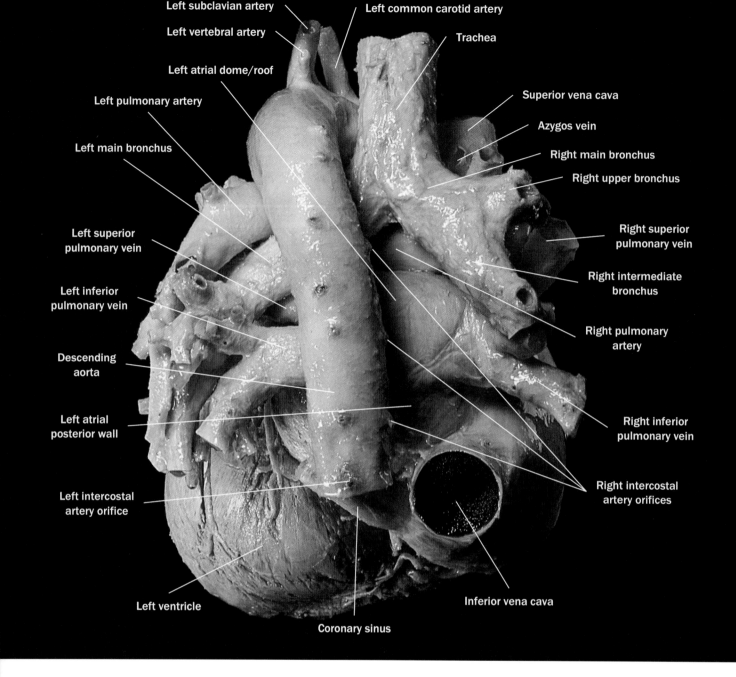

Left subclavian artery
Left common carotid artery
Left vertebral artery
Trachea
Left atrial dome/roof
Superior vena cava
Left pulmonary artery
Azygos vein
Left main bronchus
Right main bronchus
Right upper bronchus
Left superior pulmonary vein
Right superior pulmonary vein
Right intermediate bronchus
Left inferior pulmonary vein
Descending aorta
Right pulmonary artery
Left atrial posterior wall
Right inferior pulmonary vein
Left intercostal artery orifice
Right intercostal artery orifices
Left ventricle
Inferior vena cava
Coronary sinus

Figure 93   Structural extracardiac anatomy around the pulmonary vein.[1]

The heart is viewed from the posterior direction (left). The direction of the orifice of the inferior vena cava is not vertical; rather, it has a postero-inferior direction. The aortic arch and the left pulmonary artery override the left main bronchus. Thus, the left main bronchus is described as the hyparterial long bronchus. In contrast, the right pulmonary artery does not override the right main bronchus; it is only the azygos vein that overrides the right main bronchus. Thus, the right main bronchus is referred to as the eparterial short bronchus.[7] Reflecting this difference, the initial part of the left pulmonary artery directs left postero-superior compared to the horizontal course of the right pulmonary artery directing toward the right. Due to this bilateral non-uniformity, the left superior pulmonary vein is located just anterior to the left

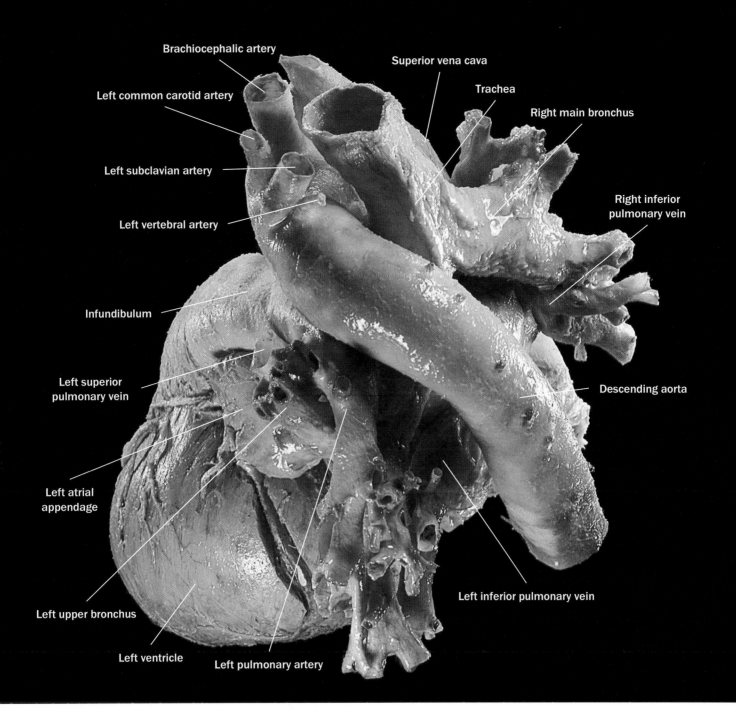

Brachiocephalic artery

Left common carotid artery

Left subclavian artery

Left vertebral artery

Superior vena cava

Trachea

Right main bronchus

Right inferior pulmonary vein

Infundibulum

Left superior pulmonary vein

Left atrial appendage

Descending aorta

Left upper bronchus

Left ventricle

Left pulmonary artery

Left inferior pulmonary vein

main bronchus. In contrast, the right pulmonary artery intervenes between the right superior pulmonary vein and the right intermediate bronchus. The tracheal carina is located superior relative to the pulmonary venous component of the left atrium. The proximity of the descending aorta to the left inferior pulmonary vein, posterior wall of the left atrium, coronary sinus, and basal infero-lateral left ventricle is noted.[8] The orifices of the right intercostal arteries at the descending aorta are also adjacent to the pulmonary venous component and posterior wall of the left atrium. The right image is the heart viewed from the left postero-superior direction.

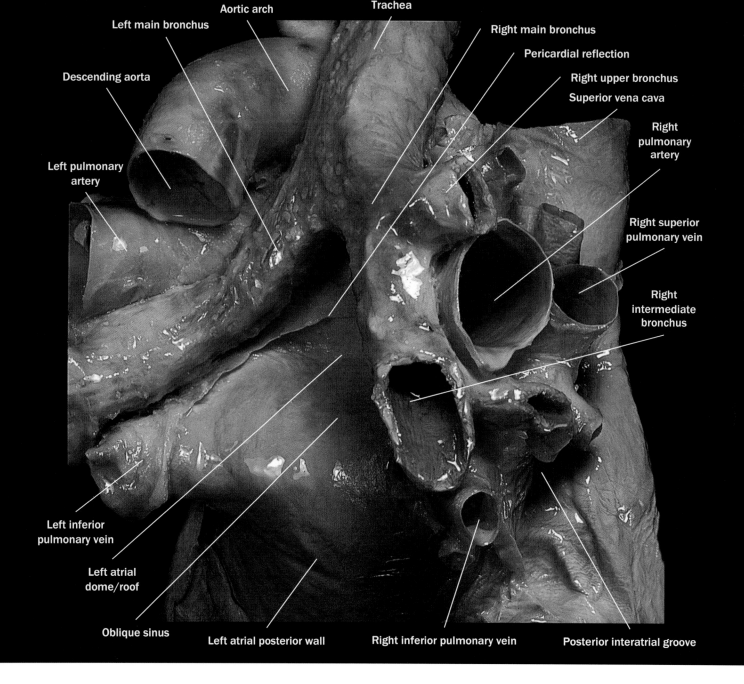

Figure 94 Structural anatomy around the pulmonary vein.[1]

Posterior to the superior vena cava, the right superior pulmonary vein is located followed by the right pulmonary artery and the right intermediate bronchus. The left main bronchus is located under the aortic arch and the left pulmonary artery, as they override the left main bronchus. The left main bronchus lies just posterior to the orifice of the left superior pulmonary vein. This structural anatomy explains why thermal bronchial injury is common at the left superior pulmonary venous

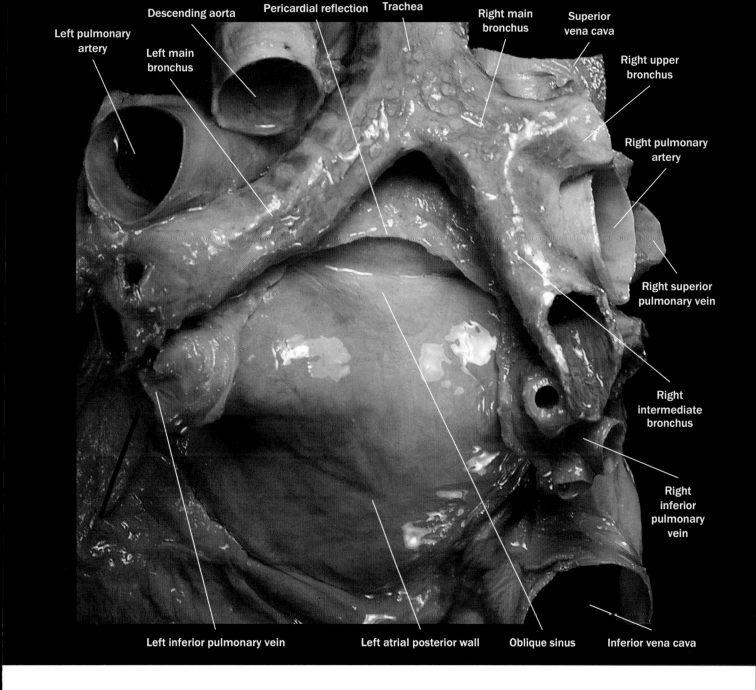

Left pulmonary artery

Descending aorta

Pericardial reflection

Trachea

Right main bronchus

Superior vena cava

Left main bronchus

Right upper bronchus

Right pulmonary artery

Right superior pulmonary vein

Right intermediate bronchus

Right inferior pulmonary vein

Left inferior pulmonary vein

Left atrial posterior wall

Oblique sinus

Inferior vena cava

isolation compared to the right superior pulmonary venous isolation.[9] The pericardial reflection at the apex of the oblique sinus is shown inferior to the tracheal carina and right pulmonary artery. Thus, the bilateral pulmonary arteries are extra-pericardial structures, above the oblique sinus.[10] The extracardiac space between the tracheal carina and pulmonary bifurcation is the location of the deep cardiac plexus of the autonomic nerves innervating to the heart. Refer to Figure 168.

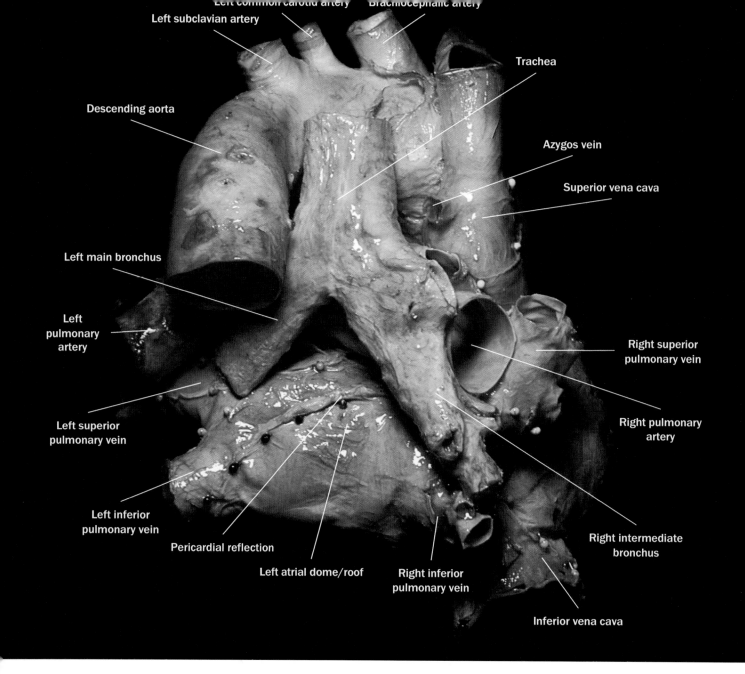

Left common carotid artery   Brachiocephalic artery

Left subclavian artery

Trachea

Descending aorta

Azygos vein

Superior vena cava

Left main bronchus

Left pulmonary artery

Right superior pulmonary vein

Left superior pulmonary vein

Right pulmonary artery

Left inferior pulmonary vein

Right intermediate bronchus

Pericardial reflection

Left atrial dome/roof

Right inferior pulmonary vein

Inferior vena cava

Figure 95   The pulmonary veins viewed from the postero-superior direction.[1]

The trachea and bronchi in the left image are removed in the right image. In the setting of normal arrangement, the left pulmonary artery overrides the left main bronchus whereas the right pulmonary artery does not override the right main bronchus.[11] Thus, the right pulmonary artery is located anterior to the right bronchus. The tracheal carina is commonly located superior to the left atrial roof. The pulmonary bifurcation and the right pulmonary artery lie on the left atrial roof.

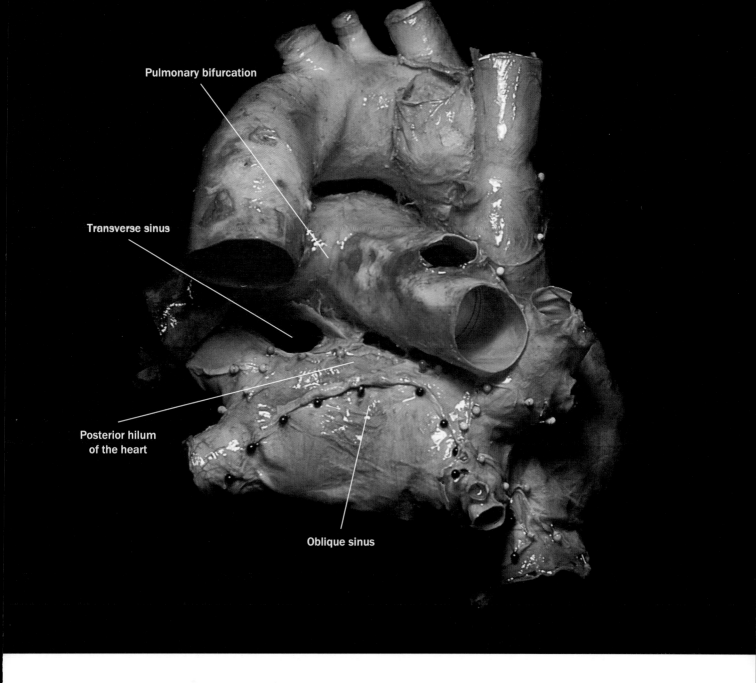

Pulmonary bifurcation

Transverse sinus

Posterior hilum
of the heart

Oblique sinus

Reflecting this anatomy, the left bronchus is located posterior to the orifice of the left superior pulmonary vein, whereas the right pulmonary artery is located posterior to the orifice of the right superior pulmonary vein. The esophagus descends posterior to the trachea. The pericardial reflection at the apex of the oblique sinus is observed at left atrial dome/roof, inferior to the tracheal carina and right pulmonary artery.

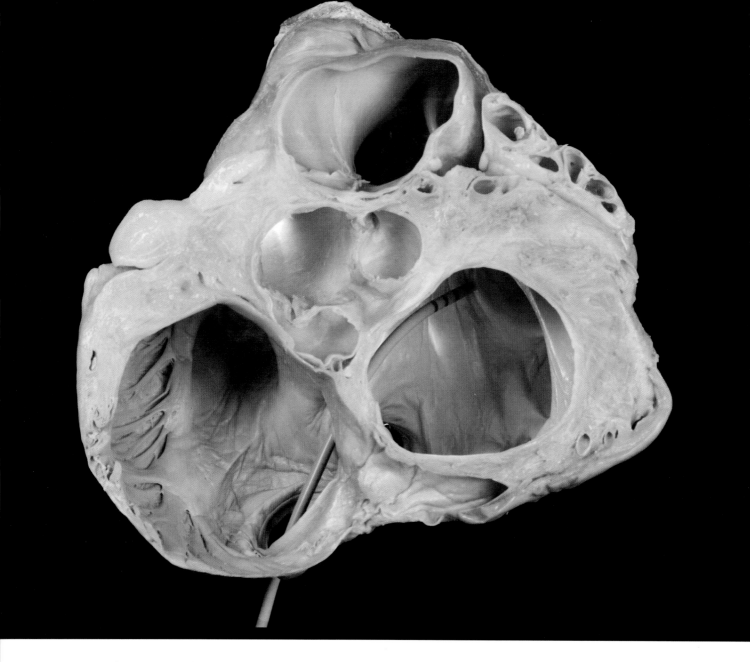

Figure 96 The transseptal approach and left pulmonary venous isolation.

The images are viewed from the left anterior oblique direction. The catheter is placed at the posterior antrum of the left superior pulmonary vein (left) and anterior antrum (right) posterior to the warfarin (Coumadin) ridge between the left pulmonary vein and left atrial appendage.

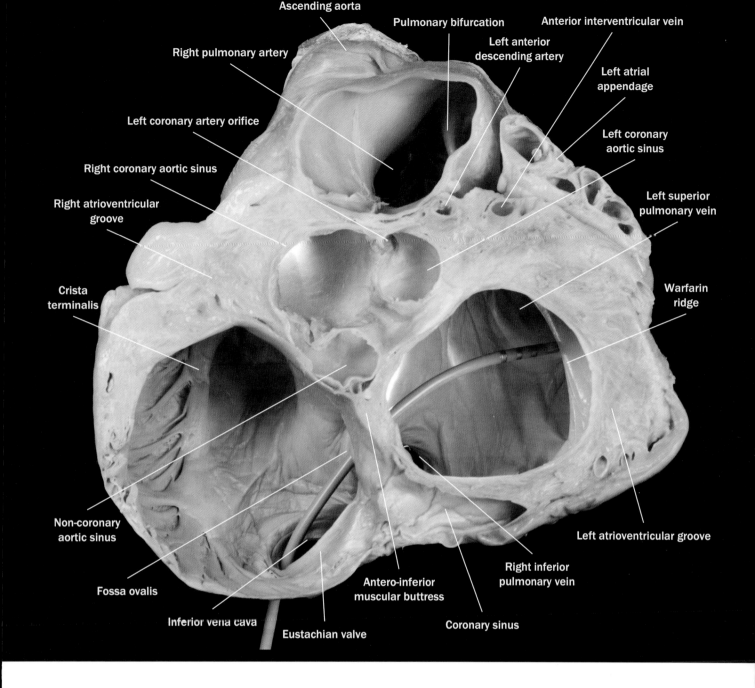

Ascending aorta

Pulmonary bifurcation

Anterior interventricular vein

Right pulmonary artery

Left anterior
descending artery

Left atrial
appendage

Left coronary artery orifice

Left coronary
aortic sinus

Right coronary aortic sinus

Right atrioventricular
groove

Left superior
pulmonary vein

Crista
terminalis

Warfarin
ridge

Non-coronary
aortic sinus

Left atrioventricular groove

Fossa ovalis

Right inferior
pulmonary vein

Antero-inferior
muscular buttress

Inferior vena cava

Coronary sinus

Eustachian valve

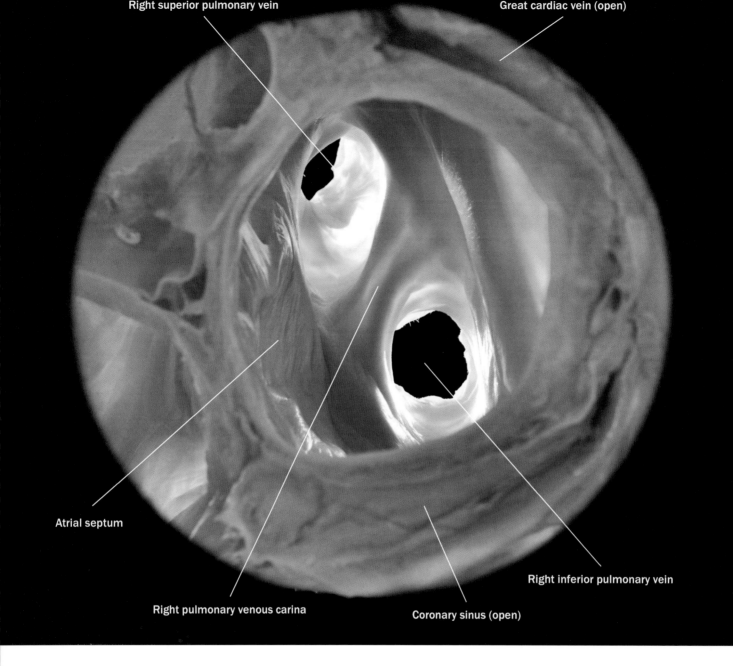

Right superior pulmonary vein

Great cardiac vein (open)

Atrial septum

Right pulmonary venous carina

Coronary sinus (open)

Right inferior pulmonary vein

Figure 97 The inner aspects of the orifices of the right and left pulmonary veins. 🕶 Anaglyph 16.

The images are viewed from the left anterior oblique direction (left) and right lateral direction (right). Between the left pulmonary veins and left atrial appendage, the fold creates the left atrial ridge, also referred to as the warfarin (Coumadin) ridge.[11] Within this fold, the vein/ligament of Marshall, patent left superior vena cava, and sinuatrial nodal artery originating from the left circumflex artery with posterior course[12] run through. Anterior antrum of the right pulmonary veins is in

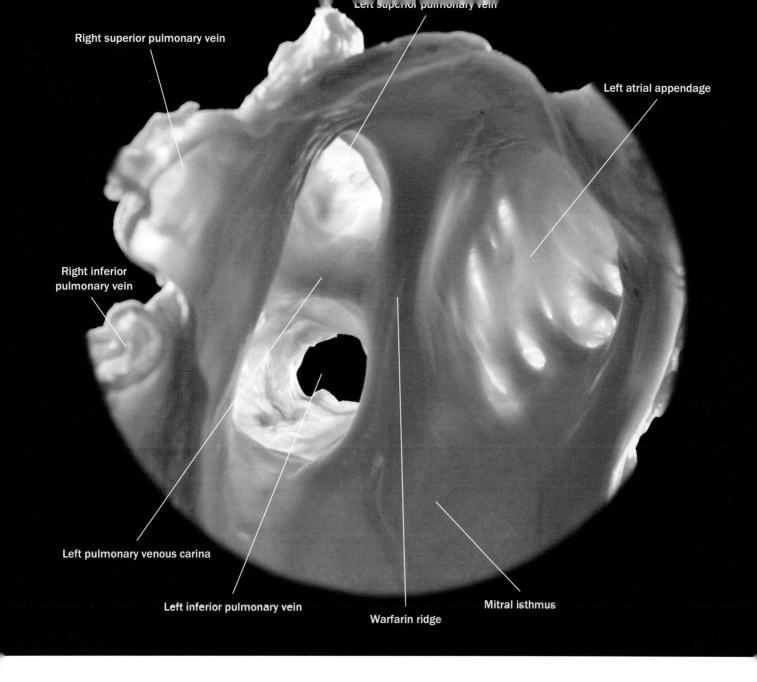

Right superior pulmonary vein

Left superior pulmonary vein

Left atrial appendage

Right inferior
pulmonary vein

Left pulmonary venous carina

Left inferior pulmonary vein

Warfarin ridge

Mitral isthmus

continuity with the posterior interatrial fold, corresponding to the Waterston's groove, or Sondergaard's groove.[8] Due to this close proximity, the epicardial interatrial muscle bundle bridging the posterior interatrial fold can connect the sinus venarum with the anterior antrum of the right pulmonary veins.[13] The orifice of the left atrial appendage is closer to the orifice of the left superior pulmonary vein than that of the left inferior pulmonary vein.

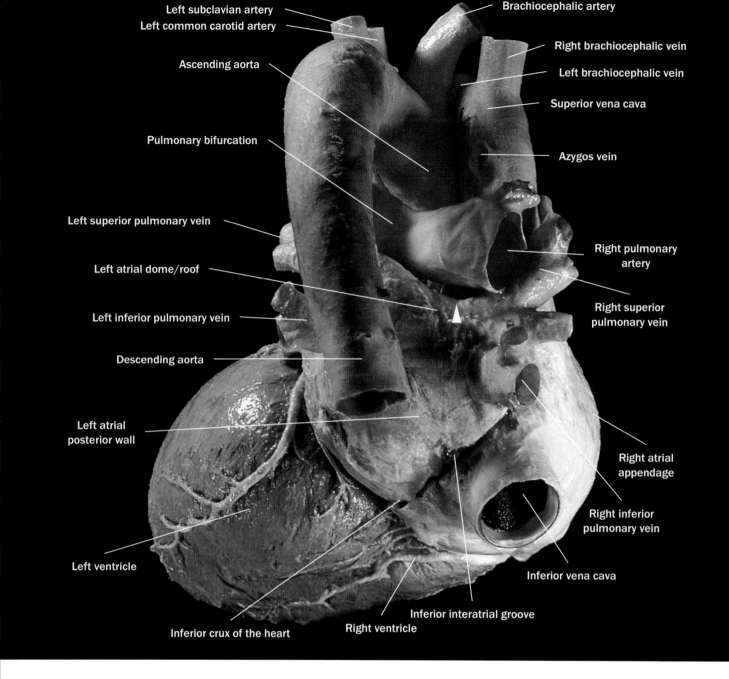

Left subclavian artery

Left common carotid artery

Ascending aorta

Pulmonary bifurcation

Left superior pulmonary vein

Left atrial dome/roof

Left inferior pulmonary vein

Descending aorta

Left atrial posterior wall

Left ventricle

Inferior crux of the heart

Right ventricle

Inferior interatrial groove

Inferior vena cava

Right inferior pulmonary vein

Right atrial appendage

Right superior pulmonary vein

Right pulmonary artery

Azygos vein

Superior vena cava

Left brachiocephalic vein

Right brachiocephalic vein

Brachiocephalic artery

Figure 98 The posterior view of the heart.[1]

The pulmonary venous component, the area surrounded by the four pulmonary veins, is located superior within the entire left atrium.[2] Therefore, this pulmonary venous component corresponds to the dome or the roof of the left atrium, relative to the true posterior wall of the left atrium extending inferior. The left atrial dome/roof is located inferior to the aortic arch and pulmonary arteries. The orifices of the inferior pulmonary veins are located infero-posterior relative to the orifices of the superior pulmonary veins. This is because the left atrial dome/roof tilt anterior. As the pulmonary trunk is located left to the ascending aorta, it is the right pulmonary artery that runs through the space beneath the aortic arch on the dome/roof of the left atrium. The V-shaped dimple (arrowhead) occasionally found at the left atrial roof between the bilateral superior pulmonary veins[14] corresponds to the location where the right pulmonary artery sits. The phrenic nerves descend anterior to the pulmonary hila.[15] Thus, in addition to the crista terminalis and postero-lateral sinus venarum, the anterior regions of the right pulmonary veins are close to the right phrenic nerve.[16] Ablation to the right pulmonary veins can induce transient or persistent right phrenic nerve injury.[17]

References

1. McAlpine WA. Digitized collection of all the images created by Dr. McAlpine at UCLA. Copyright UCLA Cardiac Arrhythmia Center. Part of this collection appeared in *Heart and Coronary Arteries: An Anatomical Atlas for Clinical Diagnosis, Radiological Investigation, and Surgical Treatment*. New York: Springer-Verlag; 1975.

2. Elbatran AI, Anderson RH, Mori S, et al. The rationale for isolation of the left atrial pulmonary venous component to control atrial fibrillation: A review article. *Heart Rhythm*. 2019;16:1392–1398.

3. Kottkamp H, Piorkowski C, Tanner H, et al. Topographic variability of the esophageal left atrial relation influencing ablation lines in patients with atrial fibrillation. *J Cardiovasc Electrophysiol*. 2005;16:146–150.

4. Ho SY, Anderson RH, Sánchez-Quintana D. Atrial structure and fibres: Morphologic bases of atrial conduction. *Cardiovasc Res*. 2002;54:325–336.

5. Silbiger JJ. The anatomy of the Coumadin ridge. *J Am Soc Echocardiogr*. 2019;32:912–913.

6. Becker AE. Left atrial isthmus: Anatomic aspects relevant for linear catheter ablation procedures in humans. *J Cardiovasc Electrophysiol*. 2004;15:809–812.

7. Mori S, Anderson RH, Nishii T, et al. Isomerism in the setting of the so-called "heterotaxy": The usefulness of computed tomographic analysis. *Ann Pediatr Cardiol*. 2017;10:175–186.

8. Konishi H, Mori S, Nishii T, et al. Extracardiac compression of the inferolateral branch of the coronary vein by the descending aorta in a patient with dilated cardiomyopathy. *J Arrhythm*. 2017;33:646–648.

9. Bellmann B, Hübner RH, Lin T, et al. Bronchial injury after atrial fibrillation ablation using the second-generation cryoballoon. *Circ Arrhythm Electrophysiol*. 2018;11:e005925.

10. Mori S, Hanna P, Dacey MJ, et al. Comprehensive anatomy of the pericardial space and the cardiac hilum: Anatomical dissections with intact pericardium. *JACC Cardiovasc Imaging*. 2021. DOI: 10.1016/j.jcmg.2021.04.016. Online ahead of print.

11. Piątek-Koziej K, Hołda J, Tyrak K, et al. Anatomy of the left atrial ridge (Coumadin ridge) and possible clinical implications for cardiovascular imaging and invasive procedures. *J Cardiovasc Electrophysiol*. 2020;31:220–226.

12. Zhang LJ, Wang YZ, Huang W, et al. Anatomical investigation of the sinus node artery using dual-source computed tomography. *Circ J*. 2008;72:1615–1620.

13. Ho SY, Cabrera JA, Sánchez-Quintana D. Left atrial anatomy revisited. *Circ Arrhythm Electrophysiol*. 2012;5:220–228.

14. Matsumoto A, Fukuzawa K, Kiuchi K, et al. Characteristics of residual atrial posterior wall and roof-dependent atrial tachycardias after pulmonary vein isolation. *Pacing Clin Electrophysiol*. 2016;39:1090–1098.

15. Sánchez-Quintana D, Cabrera JA, Climent V, Farré J, Weiglein A, Ho SY. How close are the phrenic nerves to cardiac structures? Implications for cardiac interventionalists. *J Cardiovasc Electrophysiol*. 2005;16:309–313.

16. Roka A, Heist EK, Refaat M, et al. Novel technique to prevent phrenic nerve injury during pulmonary vein isolation using preprocedural imaging. *J Cardiovasc Electrophysiol*. 2015;26:1057–1062.

17. Tokuda M, Yamashita S, Sato H, et al. Long-term course of phrenic nerve injury after cryoballoon ablation of atrial fibrillation. *Sci Rep*. 2021;11:6226.

15

Left Atrium

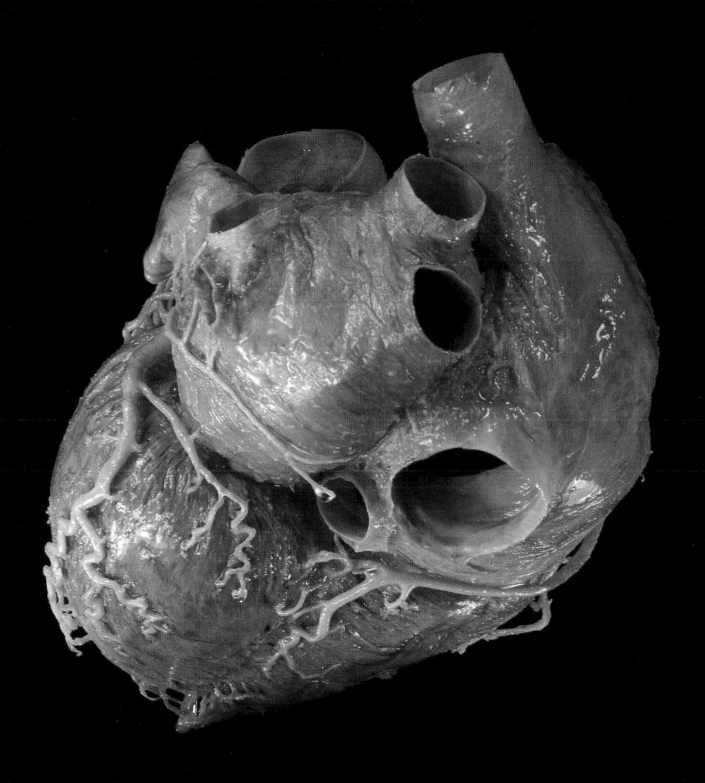

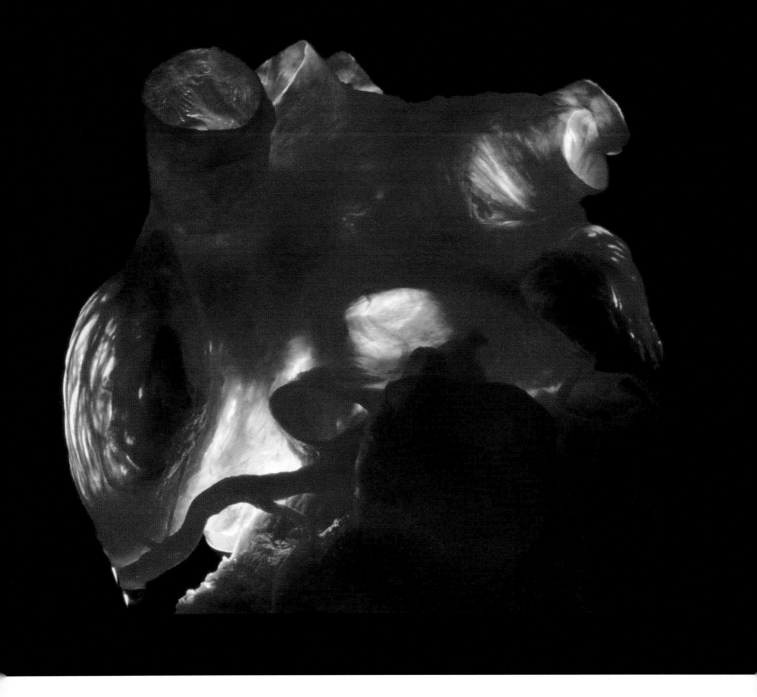

Figure 99   The transilluminated left and right atria viewed from the antero-superior direction.[1]

The Bachmann's bundle, the thick subepicardial interatrial muscular connection, is facing toward the transverse sinus between the arterial trunks and anterior wall of the atria.[2] The distal part of the bundle divides to surround the base of both appendages. At the right atrium, superior part of the Bachmann's bundle is confluent with the precaval bundle of the crista terminalis. At the left atrium, superior part of the Bachmann's bundle is in continuity with the fold between the left pulmonary veins and the left atrial appendage, also referred to as the left atrial ridge or warfarin (Coumadin) ridge.[3]

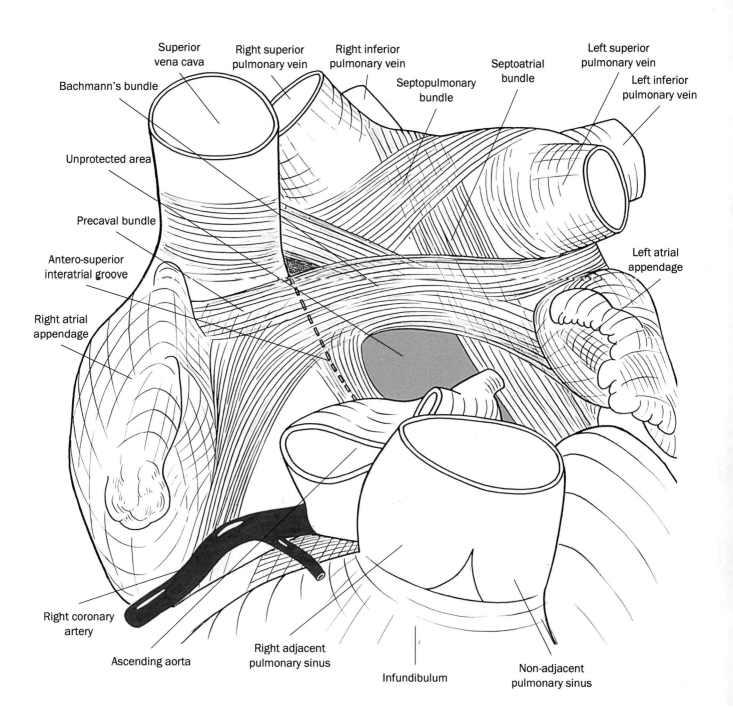

Superior
vena cava

Bachmann's bundle

Right superior
pulmonary vein

Right inferior
pulmonary vein

Septopulmonary
bundle

Septoatrial
bundle

Left superior
pulmonary vein

Left inferior
pulmonary vein

Unprotected area

Precaval bundle

Antero-superior
interatrial groove

Right atrial
appendage

Left atrial
appendage

Right coronary
artery

Ascending aorta

Right adjacent
pulmonary sinus

Infundibulum

Non-adjacent
pulmonary sinus

Inferior to the Bachmann's bundle, the anterior wall of the left atrium and right atrium divided by the antero-superior interatrial groove is so thin that the regions are transilluminated posterior to the aortic root. McAlpine referred to this thin region in the left atrium as the unprotected area.[1] Both regions correspond to the right and left aortic mound observed in the antero-medial part of the right and left atrium, as the aortic imprint into the atrium.[4] The subepicardial septopulmonary bundle and subendocardial septoatrial bundle is observed.[5]

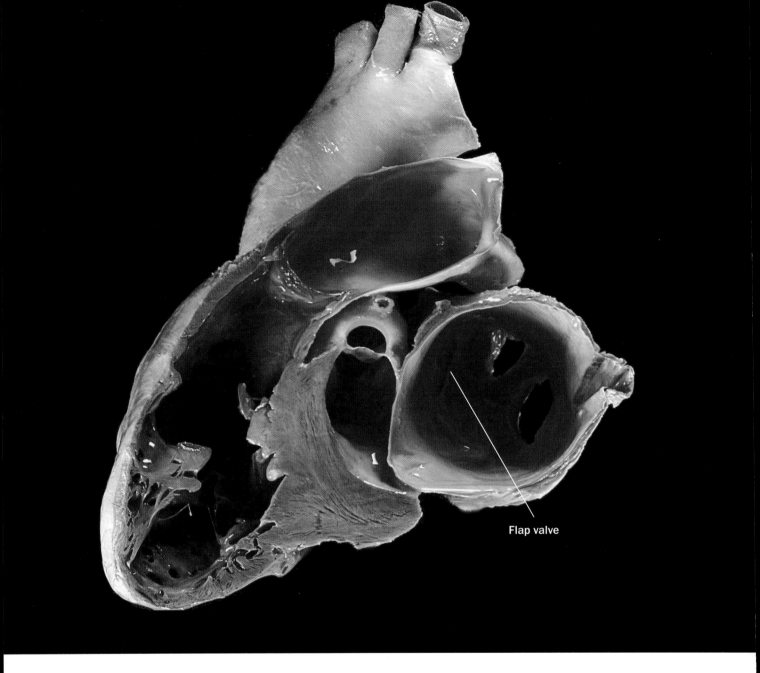

Flap valve

Figure 100   The sagittal section of the heart viewed from the left lateral direction.[1]

The pulmonary bifurcation and the right pulmonary artery lie on the roof of the left atrium, after the pulmonary trunk overriding the left coronary aortic sinus and the left main trunk of the left coronary artery. This part of the left atrial roof, although variable, corresponds to the posterior hilum of the heart without pericardium between the transverse sinus and the oblique sinus.[6] Refer to Figure 156. The fossa ovalis itself cannot be seen from the left side, but the flap valve can be observed at the left side atrial septum.[7] The patent foramen ovale is commonly located at the antero-superior margin of the fossa ovalis,[7] and the probe passing through the patent foramen ovale from the right atrium to the left atrium directs to the aortic

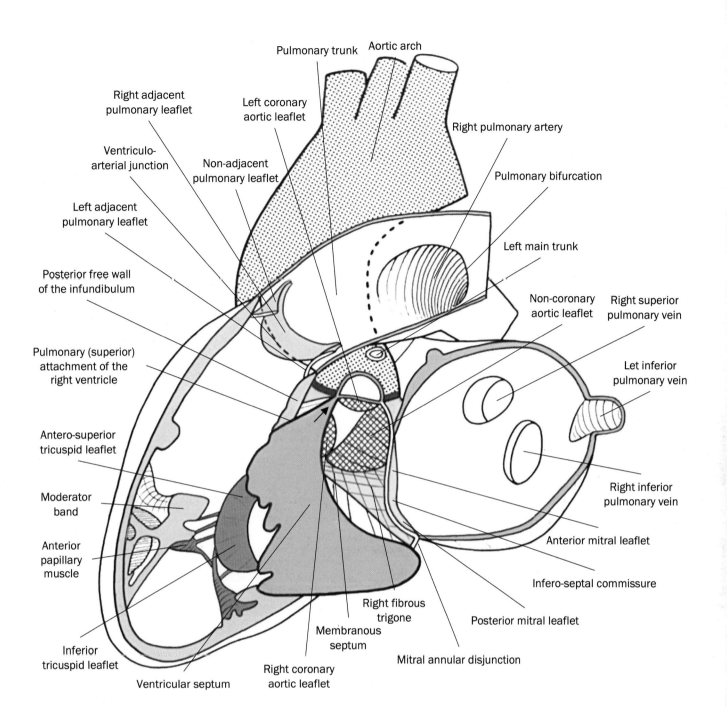

Pulmonary trunk

Aortic arch

Right adjacent
pulmonary leaflet

Left coronary
aortic leaflet

Ventriculo-
arterial junction

Non-adjacent
pulmonary leaflet

Right pulmonary artery

Left adjacent
pulmonary leaflet

Pulmonary bifurcation

Posterior free wall
of the infundibulum

Left main trunk

Non-coronary
aortic leaflet

Right superior
pulmonary vein

Pulmonary (superior)
attachment of the
right ventricle

Let inferior
pulmonary vein

Antero-superior
tricuspid leaflet

Moderator
band

Right inferior
pulmonary vein

Anterior
papillary
muscle

Anterior mitral leaflet

Infero-septal commissure

Right fibrous
trigone

Posterior mitral leaflet

Inferior
tricuspid leaflet

Membranous
septum

Mitral annular disjunction

Ventricular septum

Right coronary
aortic leaflet

root via the opening of this flap valve. The orifices of the right pulmonary veins and left inferior pulmonary vein are visualized in this section. On this plane, the left inferior pulmonary vein is located most posterior. The mitral annular disjunction
can be also appreciated at the attachment of the medial scallop of the posterior mitral leaflet.[8] The posterior free wall of the
right ventricular outflow tract is observed in this section, anterior to the left coronary aortic sinus, apart from the left ventricular free wall. Note the beak-shaped thin left ventricular free wall myocardium supporting the left coronary aortic sinus
(black arrow).[9] The paired section of this image is Figure 87.

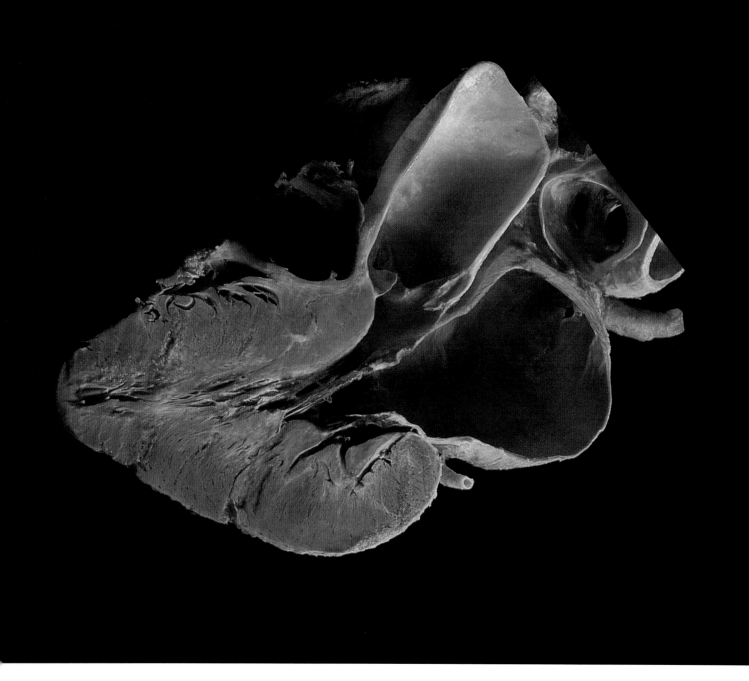

Figure 101   The section corresponding to the parasternal left ventricular long-axis view.[1]

The heart is viewed from the left postero-superior direction, showing the section corresponding to the parasternal left ventricular long-axis image. The uneven thickness of the left atrial wall is noted. The Bachmann's bundle is observed at the thickening of the superior part of the left atrial anterior wall. The Bachmann's bundle faces to the ascending aorta. Inferior to the Bachmann's bundle, the left atrial anterior wall is thin, as is the postero-inferior wall of the left atrium. This

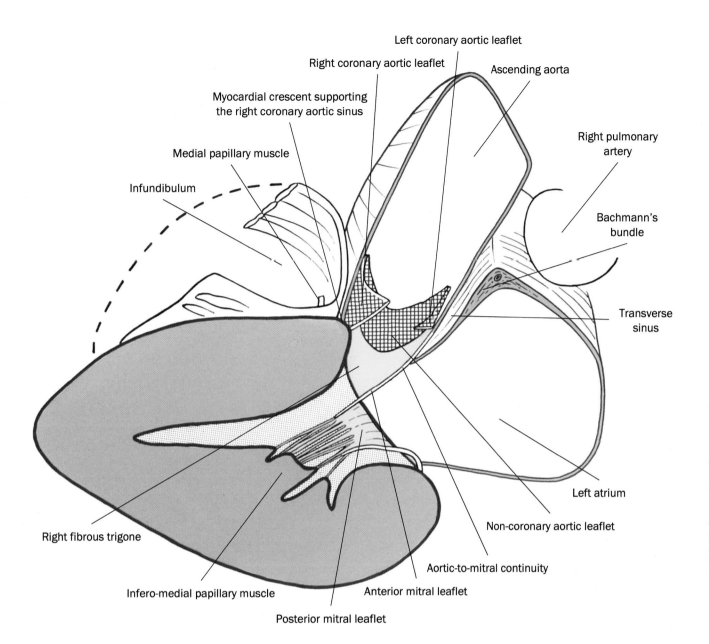

Left coronary aortic leaflet

Right coronary aortic leaflet

Ascending aorta

Myocardial crescent supporting
the right coronary aortic sinus

Right pulmonary
artery

Medial papillary muscle

Bachmann's
bundle

Infundibulum

Transverse
sinus

Left atrium

Non-coronary aortic leaflet

Right fibrous trigone

Aortic-to-mitral continuity

Infero-medial papillary muscle

Anterior mitral leaflet

Posterior mitral leaflet

thin anterior wall is facing to the non-coronary and left coronary aortic sinuses, intervened by the transverse sinus. In contrast to the separated relationship of the pulmonary valve and tricuspid valve, the aortic valve and mitral valve are in fibrous continuity through the aortic-to-mitral (aortomitral) continuity. The infero-medial papillary muscle anchors the medial part of the mitral leaflets. The paired section of this image is Figure 102.

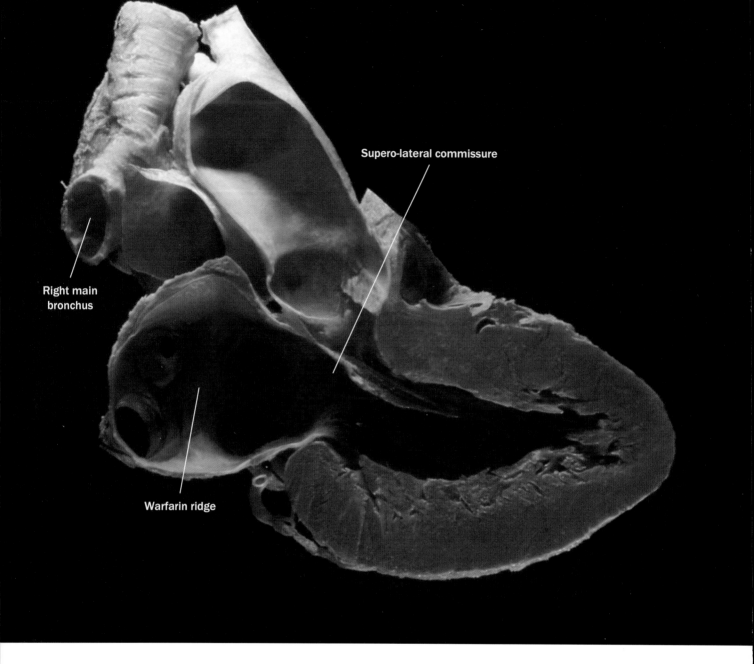

Figure 102   The paired section of the parasternal left ventricular long-axis view.[1]

The heart is viewed from the right antero-inferior direction. The thick muscle bundle at the superior part of the left atrial anterior wall is the Bachmann's bundle. The Bachmann's bundle traverses the both atria between the precaval bundle of the crista terminalis and the left atrial ridge. The left atrial ridge is also referred to as the warfarin (Coumadin) ridge between the left pulmonary veins and left atrial appendage.[3] The right pulmonary artery lies on the left atrial roof, located

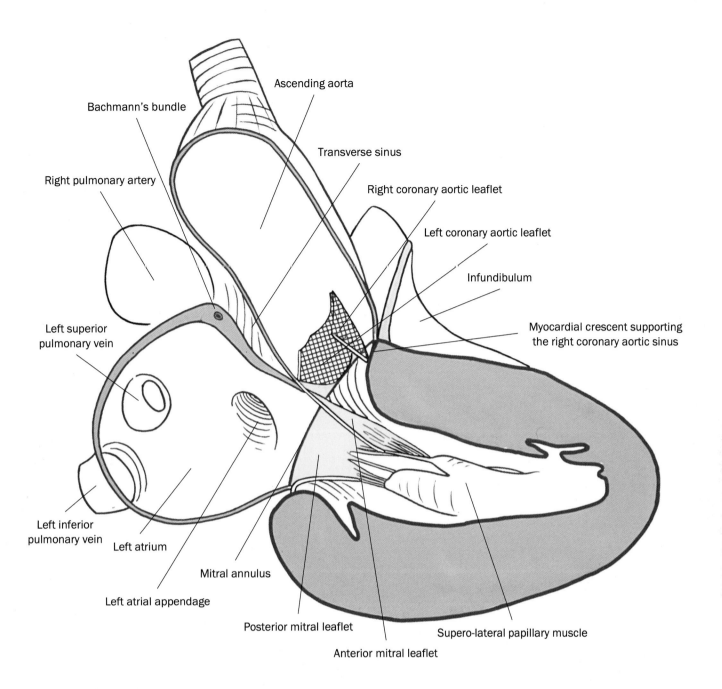

Bachmann's bundle

Ascending aorta

Transverse sinus

Right coronary aortic leaflet

Right pulmonary artery

Left coronary aortic leaflet

Infundibulum

Myocardial crescent supporting
the right coronary aortic sinus

Left superior
pulmonary vein

Left inferior
pulmonary vein

Left atrium

Left atrial appendage

Mitral annulus

Posterior mitral leaflet

Supero-lateral papillary muscle

Anterior mitral leaflet

anterior to the right main bronchus. The orifice of the left atrial appendage is located between the mitral annulus and left pulmonary veins, posterior to the supero-lateral commissure. The orifice of the left atrial appendage is closer to the orifice of the left superior pulmonary vein than that of the left inferior pulmonary vein. The supero-lateral papillary muscle anchors supero-lateral commissure and the lateral part of the mitral leaflets. The paired section of this image is Figure 101.

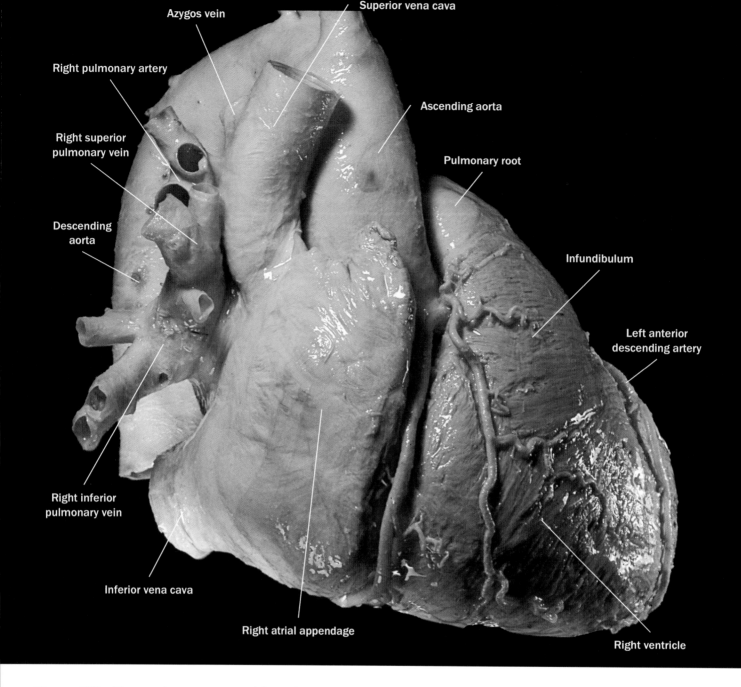

Azygos vein

Superior vena cava

Right pulmonary artery

Ascending aorta

Right superior
pulmonary vein

Pulmonary root

Descending
aorta

Infundibulum

Left anterior
descending artery

Right inferior
pulmonary vein

Inferior vena cava

Right atrial appendage

Right ventricle

Figure 103   The atrial septum viewed from the right anterior oblique direction.[1]

The right atrial components in the left image are removed in the right image. Red and blue beads mark the area where the right atrium faces the left atrium. Within this area, only the primary septum at the floor of the fossa ovalis and antero-inferior muscular buttress at the anterior limbus of the fossa ovalis is the true atrial septum. The antero-inferior muscular buttress is the muscular component of the atrial septum found between the fossa ovalis and central fibrous body. Anterior, superior, posterior, and inferior regions relative to the fossa ovalis are the interatrial grooves.[4] The aortic root is transilluminated in the right image. The non-coronary aortic sinus is wedged into the antero-superior interatrial groove between

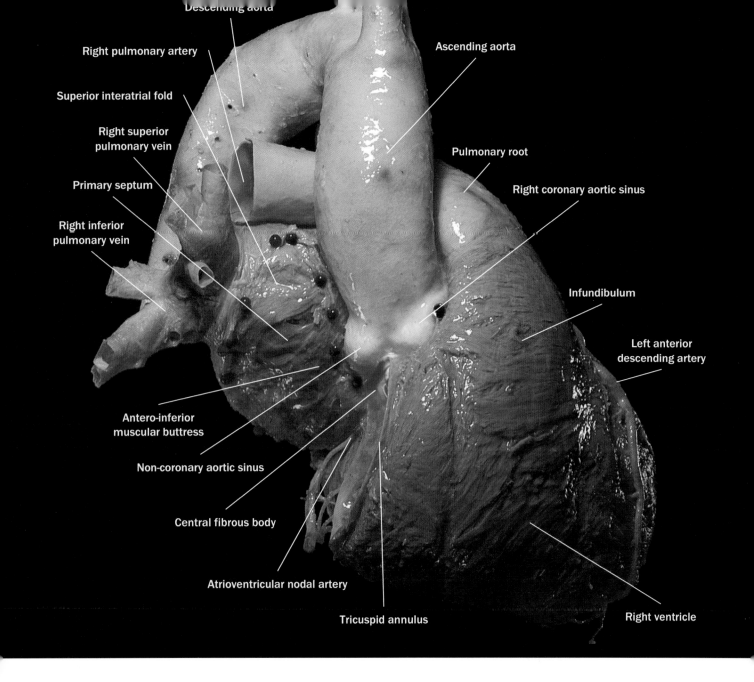

Descending aorta

Right pulmonary artery

Superior interatrial fold

Right superior
pulmonary vein

Primary septum

Right inferior
pulmonary vein

Antero-inferior
muscular buttress

Non-coronary aortic sinus

Central fibrous body

Atrioventricular nodal artery

Tricuspid annulus

Ascending aorta

Pulmonary root

Right coronary aortic sinus

Infundibulum

Left anterior
descending artery

Right ventricle

the right and left atria. As the aortic root is deeply wedged into the ventricular base, the left atrial roof is located way superior than the sinutubular junction.[10] The floor of the left atrium is located superior to the floor of the right atrium. The right superior pulmonary vein is located posterior to the superior vena cava close to its junction to the right atrium. The right pulmonary artery lies on the left atrial roof under the aortic arch and directs posterior to the right superior pulmonary vein.

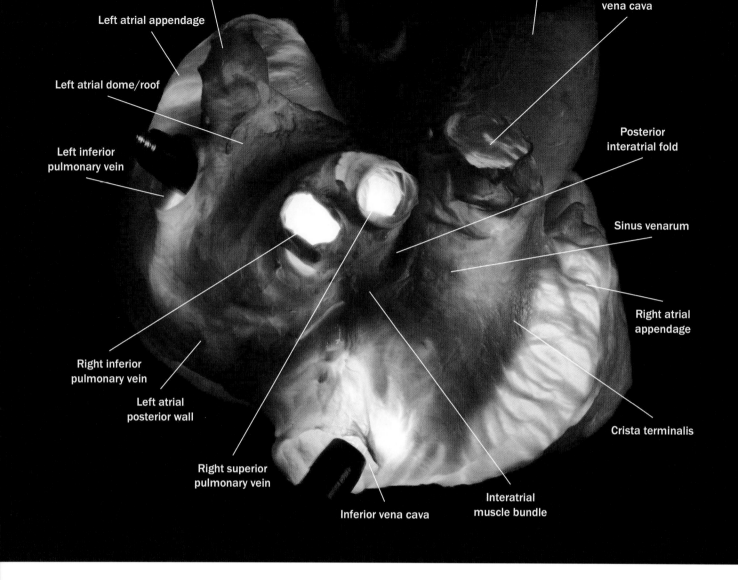

Figure 104 The transilluminated right and left atrium.

The hearts are viewed from right posterior (left) and left superior (right) directions. Compared to the extent of the pectinate muscles of the right atrial appendage surrounding the tricuspid annulus, except its medial side, the extent of the pectinate muscles of the left atrial appendage is confined at the supero-lateral region of the left atrial vestibule, left anterior to the left superior pulmonary vein (left). The epicardial interatrial muscle bundle bridges the posterior interatrial fold, between

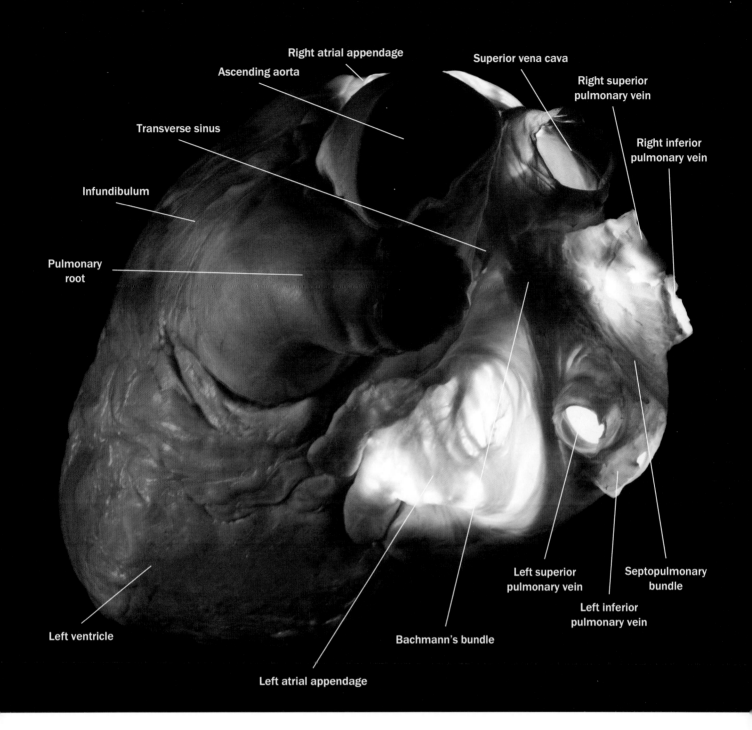

Right atrial appendage

Ascending aorta

Superior vena cava

Right superior
pulmonary vein

Transverse sinus

Right inferior
pulmonary vein

Infundibulum

Pulmonary
root

Left superior
pulmonary vein

Septopulmonary
bundle

Left inferior
pulmonary vein

Left ventricle

Bachmann's bundle

Left atrial appendage

the medial antrum of the right pulmonary veins and the sinus venarum. The subepicardial septopulmonary bundle descends the left atrial roof to the left atrial posterior wall between the pulmonary veins. In the right image, the left lateral end of the Bachmann's bundle continues to the fold between the left atrial appendage and left pulmonary veins.

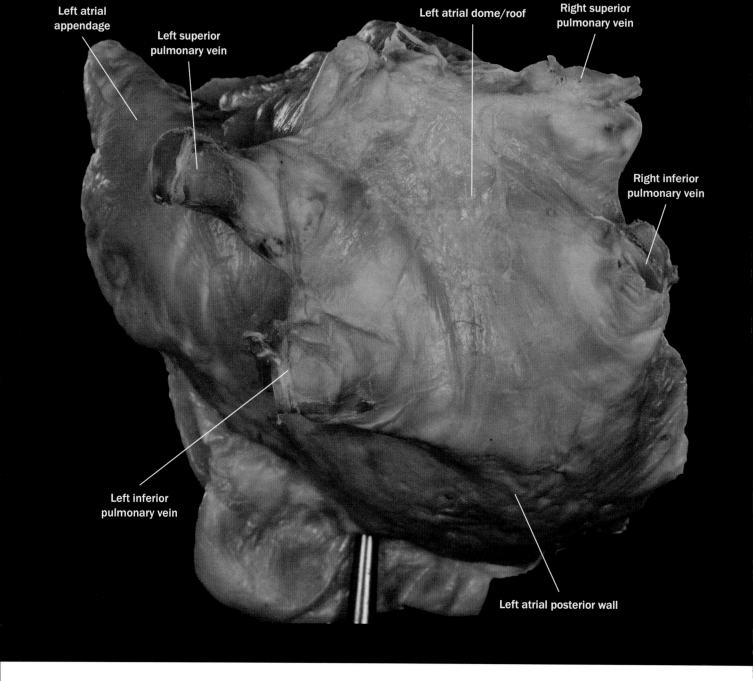

Left atrial
appendage

Left superior
pulmonary vein

Left atrial dome/roof

Right superior
pulmonary vein

Right inferior
pulmonary vein

Left inferior
pulmonary vein

Left atrial posterior wall

Figure 105 The septopulmonary bundle.

The pulmonary venous component of the left atrium is viewed from the postero-superior direction. Transillumination (right) reveals the subepicardial septopulmonary bundle descending between the bilateral pulmonary veins. The septopulmonary bundle is confluent with the subepicardial circumferential band surrounding the inferior part of the left atrial

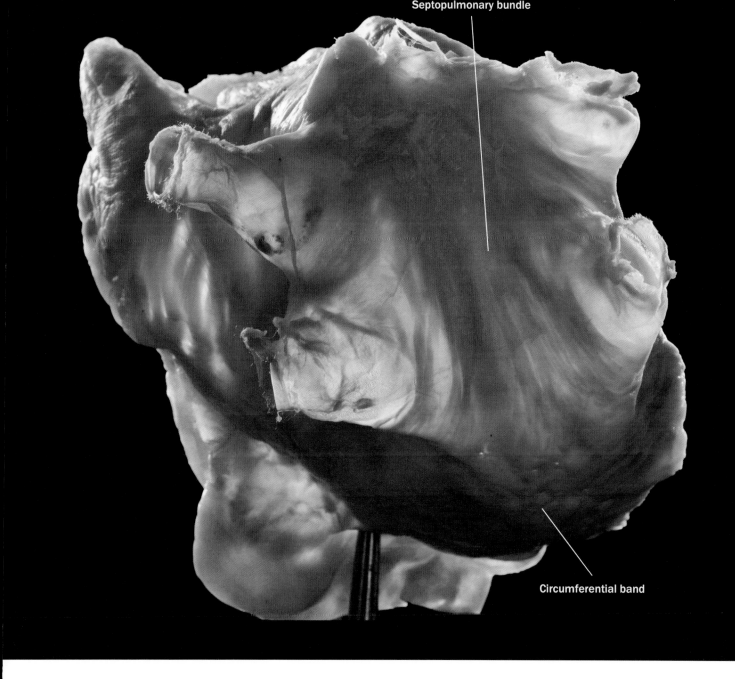

Septopulmonary bundle

Circumferential band

posterior wall.[2] Alignment of the myocardial fibers at the antrum of each pulmonary vein is non-uniform. The myocardial fibers are absent inside the pulmonary veins and the area superior to the orifice of the left inferior pulmonary vein.

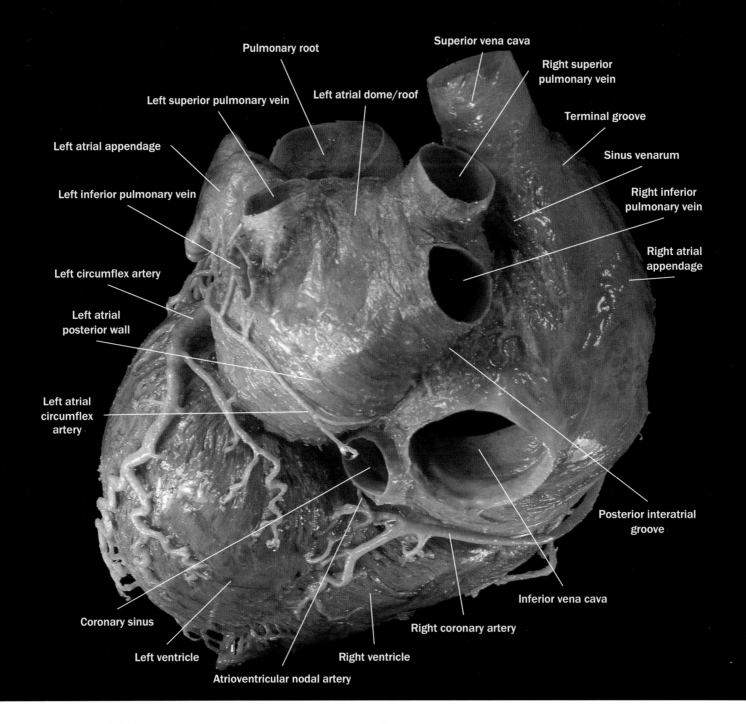

Figure 106 The left atrium viewed from the posterior direction.[1]

The heart is viewed from the posterior direction. The left atrial appendage is located left anterior to the left superior pulmonary vein, lateral to the pulmonary root. The inferior pulmonary veins are located infero-posterior to the superior pulmonary veins, reflecting the anterior tilt of the pulmonary venous component at the left atrial dome/roof. The posterior interatrial fold is not aligned in vertical fashion but tilts toward the right direction. Thus, the orifice of the superior vena cava is lateral to the orifice of the inferior vena cava. The atrial branch of the circumflex artery runs on the left atrial posterior wall located inferior to the pulmonary venous component. Whereas the pulmonary venous component surrounded by the four pulmonary veins, corresponding to the left atrial dome/roof, is nearly parallel to the frontal plane except its slight anterior tilt, the mitral orifice faces left antero-inferior direction as it is parallel to the atrioventricular plane. Thus, septal distance between the right pulmonary veins to the medial mitral orifice is longer than lateral distance between the left pulmonary veins to the lateral mitral orifice. The coronary sinus orifice is located at the inferior crux of the heart. Anterior to the coronary sinus orifice, the atrioventricular nodal artery ascends within the inferior pyramidal space toward the central fibrous body.[11]

References

1. McAlpine WA. Digitized collection of all the images created by Dr. McAlpine at UCLA. Copyright UCLA Cardiac Arrhythmia Center. Part of this collection appeared in *Heart and Coronary Arteries: An Anatomical Atlas for Clinical Diagnosis, Radiological Investigation, and Surgical Treatment.* New York: Springer-Verlag; 1975.

2. Ho SY, Sánchez-Quintana D. The importance of atrial structure and fibers. *Clin Anat.* 2009;22:52–63.

3. Silbiger JJ. The anatomy of the Coumadin ridge. *J Am Soc Echocardiogr.* 2019;32:912–913.

4. Mori S, Nishii T, Tretter JT, et al. Demonstration of living anatomy clarifies the morphology of interatrial communications. *Heart.* 2018;104:2003–2009.

5. Ho SY, Anderson RH, Sánchez-Quintana D. Atrial structure and fibres: Morphologic bases of atrial conduction. *Cardiovasc Res.* 2002;54:325–336.

6. Mori S, Hanna P, Dacey MJ, et al. Comprehensive anatomy of the pericardial space and the cardiac hilum: Anatomical dissections with Intact pericardium. *JACC Cardiovasc Imaging.* 2021. DOI: 10.1016/j.jcmg.2021.04.016. Online ahead of print.

7. Ho SY, Cabrera JA, Sánchez-Quintana D. Left atrial anatomy revisited. *Circ Arrhythm Electrophysiol.* 2012;5:220–228.

8. Toh H, Mori S, Izawa Y, et al. Prevalence and extent of mitral annular disjunction in structurally normal hearts: Comprehensive 3D analysis using cardiac computed tomography. *Eur Heart J Cardiovasc Imaging.* 2021;22:614–622.

9. Toh H, Mori S, Tretter JT, et al. Living anatomy of the ventricular myocardial crescents supporting the coronary aortic sinuses. *Semin Thorac Cardiovasc Surg.* 2020;32:230–241.

10. Mori S, Anderson RH, Takaya T, et al. The association between wedging of the aorta and cardiac structural anatomy as revealed using multidetector-row computed tomography. *J Anat.* 2017;231:110–120.

11. Mori S, Nishii T, Takaya T, et al. Clinical structural anatomy of the inferior pyramidal space reconstructed from the living heart: Three-dimensional visualization using multidetector-row computed tomography. *Clin Anat.* 2015;28:878–887.

16

Left Atrial Appendage

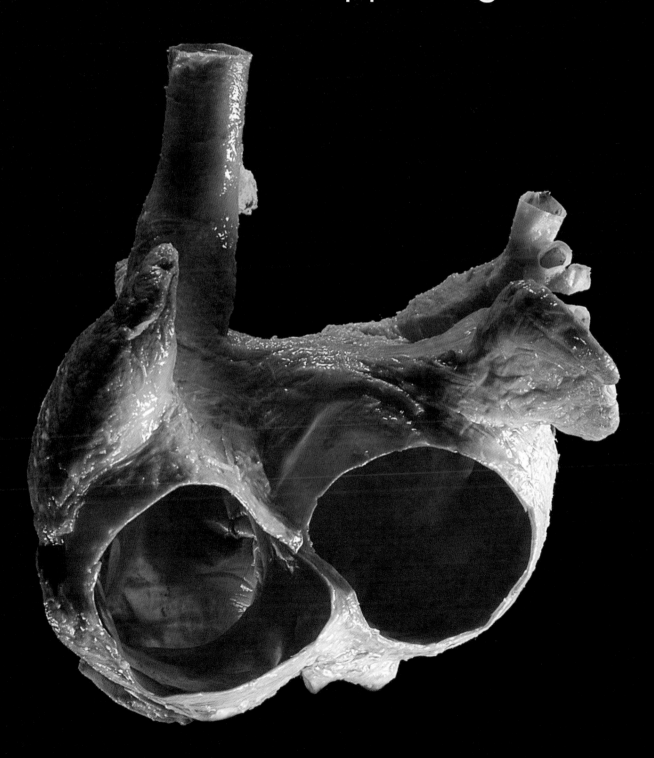

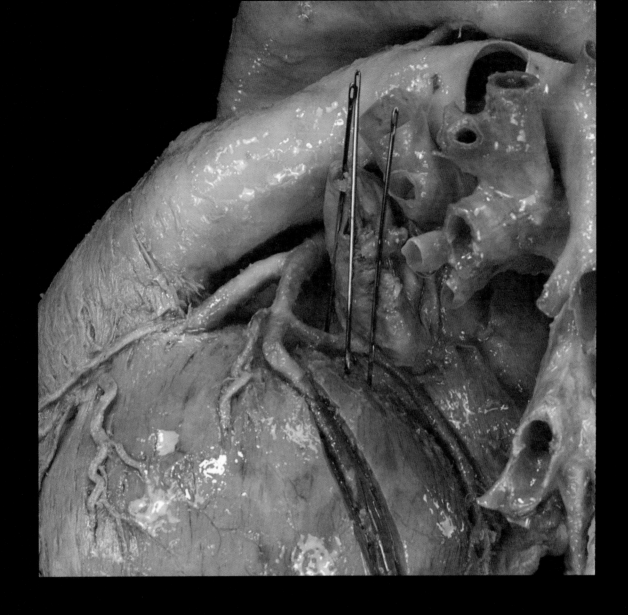

Figure 107 The relationship between the left atrial appendage, left coronary artery, left ventricular summit, and the pulmonary root and trunk.[1]

The heart is viewed from the left lateral direction. The left atrial appendage is located lateral to the pulmonary root/trunk, covering the proximal left coronary artery running on the left ventricular summit.[2] The left atrial appendage guards the

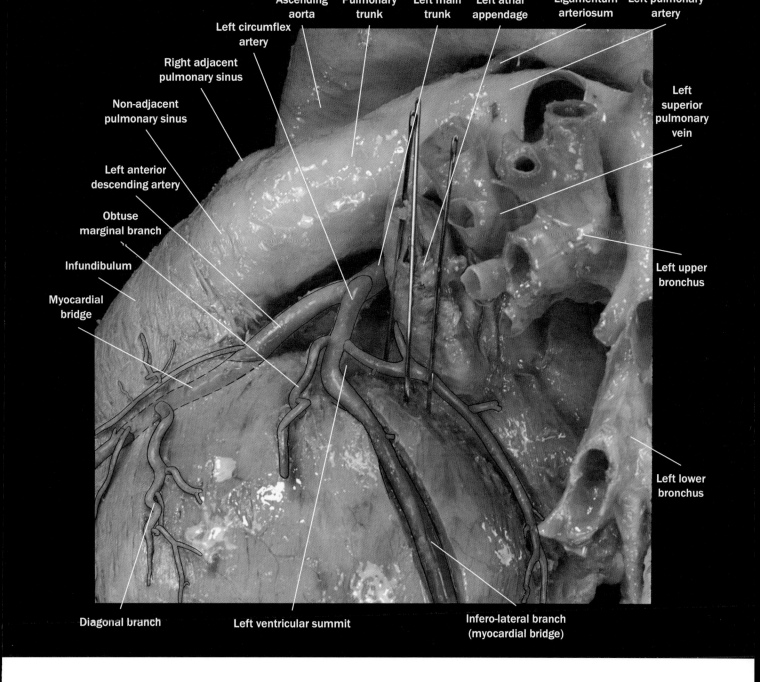

Ascending aorta

Pulmonary trunk

Left main trunk

Left atrial appendage

Ligamentum arteriosum

Left pulmonary artery

Left circumflex artery

Right adjacent pulmonary sinus

Non-adjacent pulmonary sinus

Left anterior descending artery

Obtuse marginal branch

Infundibulum

Myocardial bridge

Left superior pulmonary vein

Left upper bronchus

Left lower bronchus

Diagonal branch

Left ventricular summit

Infero-lateral branch (myocardial bridge)

left lateral entrance/exit of the transverse sinus. The proximal-mid left anterior descending artery and infero-lateral branch show myocardial bridge. Refer to Figure 88.

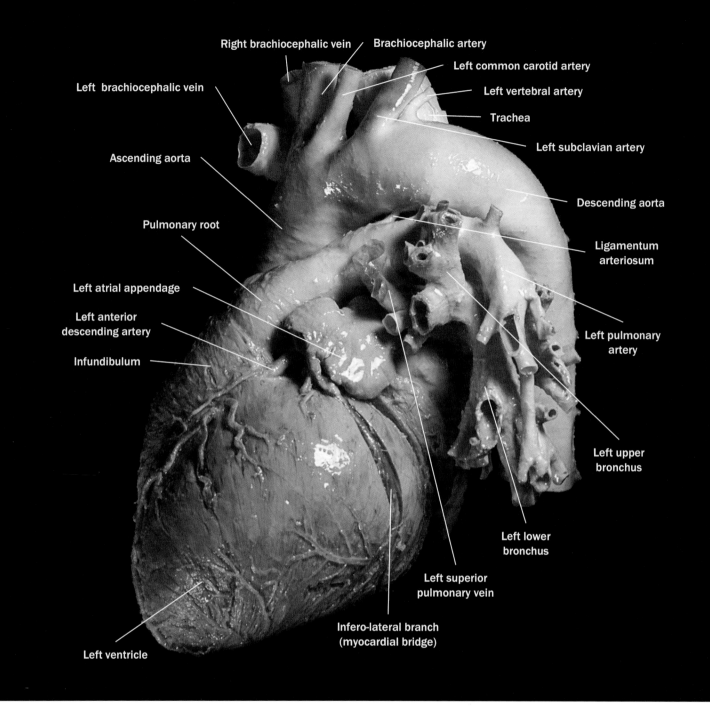

Right brachiocephalic vein   Brachiocephalic artery

Left common carotid artery

Left brachiocephalic vein

Left vertebral artery

Trachea

Ascending aorta

Left subclavian artery

Descending aorta

Pulmonary root

Ligamentum
arteriosum

Left atrial appendage

Left anterior
descending artery

Left pulmonary
artery

Infundibulum

Left upper
bronchus

Left lower
bronchus

Left superior
pulmonary vein

Infero-lateral branch
(myocardial bridge)

Left ventricle

Figure 108   The location of the left atrial appendage.[1]

The hearts are viewed from the left lateral direction. The left atrial appendage is located superior to the supero-lateral region of the basal left ventricle. Posterior to the left atrial appendage, the left superior pulmonary vein, left main bronchus, and the left pulmonary artery overriding the left main bronchus are aligned in order (left). This is not the case in the right side, where the right pulmonary artery is located anterior to the right intermediate bronchus. Refer to Figure 94. The apex of the left atrial appendage is free within the pericardial space. The superior vena cava, brachiocephalic veins, distal pulmonary artery, and trachea and bronchus are removed in the right image. When the atrial appendage is lifted

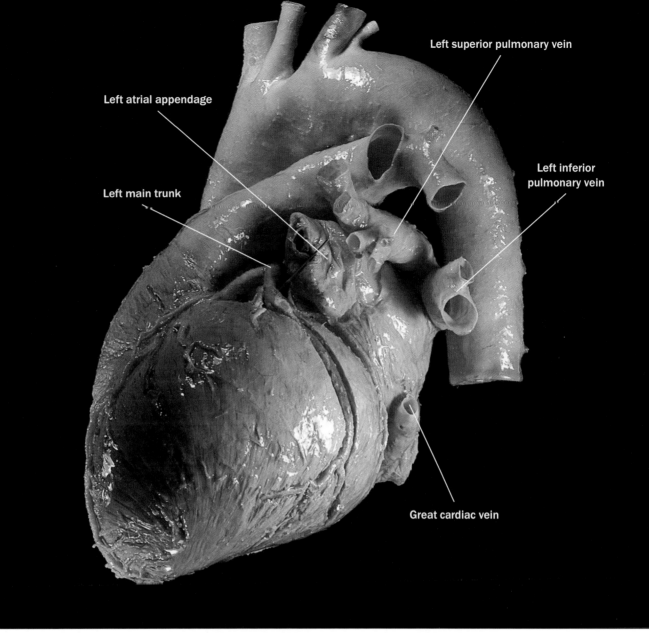

Left superior pulmonary vein

Left atrial appendage

Left inferior pulmonary vein

Left main trunk

Great cardiac vein

up by the pin stuck on the left ventricular summit, the proximal coronary artery lying on the left ventricular summit can be observed. The left circumflex artery runs beneath the left atrial appendage. As shown in this image, the proximal left coronary artery is located in the compartment surrounded by the pulmonary root/trunk antero-superior, aortic root medially, left ventricular summit inferior, and the left atrial appendage supero-lateral. This compartment is filled with the epicardial adipose tissue that is removed in this heart. This region is also the left-side entrance/exit of the transverse sinus. Refer to Figures 88 and 107.

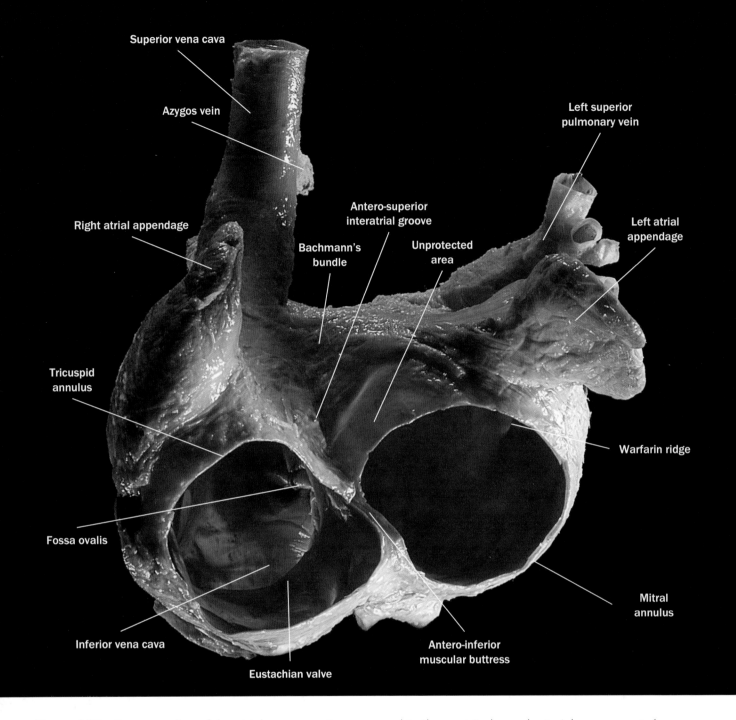

Figure 109 Segmentation of the atrial component as opposed to the ventricular and arterial components.[1]

The heart is separated into atrial components (left) and ventricular/arterial components (right). The orifice of the left atrial appendage is narrower than the orifice of the right atrial appendage. It is superior to supero-lateral part of the left atrial vestibule. The right and left atrial appendages cover the proximal aorta and pulmonary root/trunk, respectively. The medial

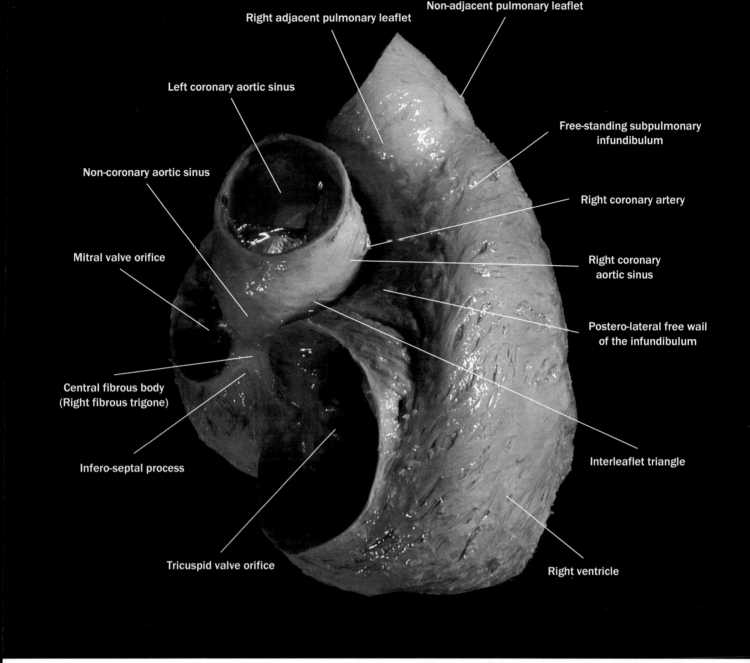

Non-adjacent pulmonary leaflet

Right adjacent pulmonary leaflet

Left coronary aortic sinus

Non-coronary aortic sinus

Mitral valve orifice

Central fibrous body
(Right fibrous trigone)

Infero-septal process

Tricuspid valve orifice

Free-standing subpulmonary
infundibulum

Right coronary artery

Right coronary
aortic sinus

Postero-lateral free wail
of the infundibulum

Interleaflet triangle

Right ventricle

anterior wall of the left atrium is thin at the region adjacent to the antero-superior interatrial groove. This unprotected area[1] has a paucity of muscle fibers, posterior to the aortic root and inferior to the Bachmann's bundle. Refer to Figure 99.

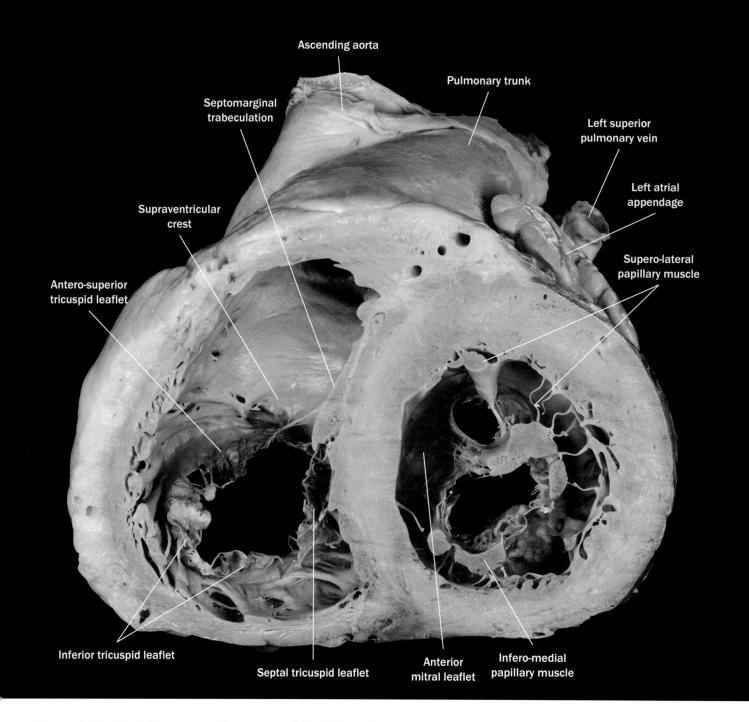

Figure 110 The left anterior oblique view of the left atrial appendage.

The left and right images show the sections at the tricuspid valve and mitral valve levels, respectively. When viewed from this direction, the left atrial appendage extends from the left superior to supero-lateral epicardial region at the basal left ventricle. The supero-medial part of the left atrial appendage is adjacent to the lateral pulmonary root/trunk, covering the

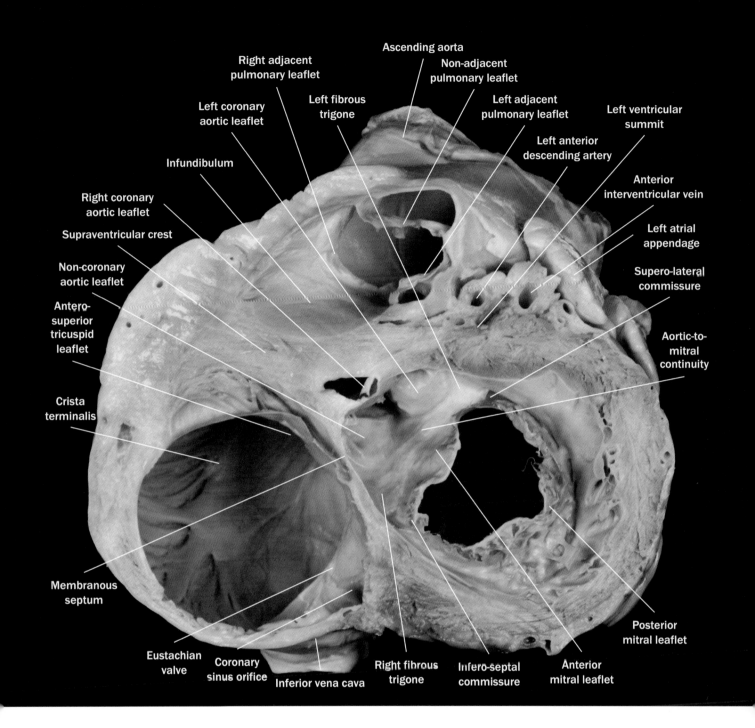

Right adjacent
pulmonary leaflet

Ascending aorta

Non-adjacent
pulmonary leaflet

Left coronary
aortic leaflet

Left fibrous
trigone

Left adjacent
pulmonary leaflet

Left ventricular
summit

Infundibulum

Left anterior
descending artery

Anterior
interventricular vein

Right coronary
aortic leaflet

Left atrial
appendage

Supraventricular crest

Supero-lateral
commissure

Non-coronary
aortic leaflet

Antero-
superior
tricuspid
leaflet

Aortic-to-
mitral
continuity

Crista
terminalis

Membranous
septum

Posterior
mitral leaflet

Eustachian
valve

Coronary
sinus orifice

Inferior vena cava

Right fibrous
trigone

Infero-septal
commissure

Anterior
mitral leaflet

proximal left coronary artery. The infero-lateral part of the left atrial appendage attaches to the supero-lateral basal left ventricle. Regarding the relationship with the mitral valve leaflet, the left atrial appendage extends at the direction between the supero-lateral commissure and lateral scallop of the posterior mitral leaflet.

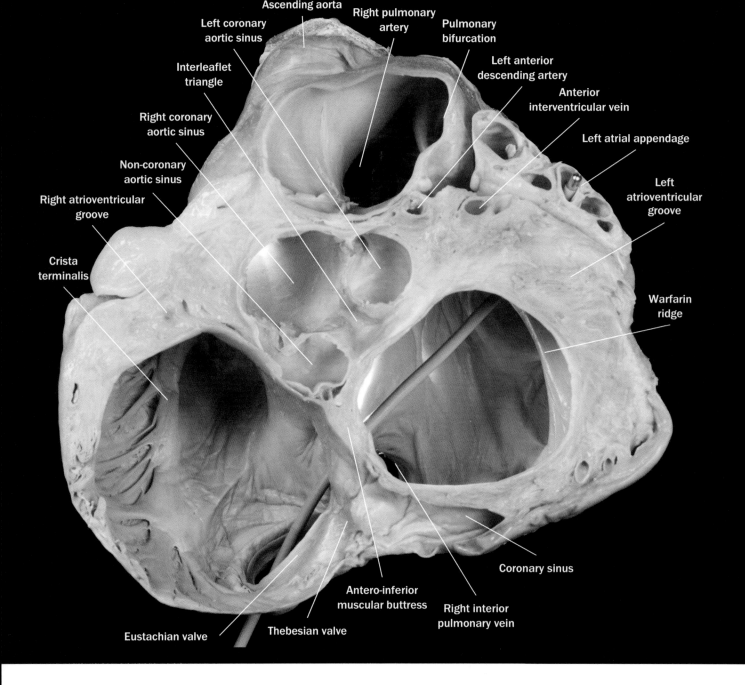

Ascending aorta

Left coronary
aortic sinus

Right pulmonary
artery

Pulmonary
bifurcation

Interleaflet
triangle

Left anterior
descending artery

Right coronary
aortic sinus

Anterior
interventricular vein

Non-coronary
aortic sinus

Left atrial appendage

Right atrioventricular
groove

Left
atrioventricular
groove

Crista
terminalis

Warfarin
ridge

Coronary sinus

Antero-inferior
muscular buttress

Right interior
pulmonary vein

Eustachian valve

Thebesian valve

Figure 111 The left anterior oblique view of the catheter placed in the left atrial appendage.

The left image is the section at the left atrioventricular groove level. The catheter is placed in the left atrial appendage via transseptal puncture. The entrance of the appendage is located in front of the fold between the left atrial appendage and left pulmonary veins, referred to as the left atrial ridge or warfarin (Coumadin) ridge.[3] The right image is the internal aspect of the left atrial appendage viewed from its orifice. The dense pectinate muscle jungle and complicated lobulations with narrow entrances do not always allow the catheter to reach the apical part of each lobulation. This complicated anatomy

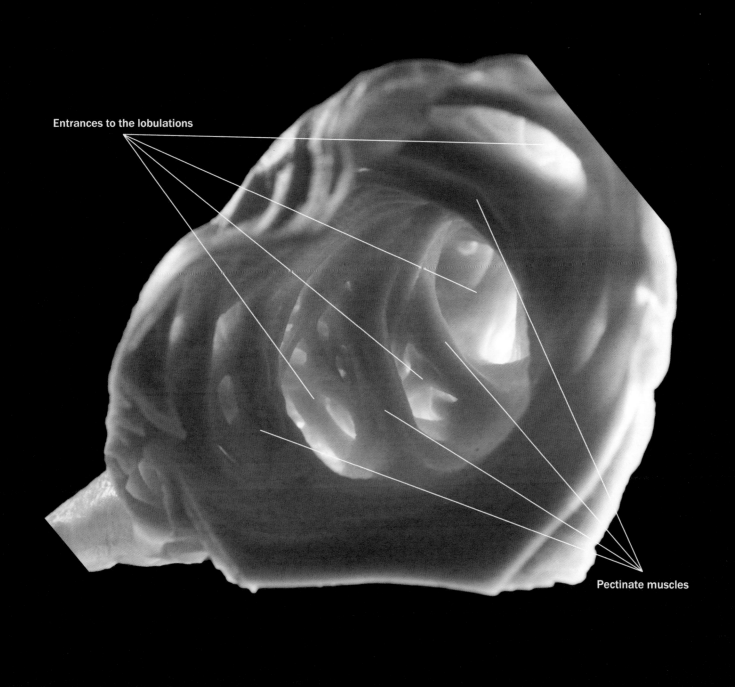

Entrances to the lobulations

Pectinate muscles

can explain why sometimes an endocardial approach is ineffective to ablate an atrial arrhythmia originating from the left atrial appendage. In such cases, an alternative approach involves the epicardial ablation[4] or surgical option to treat the atrial arrhythmia originating from the left atrial appendage.[5] When ablating the left atrial appendage, care for the left phrenic nerve is necessary,[6] as it generally descends alongside the pericardium close to the left atrial appendage.[7]

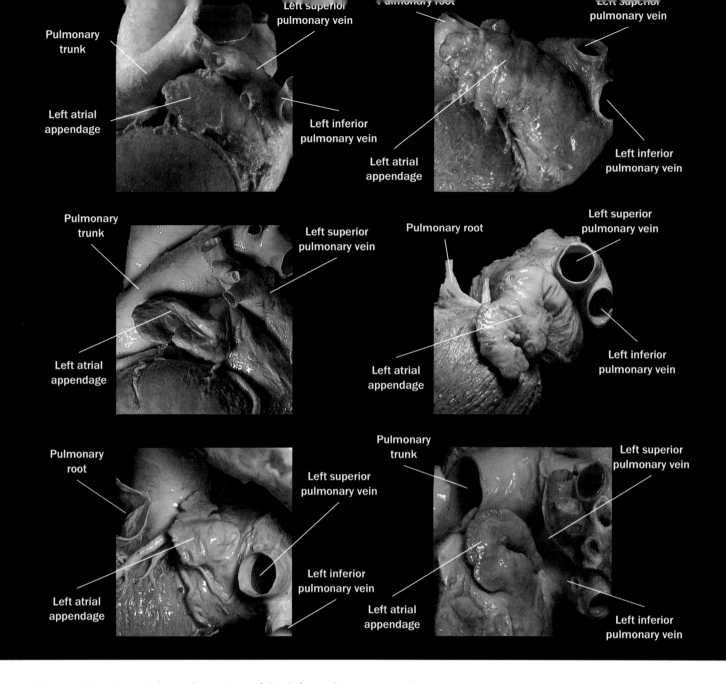

Figure 112   Morphological variation of the left atrial appendage.[1]

The shape, lobulation, and size of the left atrial appendage, as well as its spatial relationships with the pulmonary root/trunk, left pulmonary veins, left coronary artery, and left ventricular base, are quite variable.[8]

References

1. McAlpine WA. Digitized collection of all the images created by Dr. McAlpine at UCLA. Copyright UCLA Cardiac Arrhythmia Center. Part of this collection appeared in *Heart and Coronary Arteries: An Anatomical Atlas for Clinical Diagnosis, Radiological Investigation, and Surgical Treatment*. New York: Springer-Verlag; 1975.

2. Yamada T, McElderry HT, Doppalapudi H, et al. Idiopathic ventricular arrhythmias originating from the left ventricular summit: Anatomic concepts relevant to ablation. *Circ Arrhythm Electrophysiol*. 2010;3:616–623.

3. Piątek-Koziej K, Hołda J, Tyrak K, et al. Anatomy of the left atrial ridge (coumadin ridge) and possible clinical implications for cardiovascular imaging and invasive procedures. *J Cardiovasc Electrophysiol*. 2020;31:220–226.

4. Khakpour H, Hayase JH, Bradfield JS, et al. Atrial tachycardia arising from the distal left atrial appendage requiring high-power endocardial and epicardial ablation. *Heart Rhythm Case Rep*. 2020;7:157–161.

5. Yamada Y, Ajiro Y, Shoda M, et al. Video-assisted thoracoscopy to treat atrial tachycardia arising from left atrial appendage. *J Cardiovasc Electrophysiol*. 2006;17:895–898.

6. Sato T, Miyamoto K, Nishii T, et al. Pace-and-ablate technique for atrial tachycardia originating from the left atrial appendage. *Circ J*. 2020;84:1046.

7. Mori S, Hanna P, Dacey MJ, et al. Comprehensive anatomy of the pericardial space and the cardiac hilum: Anatomical dissections with intact pericardium. *JACC Cardiovasc Imaging*. 2021. DOI: 10.1016/j.jcmg.2021.04.016. Online ahead of print.

8. Di Biase L, Santangeli P, Anselmino M, et al. Does the left atrial appendage morphology correlate with the risk of stroke in patients with atrial fibrillation? Results from a multicenter study. *J Am Coll Cardiol*. 2012;60:531–538.

17

Mitral Valve, Left Ventricular Inflow

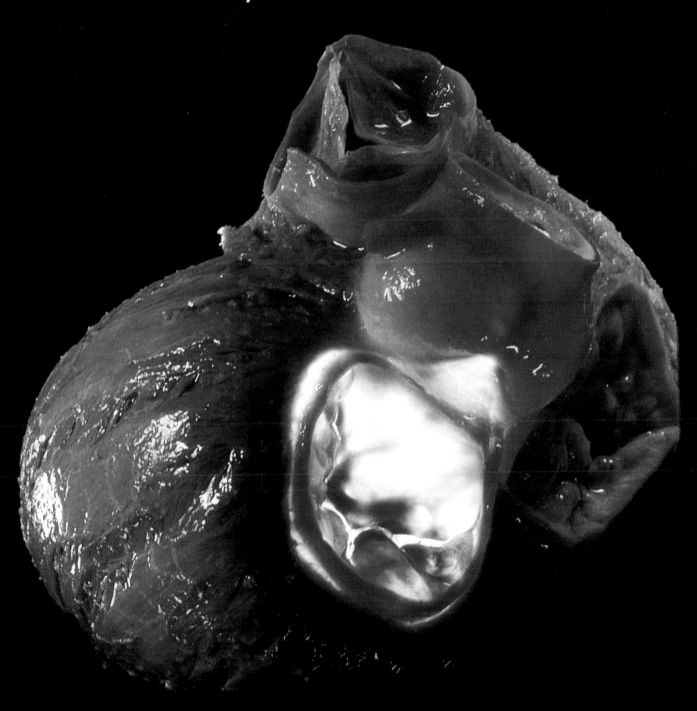

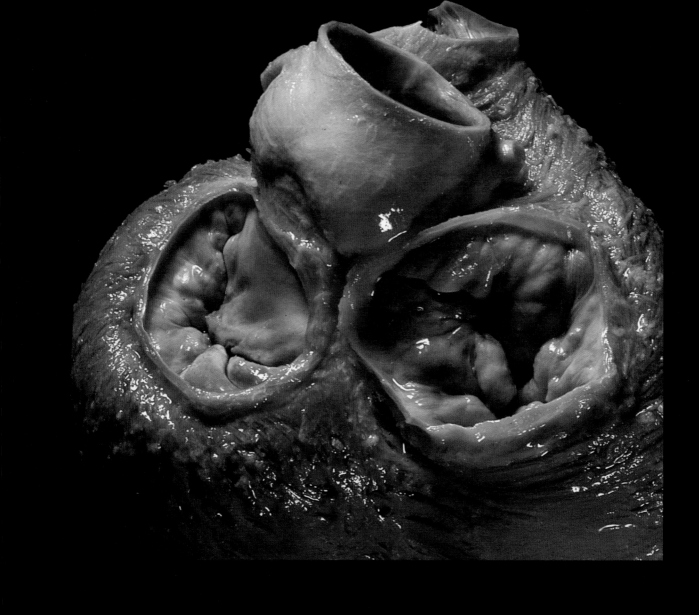

Figure 113   The atrioventricular junction viewed from the right posterior direction.[1]

The aortic root, specifically the non-coronary aortic sinus, wedges between the mitral and tricuspid valves. The tricuspid annulus is located apical relative to the mitral annulus. Thus, the triangular left ventricular free wall between the mitral and tricuspid annuli faces to the right atrium, intervened by the inferior pyramidal space.[2] This part of the basal medial left ventricle is referred to as the infero-septal process of the left ventricle.[3] The anterior mitral leaflet, also referred to as the aortic leaflet of the mitral valve, is in continuity with the aortic root via the aortic-to-mitral (aortomitral) continuity, specifically with the interleaflet triangle between the left and non-coronary aortic sinuses. Although there is no anatomical boundary between them when viewed from the ventricular side, the attachment of the left atrial anterior wall divides the interleaflet triangle from the aortic-to-mitral continuity when viewed from the atrial side. In this regard, the interleaflet triangle faces to the left ventricular outflow tract and transverse sinus, but the aortic-to-mitral continuity faces to the left

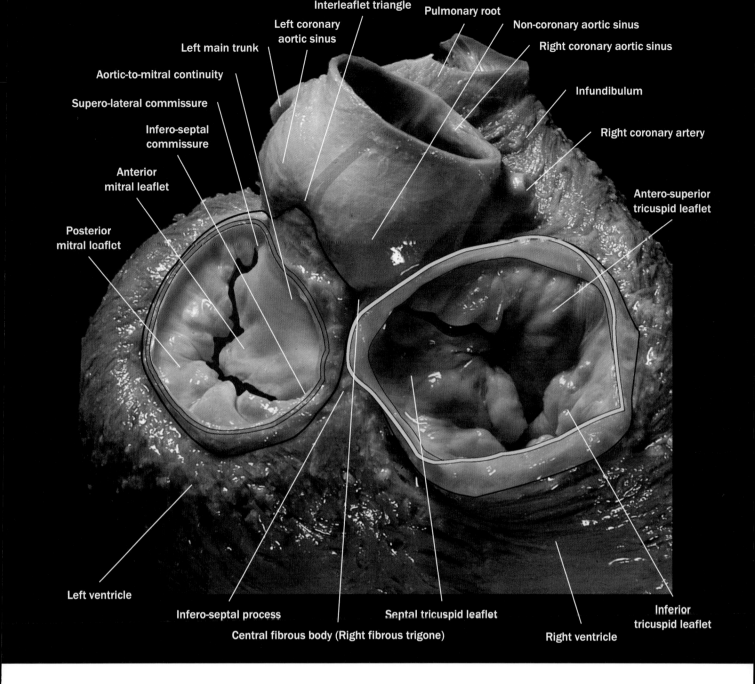

Interleaflet triangle
Pulmonary root
Left coronary aortic sinus
Non-coronary aortic sinus
Left main trunk
Right coronary aortic sinus
Aortic-to-mitral continuity
Supero-lateral commissure
Infundibulum
Infero-septal commissure
Right coronary artery
Anterior mitral leaflet
Antero-superior tricuspid leaflet
Posterior mitral leaflet
Left ventricle
Infero-septal process
Septal tricuspid leaflet
Inferior tricuspid leaflet
Central fibrous body (Right fibrous trigone)
Right ventricle

ventricular outflow tract and internal left atrium. The posterior mitral leaflet, also referred to as the mural leaflet of the mitral valve, arises from the basal left ventricular free wall mass. The supero-lateral commissure is close to the nadir of the left coronary aortic sinus, whereas the infero-septal commissure is close to the nadir of the non-coronary aortic sinus. The strong fibrous tissues supporting the lateral and medial part of the anterior mitral leaflet are the left and right fibrous trigones, respectively.[4] The left fibrous trigone extends from the nadir of the left coronary aortic sinus toward the supero-lateral commissure. The right fibrous trigone extends from the nadir of the non-coronary aortic sinus toward the infero-septal commissure. The right fibrous trigone is more extensive than the left fibrous trigone,[1] rendering the infero-septal commissure distant from the aortic root, compared to the distance between the aortic root to the supero-lateral commissure. The right fibrous trigone is also referred to as the central fibrous body.[1,4]

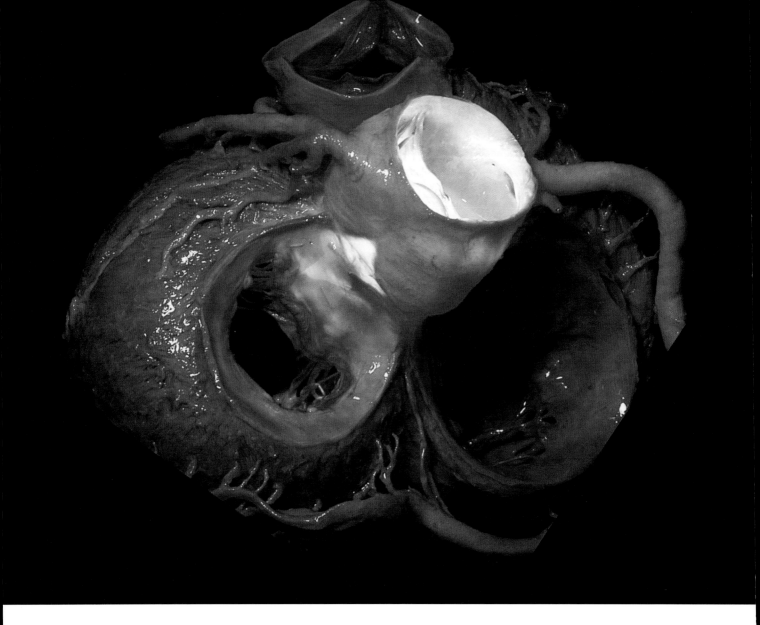

Figure 114 Atrioventricular nodal artery and the mitral valve.[1]

The atrioventricular nodal artery ascends toward the compact atrioventricular node located at the right atrial side of the central fibrous body, also referred to as the right fibrous trigone.[1,4] Thus, from the left atrial side, medial mitral annulus close to the infero-septal commissure is adjacent to the atrioventricular nodal artery and compact atrioventricular node, intervened by the central fibrous body. The atrioventricular nodal artery is located within the inferior pyramidal space, which is the sandwiched epicardial adipose tissue wedging from the inferior cardiac crux.[5] The epicardial adipose tissue is, however,

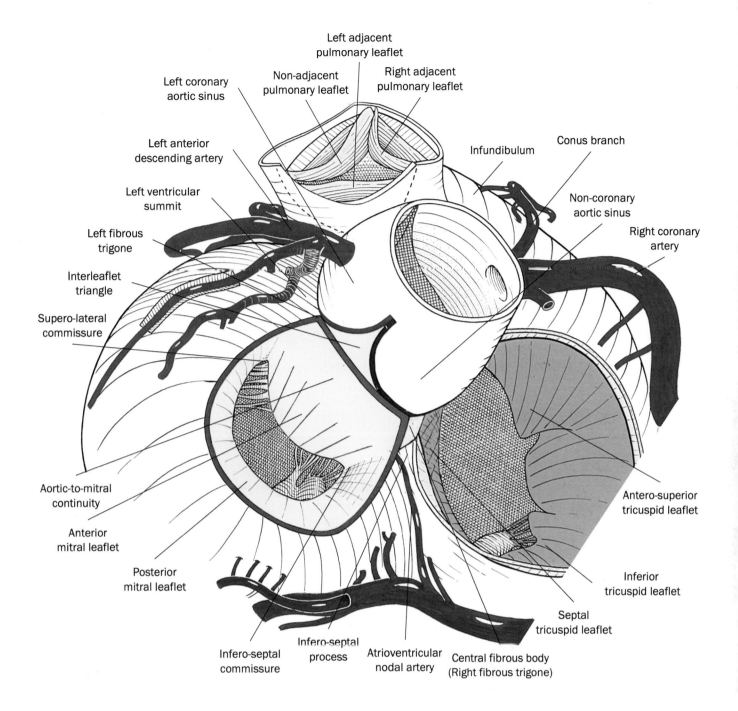

Left adjacent
pulmonary leaflet

Non-adjacent
pulmonary leaflet

Right adjacent
pulmonary leaflet

Left coronary
aortic sinus

Infundibulum

Conus branch

Left anterior
descending artery

Non-coronary
aortic sinus

Left ventricular
summit

Right coronary
artery

Left fibrous
trigone

Interleaflet
triangle

Supero-lateral
commissure

Antero-superior
tricuspid leaflet

Aortic-to-mitral
continuity

Anterior
mitral leaflet

Inferior
tricuspid leaflet

Posterior
mitral leaflet

Septal
tricuspid leaflet

Infero-septal
commissure

Infero-septal
process

Atrioventricular
nodal artery

Central fibrous body
(Right fibrous trigone)

removed in this heart. The inferior pyramidal space is located between the mitral annulus and tricuspid annulus, posterior to the infero-septal process of the left ventricle.[3] When viewed from the right atrial side, the inferior pyramidal space corresponds to the floor of the triangle of Koch.[6] Neither the supero-lateral nor the infero-septal commissure reaches to the level of the mitral annulus. The proportion of the posterior mitral leaflet within the entire circumference of the mitral annulus is larger than that of the anterior mitral leaflet, occupying two-thirds to three-fourths of the entire mitral annulus.[7]

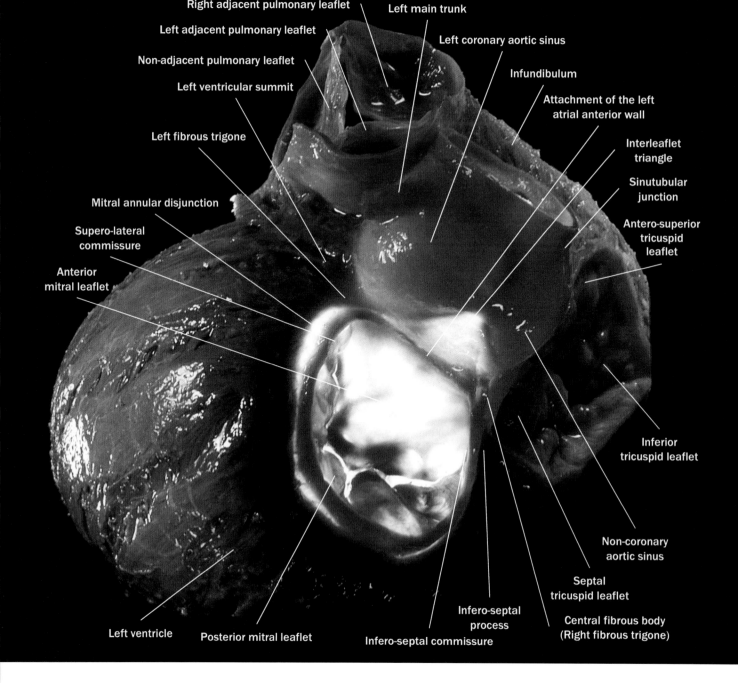

Right adjacent pulmonary leaflet

Left adjacent pulmonary leaflet

Non-adjacent pulmonary leaflet

Left ventricular summit

Left fibrous trigone

Mitral annular disjunction

Supero-lateral commissure

Anterior mitral leaflet

Left main trunk

Left coronary aortic sinus

Infundibulum

Attachment of the left atrial anterior wall

Interleaflet triangle

Sinutubular junction

Antero-superior tricuspid leaflet

Inferior tricuspid leaflet

Non-coronary aortic sinus

Septal tricuspid leaflet

Central fibrous body (Right fibrous trigone)

Left ventricle

Posterior mitral leaflet

Infero-septal commissure

Infero-septal process

Figure 115 The mitral valve showing the mitral annular disjunction.[1]

The interleaflet triangle between the left and non-coronary aortic sinuses, anterior and posterior mitral leaflets, and mitral annular disjunction are transilluminated. The mitral annular disjunction is a separation between the atrial wall-mitral valve junction and the basal left ventricular myocardium.[8] The mitral annular disjunction was initially illustrated by J. Henle with the German term meaning *fibrous ring*.[9] McAlpine refers to disjunction as the subvalvular segment of the aorto-ventricular membrane or subvalvular membrane.[1] The mitral annular disjunction is generally prominent at the attachment of the lateral (P1) and medial (P3) scallops in continuity with bilateral fibrous trigones,[7] and rarely encircles entire circumference of the attachment of the posterior mitral leaflet as demonstrated in this image.[10] It is exclusively related to the posterior mitral leaflet at its attachment, as the one of the thin fibrous anatomical structures within the normal left ventricle.[7] Thus, it should be a high-risk area during any invasive approach performed involving this region, including radiofrequency catheter ablation of the accessory pathway[11] or ventricular arrhythmia originating from the mitral annulus,[12] mitral valve surgery,[13] and transcatheter mitral valve replacement. Potential relationships between the mitral annular disjunction and mitral valve prolapse or ventricular arrhythmia[14] have been suggested. The aortic-to-mitral (aortomitral) continuity refers to the fibrous structure extending at the base of the anterior mitral leaflet between the right and left fibrous trigone. Thus, the aortic-to-mitral continuity is generally devoid of ventricular myocardium. It is the component of the virtual basal ring of the aortic root, known as the annulus of the aortic root. It extends between the superiorly located interleaflet triangle and inferiorly located anterior mitral leaflet. The left atrial attachment divides the interleaflet triangle from the aortic-to-mitral continuity. However, the aortic-to-mitral continuity is hardly distinguishable from the anterior mitral leaflet.[15] The functional differentiation of the aortic-to-mitral continuity from the anterior mitral leaflet can be made by the hingeline of the anterior mitral leaflet, as the aortic-to-mitral continuity is a not mobile structure. Thus, the height of the aortic-to-mitral continuity is seldom more than 10 mm.[15] The aortic-to-mitral continuity is also referred to as the intervalvular fibrous body,[15] or aortomitral curtain by cardiac surgeons[16] as the potential region to intervene when enlarging the annulus of the aortic root.

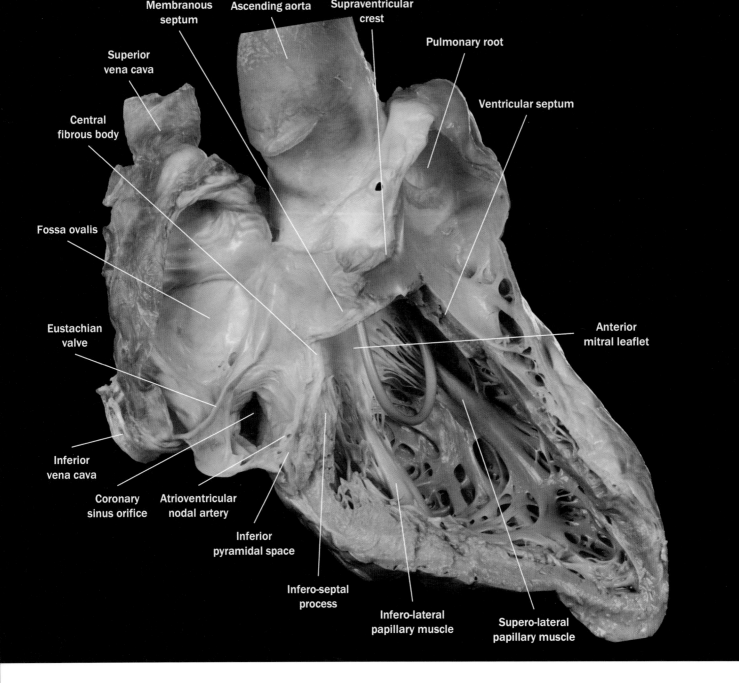

Membranous septum

Ascending aorta

Supraventricular crest

Pulmonary root

Superior vena cava

Ventricular septum

Central fibrous body

Fossa ovalis

Eustachian valve

Anterior mitral leaflet

Inferior vena cava

Coronary sinus orifice

Atrioventricular nodal artery

Inferior pyramidal space

Infero-septal process

Infero-lateral papillary muscle

Supero-lateral papillary muscle

Figure 116 The transaortic retrograde approach ablating the endocardial side of the left ventricular summit near the supero-lateral commissure.

The heart is viewed from the right anterior oblique (left) and left anterior oblique (right) directions. The left ventricular free wall supports the anterior half of the left coronary aortic sinus. The epicardial side of the left ventricular free wall is the left ventricular summit. The catheter is placed at the superior mitral annulus, corresponding to the endocardial region of the left ventricular summit. This region is located slightly apical to the supero-lateral commissure and lateral to the left fibrous trigone and aortic-to-mitral (aortomitral) continuity.[17] To reach this region, acute bend with small curve and strong counterclockwise torque is necessary. In the left image, the muscular ventricular septum is removed. The basal superior margin of the section involves the inferior margin of the membranous septum. Confusingly, in the field of electrophysiology,

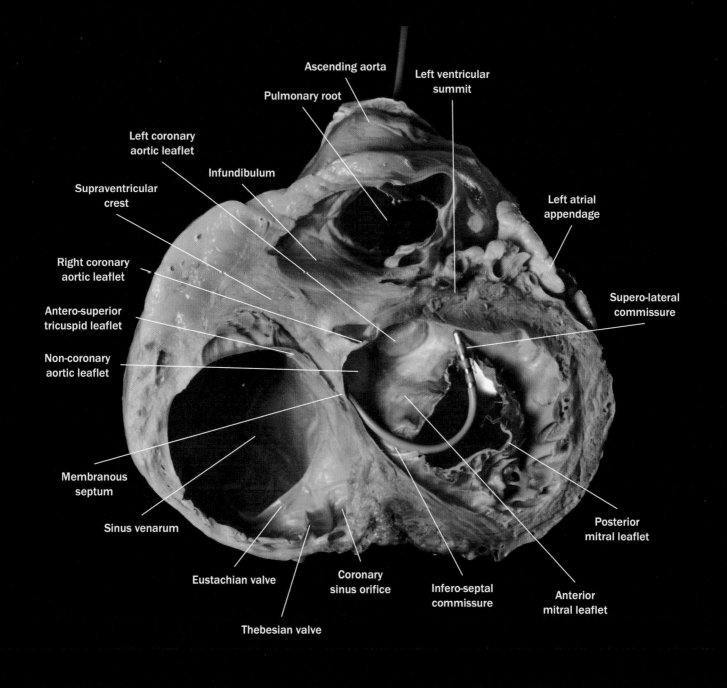

Ascending aorta

Left ventricular summit

Pulmonary root

Left coronary aortic leaflet

Infundibulum

Left atrial appendage

Supraventricular crest

Right coronary aortic leaflet

Supero-lateral commissure

Antero-superior tricuspid leaflet

Non-coronary aortic leaflet

Membranous septum

Sinus venarum

Posterior mitral leaflet

Eustachian valve

Coronary sinus orifice

Infero-septal commissure

Anterior mitral leaflet

Thebesian valve

ventricular arrhythmia originating from the aortic-to-mitral continuity generally refers to this region[18] that is close to the left fibrous trigone and left ventricular summit.[19] In fact, this region is the basal superior left ventricular free wall, or the endocardial side of the left ventricular summit, and also identical to the superior mitral annulus. This region should not be referred to as the true anatomical aortic-to-mitral continuity, which is the fibrous structure extending at the base of the anterior mitral leaflet between the right and left fibrous trigone, and between the interleaflet triangle and anterior mitral leaflet. The aortic-to-mitral continuity is generally devoid of ventricular myocardium.[20] The thickness of the left ventricular free wall myocardium supporting the left coronary aortic sinus is generally less than 3.0 mm in average.[21]

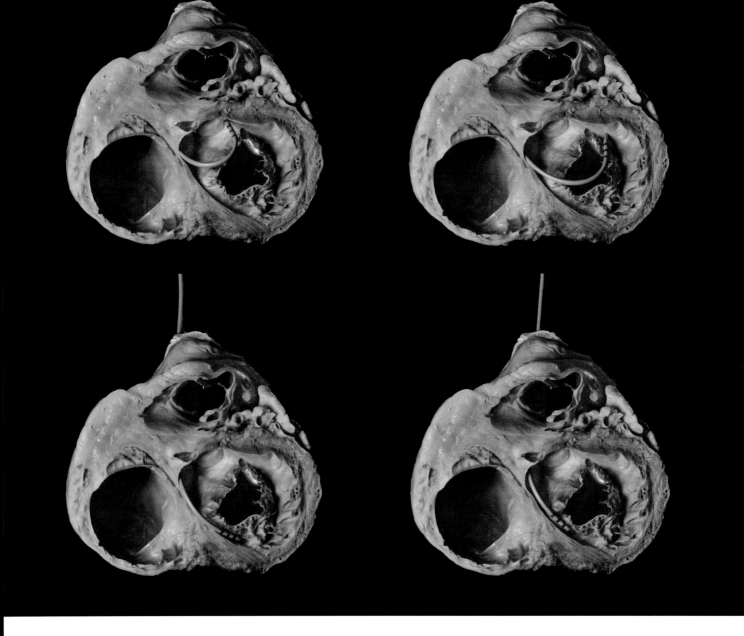

Figure 117 The transaortic retrograde approach to map the subvalvular region of the mitral valve and the infero-septal recess.

These are the sections showing the mitral valve. As the tricuspid valve is located apical to the mitral valve, the right atrium is sectioned on this plane. The mitral annulus is a potential substrate for atrial arrhythmia,[22] accessory pathway,[23] and ventricular arrhythmia.[24] Approximately, the supero-lateral commissure is located at 12 o'clock and the infero-septal commissure is located at the 9 o'clock. Description is made from the upper left image to lower right image. For the first six images, the catheter is placed at the superior, supero-lateral, lateral, infero-lateral, inferior, infero-medial mitral annulus,

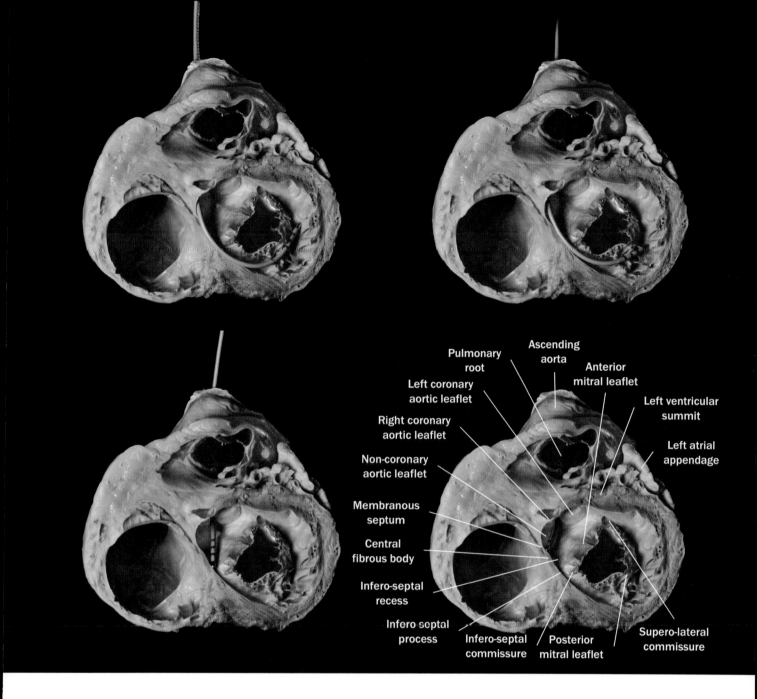

Pulmonary root

Ascending aorta

Anterior mitral leaflet

Left coronary aortic leaflet

Left ventricular summit

Right coronary aortic leaflet

Left atrial appendage

Non-coronary aortic leaflet

Membranous septum

Central fibrous body

Infero-septal recess

Infero-septal process

Infero-septal commissure

Posterior mitral leaflet

Supero-lateral commissure

respectively. The superior mitral annulus corresponds to the endocardial side of the left ventricular summit. The last two images show mapping within the infero-septal recess, the space within the inferior left ventricular outflow tract surrounded by the membranous septum and crest of the ventricular septum medially, right fibrous trigone basally, and the aortic-to-mitral (aortomitral) continuity and anterior mitral leaflet laterally. The infero-septal process, and the membranous septum is mapped. The latter position has a risk to create the infra-Hisian block by injuring the non-branching or branching portions of the atrioventricular conduction axis, or to injure the fascicles of the left bundle branch.

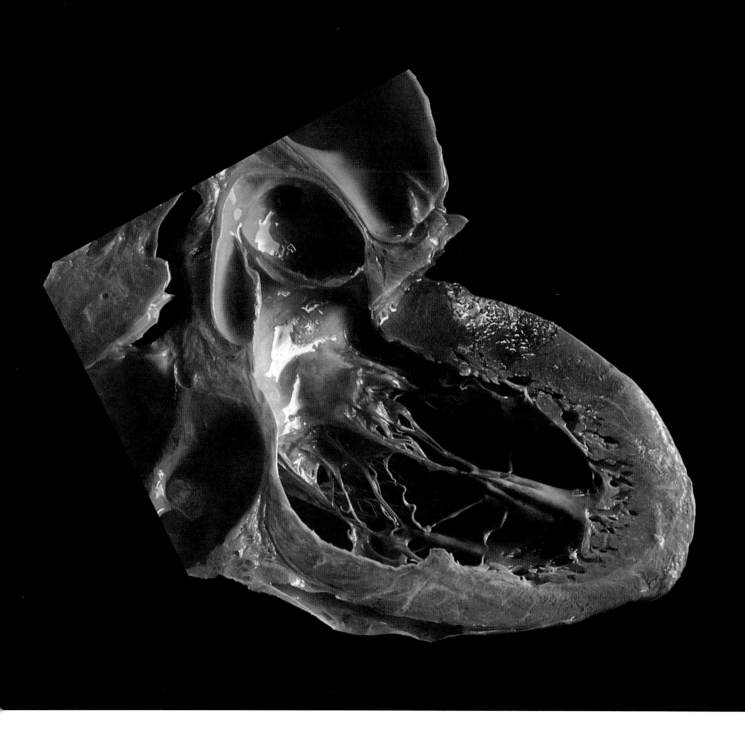

Figure 118 The mitral valve complex viewed from the right anterior oblique direction.[1]

From the ventricular septal direction, a nearly *en face* view of the opened anterior mitral leaflet is observed in front of the mitral valve orifice and the posterior mitral leaflet hidden behind the anterior mitral leaflet. The anterior mitral leaflet is related to the interleaflet triangle between the left and non-coronary aortic sinuses, connected by the aortic-to-mitral (aortomitral) continuity. From the endocardial side, no anatomical boundary can be detected between them. Lateral and medial sides of the anterior mitral leaflet are supported by the left and right fibrous trigones,[4] respectively. The infero-septal process of the left ventricle, corresponding to the basal infero-medial left ventricular wall, ascends toward the right fibrous

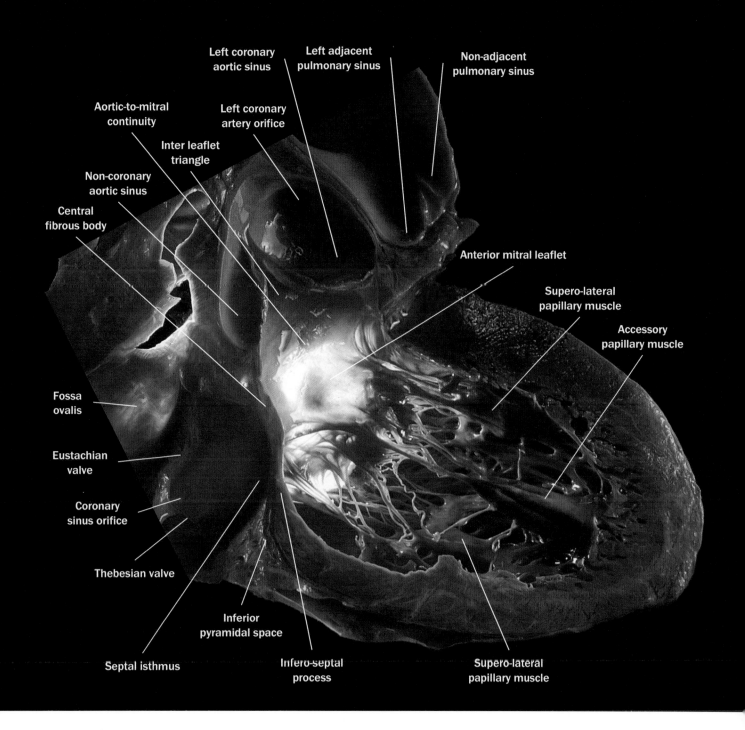

Left coronary
aortic sinus

Left adjacent
pulmonary sinus

Non-adjacent
pulmonary sinus

Aortic-to-mitral
continuity

Left coronary
artery orifice

Inter leaflet
triangle

Non-coronary
aortic sinus

Central
fibrous body

Anterior mitral leaflet

Supero-lateral
papillary muscle

Accessory
papillary muscle

Fossa
ovalis

Eustachian
valve

Coronary
sinus orifice

Thebesian valve

Inferior
pyramidal space

Septal isthmus

Infero-septal
process

Supero-lateral
papillary muscle

trigone, also referred to as the central fibrous body. The septal isthmus anterior to the coronary sinus orifice is adjacent to the infero-septal process.[3] However, the septal isthmus and the infero-septal process is intervened by the inferior pyramidal space, the epicardial fibro-adipose tissue carrying the atrioventricular nodal artery.[2] The light source in the left atrium transilluminates the mitral leaflet (right).

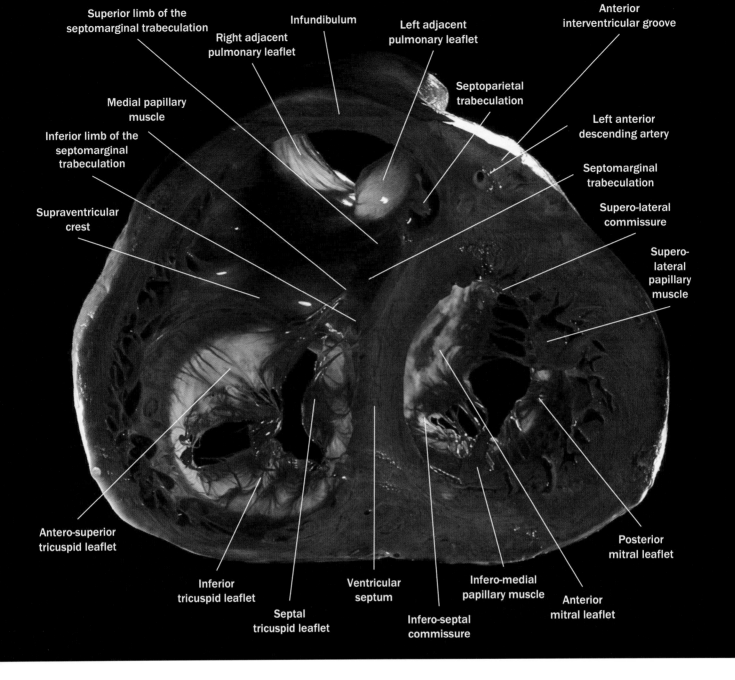

Superior limb of the septomarginal trabeculation

Infundibulum

Left adjacent pulmonary leaflet

Anterior interventricular groove

Right adjacent pulmonary leaflet

Septoparietal trabeculation

Medial papillary muscle

Left anterior descending artery

Inferior limb of the septomarginal trabeculation

Septomarginal trabeculation

Supero-lateral commissure

Supraventricular crest

Supero-lateral papillary muscle

Antero-superior tricuspid leaflet

Posterior mitral leaflet

Inferior tricuspid leaflet

Ventricular septum

Infero-medial papillary muscle

Anterior mitral leaflet

Septal tricuspid leaflet

Infero-septal commissure

Figure 119 The *en face* view of the atrioventricular junction.[1]

The *en face* view of the atrioventricular junction viewed from the ventricular side, corresponding the left antero-inferior view. The anterior mitral leaflet is located right antero-superior direction, and the posterior mitral leaflet is located in the left postero-inferior direction. Thus, the zone of coaptation is not located horizontally, but it extends supero-lateral to the infero-septal direction. Therefore, the alignment of the supero-lateral and infero-septal commissures shows the nearly parallel relationship to the alignment of supero-lateral and infero-medial papillary muscles.[25] At this sectional level, both the right and left ventricular septal surfaces show fewer trabeculations compared to both the ventricular lateral free walls. The aortic root is located behind the crest of the ventricular septum and medial part of the supraventricular crest of the right ventricle.

References

1. McAlpine WA. Digitized collection of all the images created by Dr. McAlpine at UCLA. Copyright UCLA Cardiac Arrhythmia Center. Part of this collection appeared in *Heart and Coronary Arteries: An Anatomical Atlas for Clinical Diagnosis, Radiological Investigation, and Surgical Treatment*. New York: Springer-Verlag; 1975.

2. Mori S, Nishii T, Takaya T, et al. Clinical structural anatomy of the inferior pyramidal space reconstructed from the living heart: Three-dimensional visualization using multidetector-row computed tomography. *Clin Anat*. 2015;28:878–887.

3. Li A, Zuberi Z, Bradfield JS, et al. Endocardial ablation of ventricular ectopic beats arising from the basal inferoseptal process of the left ventricle. *Heart Rhythm*. 2018;15:1356–1362.

4. Zimmerman J, Bailey CP. The surgical significance of the fibrous skeleton of the heart. *J Thorac Cardiovasc Surg*. 1962;44:701–712.

5. Kawashima T, Sato F. Clarifying the anatomy of the atrioventricular node artery. *Int J Cardiol*. 2018;269:158–164.

6. Mori S, Fukuzawa K, Takaya T, et al. Clinical structural anatomy of the Inferior pyramidal space reconstructed within the cardiac contour using multidetector-row computed tomography. *J Cardiovasc Electrophysiol*. 2015;26:705–712.

7. Toh H, Mori S, Izawa Y, et al. Prevalence and extent of mitral annular disjunction in structurally normal hearts: Comprehensive 3D analysis using cardiac computed tomography. *Eur Heart J Cardiovasc Imaging*. 2021;22:614–622.

8. Hutchins GM, Moore GW, Skoog DK. The association of floppy mitral valve with disjunction of the mitral annulus fibrosis. *N Engl J Med*. 1986;314:535–540.

9. Henle J. Handbuch der systematischen Anatomie des Menschen. v. 3 pt. 1, 1876. Germany: Vieweg; 1876. p14–20.

10. Angelini A, Ho SY, Anderson RH, et al. A histological study of the atrioventricular junction in hearts with normal and prolapsed leaflets of the mitral valve. *Br Heart J*. 1988;59:712–716.

11. Miura T, Yamazaki K, Kihara S, et al. Transatrial repair of submitral left ventricular pseudoaneurysm. *Ann Thorac Surg*. 2008;85:643–645.

12. Wang H, Zheng Z, Yao L, et al. Giant left ventricular pseudoaneurysm: a rare acute complication of radiofrequency catheter ablation for premature ventricular contraction. *J Cardiothorac Surg*. 2019;14:131.

13. Antonic M, Djordjevic A, Mohorko T, et al. Left ventricular pseudoaneurysm following atrioventricular groove rupture after mitral valve replacement. *SAGE Open Med Case Rep*. 2019;7:1–4.

14. Dejgaard LA, Skjølsvik ET, Lie ØH, et al. The mitral annulus disjunction arrhythmic syndrome. *J Am Coll Cardiol*. 2018;72:1600–1609.

15. David TE, Kuo J, Armstrong S. Aortic and mitral valve replacement with reconstruction of the intervalvular fibrous body. *J Thorac Cardiovasc Surg*. 1997;114:766–771.

16. Yang B. A novel simple technique to enlarge the aortic annulus by two valve sizes. *JTCVS Tech*. 2021;5:13–16.

17. Toh H, Mori S, Izawa Y, et al. Absence of myocardial support at the base of the left coronary aortic sinus in a patient with Ehlers-Danlos syndrome. *Circ J*. 2021;25;85:220.

18. Kumagai K, Fukuda K, Wakayama Y, et al. Electrocardiographic characteristics of the variants of idiopathic left ventricular outflow tract ventricular tachyarrhythmias. *J Cardiovasc Electrophysiol*. 2008;19:495–501.

19. Steven D, Roberts-Thomson KC, Seiler J, et al. Ventricular tachycardia arising from the aortomitral continuity in structural heart disease: Characteristics and therapeutic considerations for an anatomically challenging area of origin. *Circ Arrhythm Electrophysiol*. 2009;2:660–666.

20. Mori S, Fukuzawa K, Takaya T, et al. Optimal angulations for obtaining an *en face* view of each coronary aortic sinus and the interventricular septum: Correlative anatomy around the left ventricular outflow tract. *Clin Anat*. 2015;28:494–505.

21. Toh H, Mori S, Tretter JT, et al. Living anatomy of the ventricular myocardial crescents supporting the coronary aortic sinuses. *Semin Thorac Cardiovasc Surg*. 2020;32:230–241.

22. Nogami A, Suguta M, Tomita T, et al. Novel form of atrial tachycardia originating at the atrioventricular annulus. *Pacing Clin Electrophysiol*. 1998;21:2691–2694.

23. Fitzpatrick AP, Gonzales RP, Lesh MD, et al. New algorithm for the localization of accessory atrioventricular connections using a baseline electrocardiogram. *J Am Coll Cardiol*. 1994;23:107–116.

24. Tada H, Ito S, Naito S, et al. Idiopathic ventricular arrhythmia arising from the mitral annulus: a distinct subgroup of idiopathic ventricular arrhythmias. *J Am Coll Cardiol*. 2005;45:877–886.

25. Mori S, Fukuzawa K, Takaya T, et al. Clinical cardiac structural anatomy reconstructed within the cardiac contour using multidetector-row computed tomography: The arrangement and location of the cardiac valves. *Clin Anat*. 2016;29:364–370.

18

Left Ventricular Papillary Muscles, Left Ventricular Apex

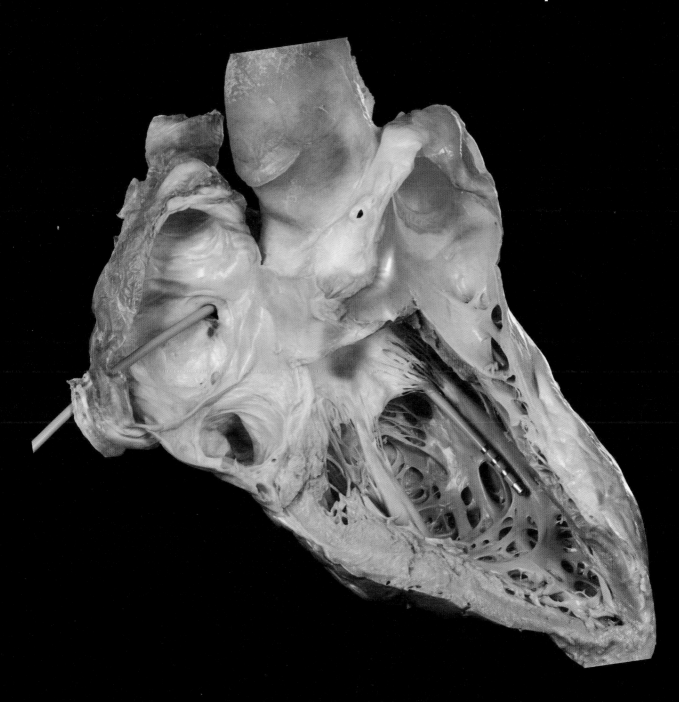

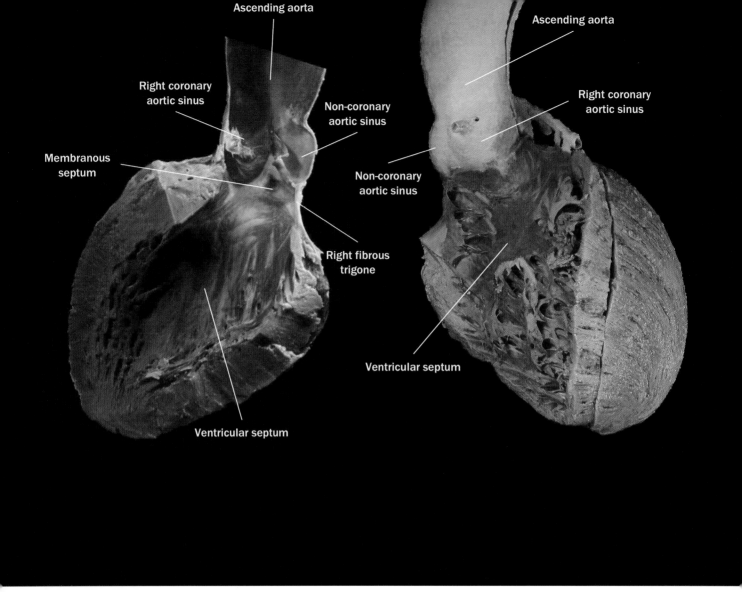

Ascending aorta

Right coronary aortic sinus

Non-coronary aortic sinus

Membranous septum

Non-coronary aortic sinus

Right fibrous trigone

Ventricular septum

Ventricular septum

Ascending aorta

Right coronary aortic sinus

Figure 120 The left ventricle divided into septal and lateral parts.[1]

The right image on the left page shows the left ventricular specimen viewed from the anterior direction showing the sectional plane. The septal part (left image on the left page) involves no papillary muscles, and related to the right coronary aortic sinus and anterior half of the non-coronary aortic sinus. The lateral part (left image on the right page) involves both infero-medial and supero-lateral papillary muscles and mitral annulus, and related to left coronary aortic sinus and

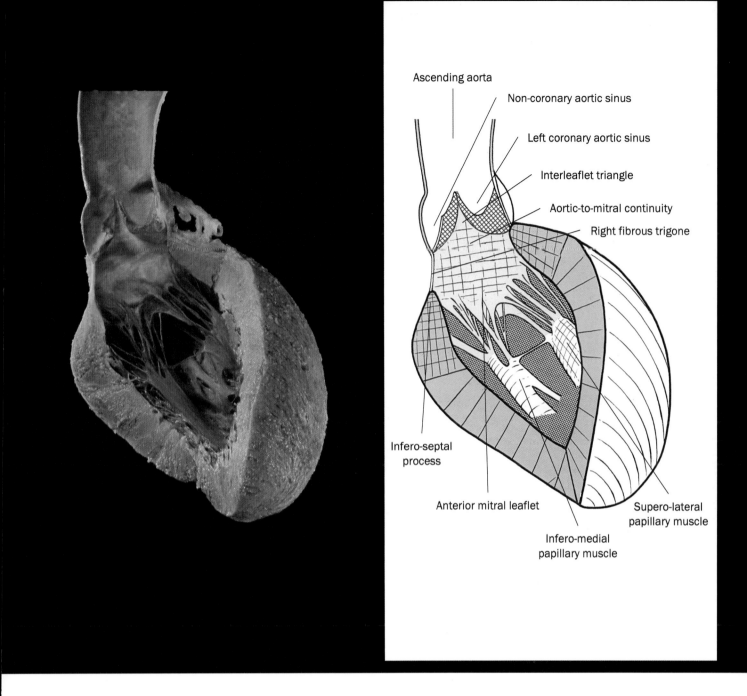

Ascending aorta

Non-coronary aortic sinus

Left coronary aortic sinus

Interleaflet triangle

Aortic-to-mitral continuity

Right fibrous trigone

Infero-septal process

Anterior mitral leaflet

Supero-lateral papillary muscle

Infero-medial papillary muscle

posterior half of the non-coronary aortic sinus.[2] The right image shows the illustration of the left image on the right page. The infero-medial and supero-lateral papillary muscles are located in vertical fashion rather than horizontal fashion.[3] Each infero-medial and supero-lateral papillary muscles give multiple chordae tendineae to the medial and lateral part of both anterior and posterior mitral leaflets, respectively. The images on the right page show the infero-septal process inferior to the central fibrous body, also referred to as the right fibrous trigone. Refer to Figure 12.

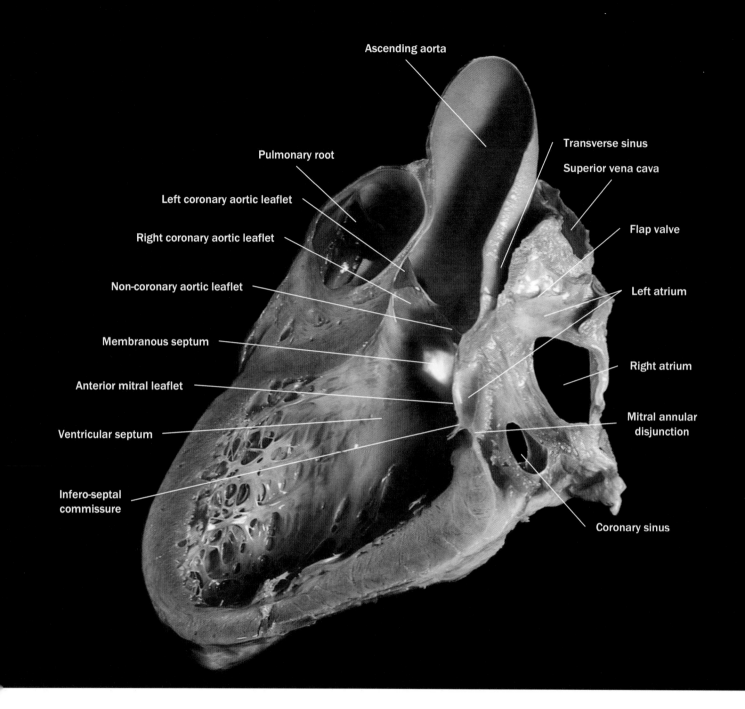

Ascending aorta

Pulmonary root

Left coronary aortic leaflet

Right coronary aortic leaflet

Non-coronary aortic leaflet

Membranous septum

Anterior mitral leaflet

Ventricular septum

Infero-septal commissure

Transverse sinus

Superior vena cava

Flap valve

Left atrium

Right atrium

Mitral annular disjunction

Coronary sinus

Figure 121   Septal and lateral surface of the left ventricle.[1]

The left and right images show the bisected left heart viewed from the left posterior oblique and right anterior oblique directions, respectively. The septal section has no papillary muscles, only showing fine apical trabeculation with smooth surface at the basal ventricular septum. The membranous septum between the right and non-coronary aortic sinuses is

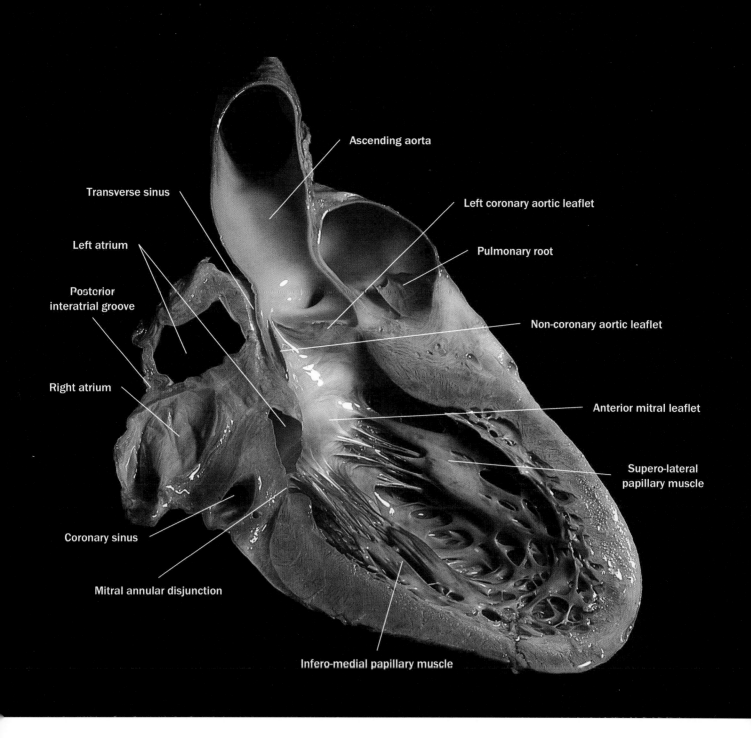

Ascending aorta

Transverse sinus

Left coronary aortic leaflet

Left atrium

Pulmonary root

Posterior interatrial groove

Non-coronary aortic leaflet

Right atrium

Anterior mitral leaflet

Supero-lateral papillary muscle

Coronary sinus

Mitral annular disjunction

Infero-medial papillary muscle

transilluminated. The free wall section involves mitral leaflets and both infero-medial and supero-lateral papillary muscles arising from the middle region of the left ventricle. The left and non-coronary aortic sinuses are observed. The trabeculations are extensive compared to the septal section.

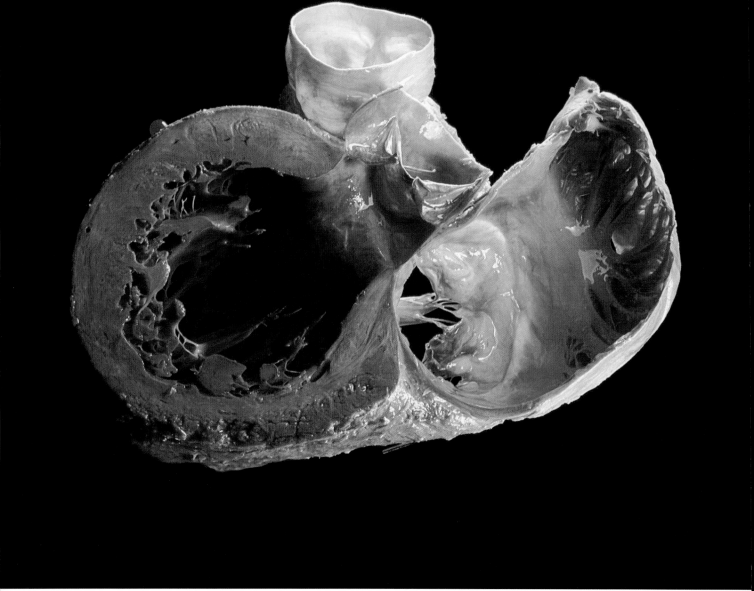

Figure 122 The frontal section of the heart viewed from the posterior direction.[1]

The heart is viewed from the posterior direction. Both papillary muscles are related to the left ventricular free wall, being located in vertical fashion. Left ventricular trabeculations are prominent in the lateral free wall rather than the septal endocardial surface. The infero-septal process of the left ventricle[4] faces to the right atrium intervened by the inferior pyramidal space.[5] The atrioventricular portion of the membranous septum tilts toward the right atrium along with the tilting of the

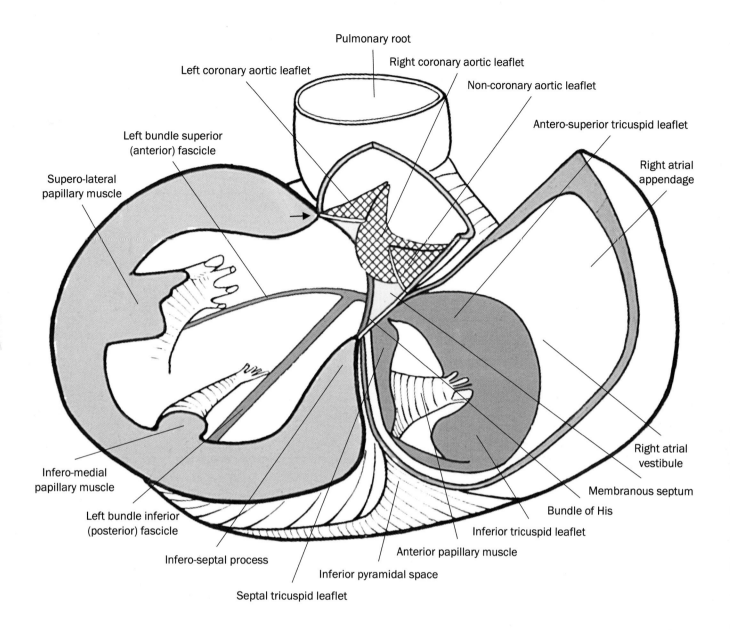

Pulmonary root

Left coronary aortic leaflet

Right coronary aortic leaflet

Non-coronary aortic leaflet

Antero-superior tricuspid leaflet

Left bundle superior
(anterior) fascicle

Right atrial
appendage

Supero-lateral
papillary muscle

Infero-medial
papillary muscle

Right atrial
vestibule

Membranous septum

Left bundle inferior
(posterior) fascicle

Bundle of His

Inferior tricuspid leaflet

Infero-septal process

Anterior papillary muscle

Inferior pyramidal space

Septal tricuspid leaflet

aortic root. This angulation is where the His catheter is fixed,[6] corresponding to the location of the penetrating bundle, the bundle of His.[7] The basal superior left ventricular muscle supports the left coronary aortic sinus. The width of the myocardium directly supporting the left coronary aortic sinus (black arrow), corresponding to the myocardial crescent, is thin.[8] The paired section of this image is Figure 30.

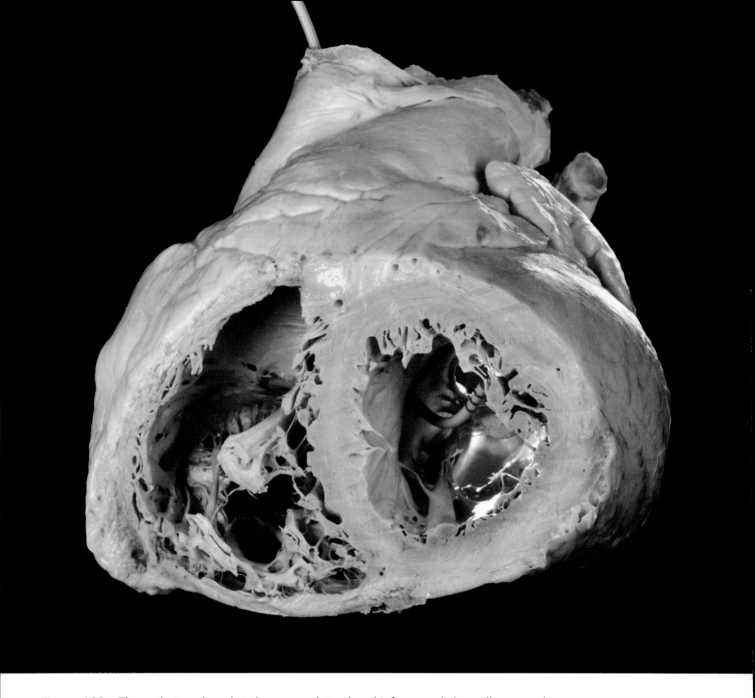

Figure 123   The catheter placed at the supero-lateral and infero-medial papillary muscles.

The heart is sectioned at the mid-ventricular level and viewed from the left anterior oblique direction. The catheter is placed at the supero-lateral (left) and infero-medial (right) papillary muscles using the transaortic retrograde approach.

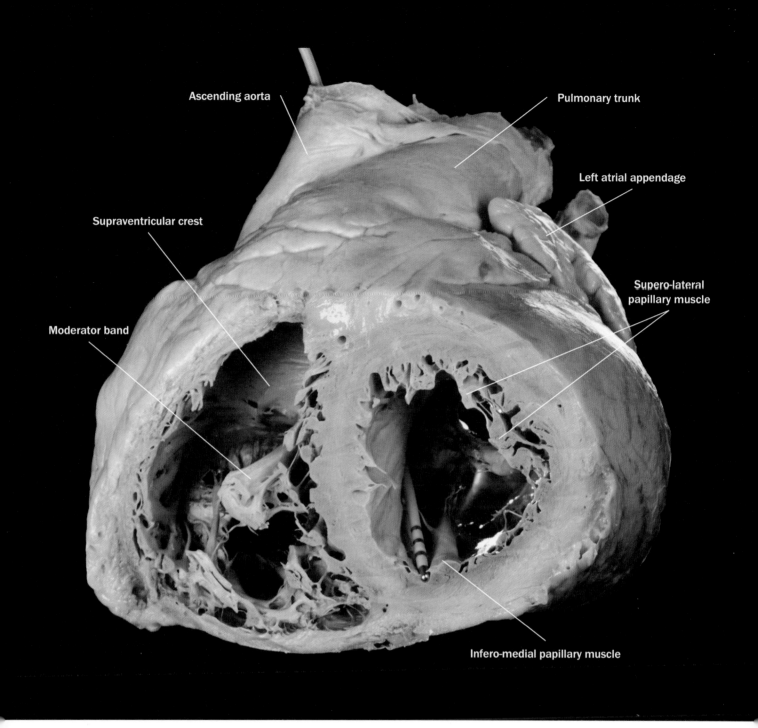

Ascending aorta

Pulmonary trunk

Left atrial appendage

Supraventricular crest

Supero-lateral
papillary muscle

Moderator band

Infero-medial papillary muscle

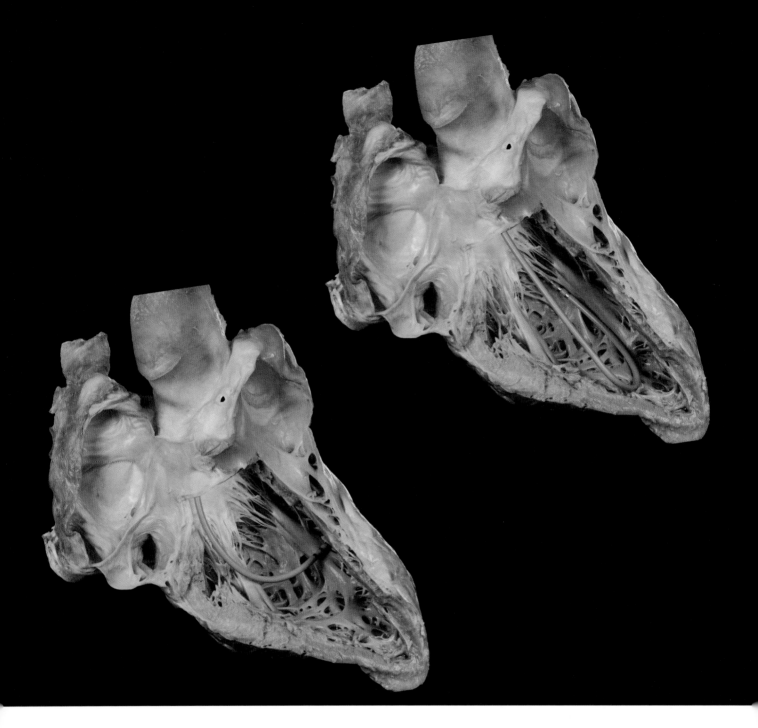

Figure 124 The catheter placed at the supero-lateral papillary muscle.

The heart is viewed from the right anterior oblique direction. The muscular ventricular septum is removed to observe the left ventricular free wall. The catheter is placed at the supero-lateral papillary muscle using the transaortic retrograde approach (lower left image on the left page), retrograde U-turn approach (upper image on the left page), and transseptal

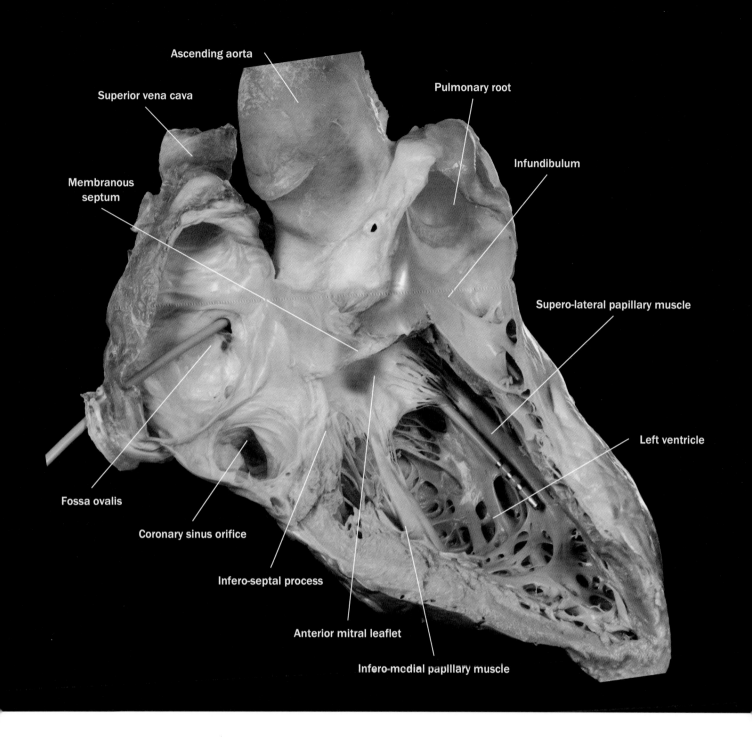

Ascending aorta

Superior vena cava

Pulmonary root

Infundibulum

Membranous
septum

Supero-lateral papillary muscle

Left ventricle

Fossa ovalis

Coronary sinus orifice

Infero-septal process

Anterior mitral leaflet

Infero-medial papillary muscle

antegrade approach (image on the right page). Note the parallel alignment to the supero-lateral papillary muscle is readily feasible using the antegrade approach, whereas the retrograde approach is not feasible unless the U-turn approach is used.

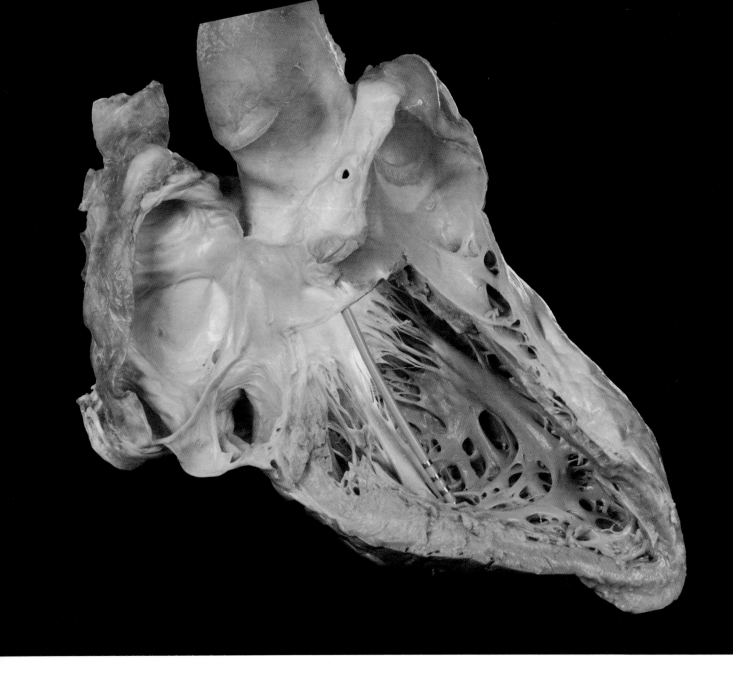

Figure 125 The catheter placed at the infero-medial papillary muscle.

The heart is viewed from the right anterior oblique direction. The muscular ventricular septum is removed to observe the left ventricular free wall. The catheter is placed at the infero-medial papillary muscle using the transaortic retrograde

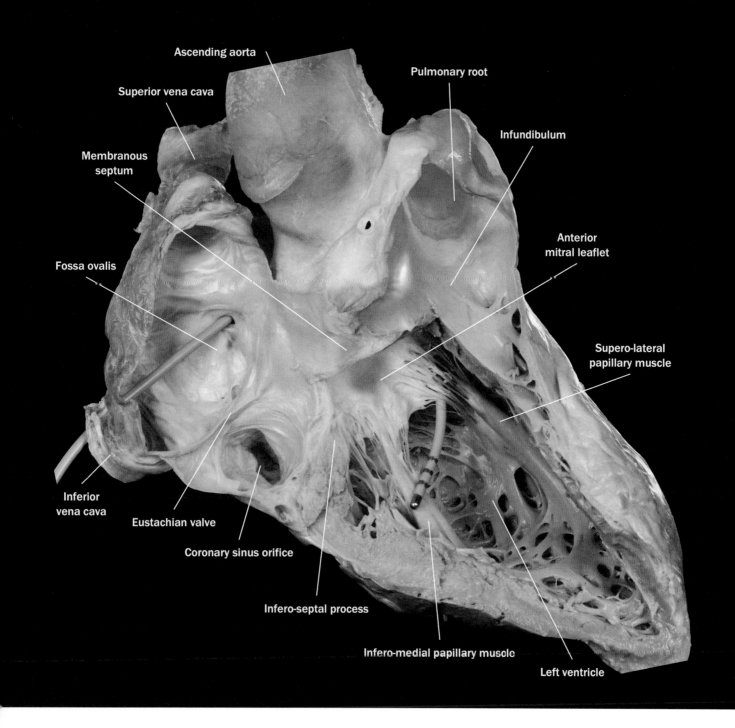

Ascending aorta

Superior vena cava

Pulmonary root

Infundibulum

Membranous
septum

Anterior
mitral leaflet

Fossa ovalis

Supero-lateral
papillary muscle

Inferior
vena cava

Eustachian valve

Coronary sinus orifice

Infero-septal process

Infero-medial papillary muscle

Left ventricle

approach (left) and transseptal antegrade approach (right). Note the parallel alignment to the infero-medial papillary muscle is readily feasible using the retrograde approach, whereas the antegrade approach is not.

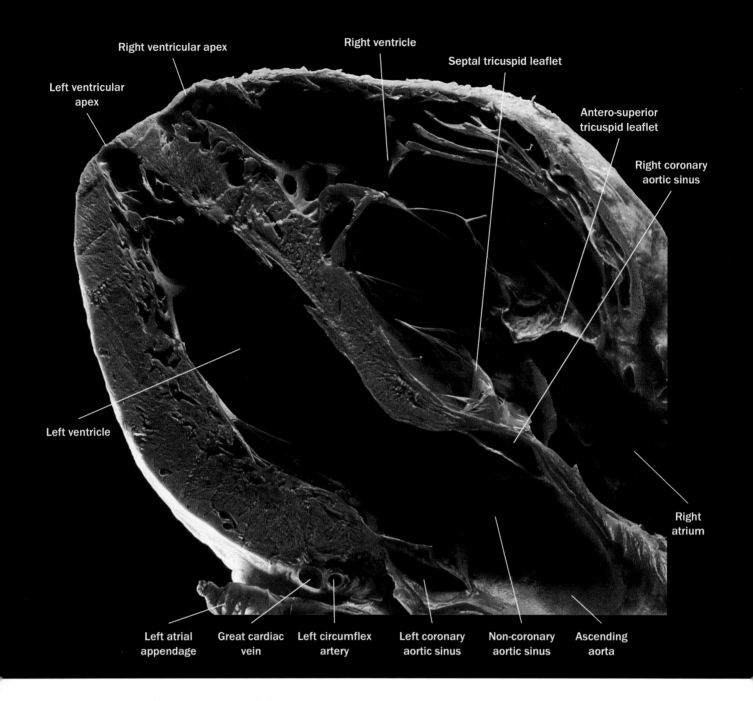

Left ventricular apex

Right ventricular apex

Right ventricle

Septal tricuspid leaflet

Antero-superior tricuspid leaflet

Right coronary aortic sinus

Left ventricle

Right atrium

Left atrial appendage

Great cardiac vein

Left circumflex artery

Left coronary aortic sinus

Non-coronary aortic sinus

Ascending aorta

Figure 126 The left ventricular apical thinning.[1]

The four-chamber cut section viewed from the superior direction (left) shows the physiological localized apical thinning of the left ventricle. When viewed from the apex (right), the clockwise vortex of the myocardial alignment is appreciated. A light source placed in the left ventricle transilluminates the localized apical thinning at the center of the vortex, lateral to

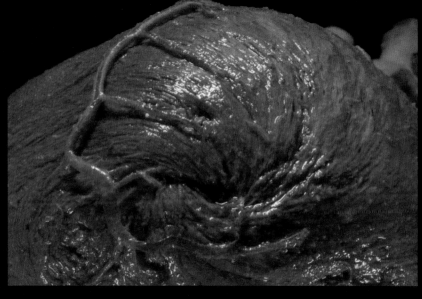

Left anterior descending artery

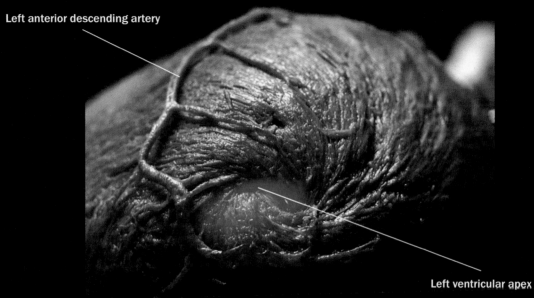

Left ventricular apex

the distal left anterior descending artery. This anatomy suggests the potential risk of apical perforation.[9] Generally, the apical thickness is less than 3.0 mm with average area of 5.0 mm^2,[10] equivalent to the cross-section area of 7.5-French catheter. Thin wall of the right ventricular apex is also appreciated.

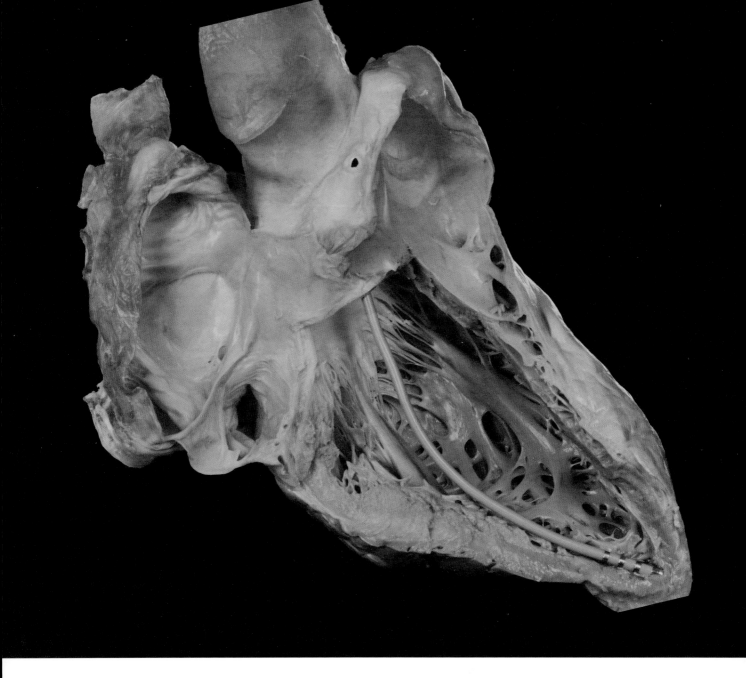

Figure 127   The catheter placed at the left ventricular apex.

The heart is viewed from the right anterior oblique direction. The muscular ventricular septum is removed to observe the left ventricular free wall. The catheter is placed at the left ventricular apex using the transaortic retrograde approach (left) and transseptal antegrade approach (right). When using the retrograde approach, the catheter runs along the infero-medial papillary muscle to reach the apex. Thus, the initial direction of the catheter toward the base of the infero-medial papillary

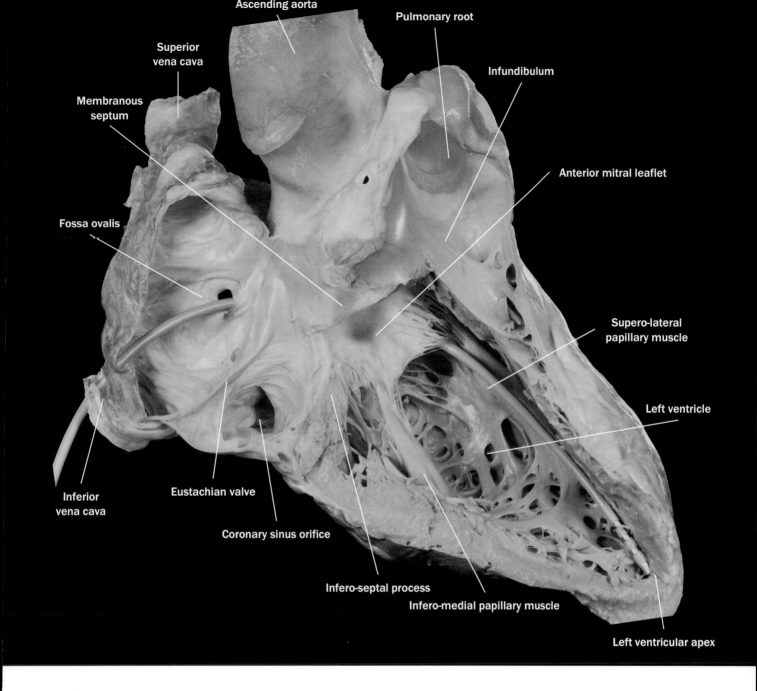

Ascending aorta

Pulmonary root

Superior
vena cava

Infundibulum

Membranous
septum

Anterior mitral leaflet

Fossa ovalis

Supero-lateral
papillary muscle

Left ventricle

Inferior
vena cava

Eustachian valve

Coronary sinus orifice

Infero-septal process

Infero-medial papillary muscle

Left ventricular apex

muscle corresponds to the mid-infero-lateral wall of the left ventricle. Therefore, during any procedures using bulky system via the retrograde approach, the brunt of rough and direct force increases the risk for harming this infero-lateral region. This is because of the physiological angulation created between the left ventricular axis and aortic axis, which are not parallel. When using the transseptal approach, the catheter runs along the supero-lateral papillary muscle to reach the apex.

References

1. McAlpine WA. Digitized collection of all the images created by Dr. McAlpine at UCLA. Copyright UCLA Cardiac Arrhythmia Center. Part of this collection appeared in *Heart and Coronary Arteries: An Anatomical Atlas for Clinical Diagnosis, Radiological Investigation, and Surgical Treatment.* New York: Springer-Verlag; 1975.

2. Mori S, Fukuzawa K, Takaya T, et al. Clinical cardiac structural anatomy reconstructed within the cardiac contour using multi-detector-row computed tomography: Left ventricular outflow tract. *Clin Anat.* 2016;29:353–363.

3. Mori S, Fukuzawa K, Takaya T, et al. Clinical cardiac structural anatomy reconstructed within the cardiac contour using multi-detector-row computed tomography: The arrangement and location of the cardiac valves. *Clin Anat.* 2016;29:364–370.

4. Li A, Zuberi Z, Bradfield JS, et al. Endocardial ablation of ventricular ectopic beats arising from the basal inferoseptal process of the left ventricle. *Heart Rhythm.* 2018;15:1356–1362.

5. Mori S, Nishii T, Takaya T, et al. Clinical structural anatomy of the inferior pyramidal space reconstructed from the living heart: Three-dimensional visualization using multidetector-row computed tomography. *Clin Anat.* 2015;28:878–887.

6. Mori S, Fukuzawa K, Takaya T, et al. Clinical structural anatomy of the Inferior pyramidal space reconstructed within the cardiac contour using multidetector-row computed tomography. *J Cardiovasc Electrophysiol.* 2015;26:705–712.

7. Anderson RH, Mori S. Wilhelm His Junior and his bundle. *J Electrocardiol.* 2016;49:637–643.

8. Toh H, Mori S, Tretter JT, et al. Living anatomy of the ventricular myocardial crescents supporting the coronary aortic sinuses. *Semin Thorac Cardiovasc Surg.* 2020;32:230–241.

9. Foerst J. Percutaneous repair of left ventricular wire perforation complicating transcatheter aortic valve replacement for aortic regurgitation. *JACC Cardiovasc Interv.* 2016;9:1410–1411.

10. Yamamoto K, Mori S, Fukuzawa K, et al. Revisiting the prevalence and diversity of localized thinning of the left ventricular apex. *J Cardiovasc Electrophysiol.* 2020;31:915–920.

19

Left Ventricular Outflow Tract

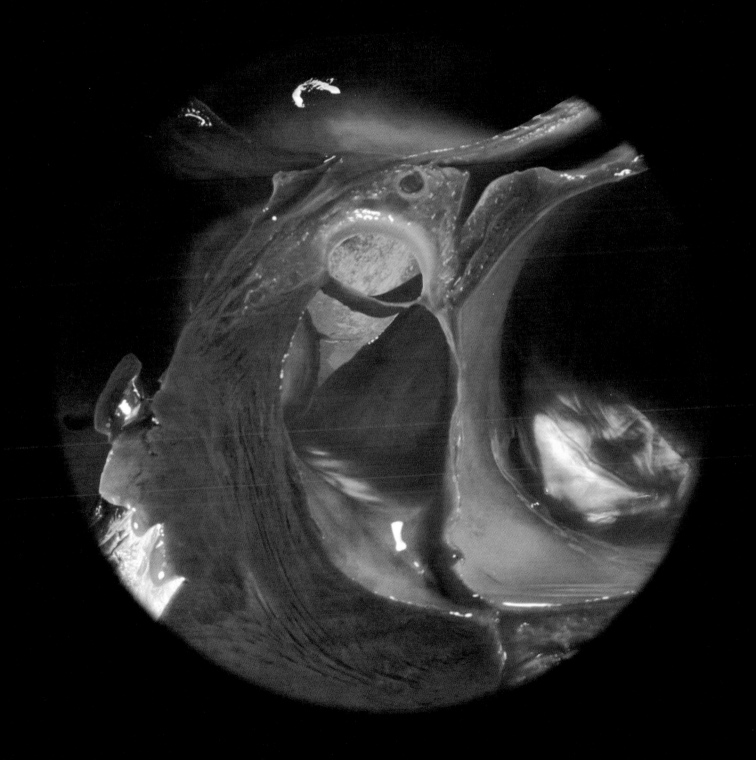

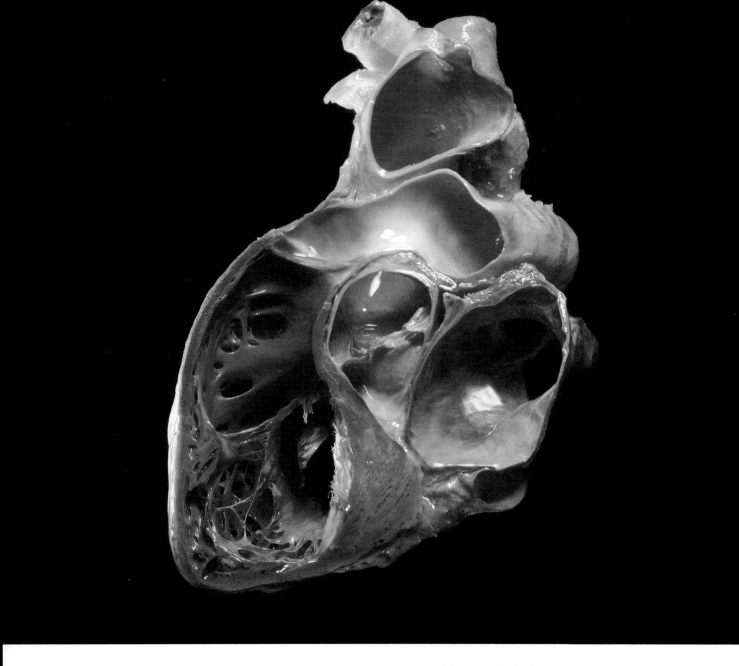

Figure 128　Sagittal section of the left ventricular outflow tract viewed from the left direction.[1]

In contrast to the right ventricular outflow tract that is uniformly encircled by the ventricular muscle, the component of the left ventricular outflow tract is not uniform.[2] Two-fifths of the circumference of the virtual basal ring is composed of the myocardial support, whereas the rest component is composed of fibrous support.[3] The muscular support involves the crest of the ventricular septum and free wall. The crest of the ventricular septum supports the right coronary aortic sinus, and the free wall supports the anterior half of the left coronary aortic sinus. The fibrous support involves the membranous septum, right fibrous trigone, aortic-to-mitral (aortomitral) continuity, and left fibrous trigone. In this section, the medial part of the left ventricular outflow tract is observed. The reversed, triangular-shaped left ventricular outflow tract is

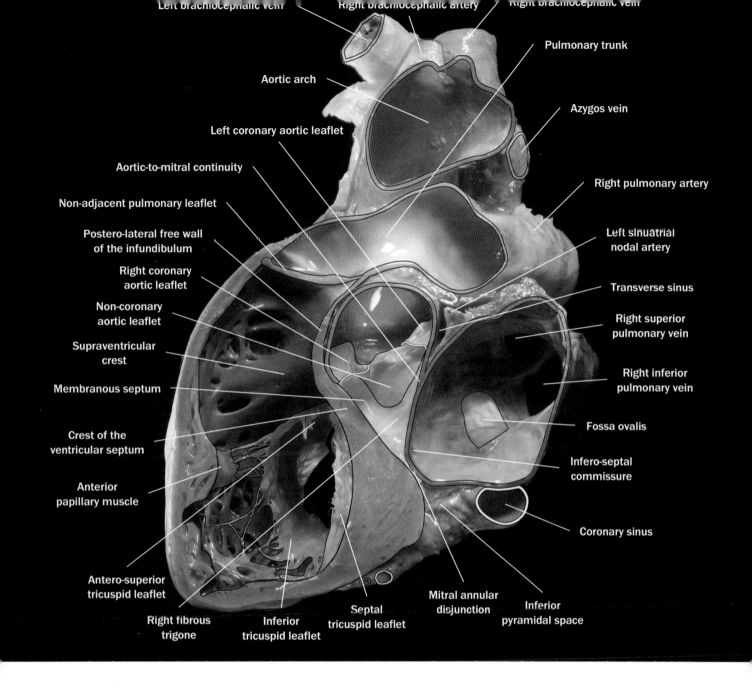

Left brachiocephalic vein
Right brachiocephalic artery
Right brachiocephalic vein
Pulmonary trunk
Aortic arch
Azygos vein
Left coronary aortic leaflet
Right pulmonary artery
Aortic-to-mitral continuity
Left sinuatrial nodal artery
Non-adjacent pulmonary leaflet
Postero-lateral free wall of the infundibulum
Transverse sinus
Right coronary aortic leaflet
Right superior pulmonary vein
Non-coronary aortic leaflet
Supraventricular crest
Right inferior pulmonary vein
Membranous septum
Fossa ovalis
Crest of the ventricular septum
Infero-septal commissure
Anterior papillary muscle
Coronary sinus
Antero-superior tricuspid leaflet
Right fibrous trigone
Inferior tricuspid leaflet
Septal tricuspid leaflet
Mitral annular disjunction
Inferior pyramidal space

observed. This anatomy is also referred to as the infero-septal recess, demarcated by the crest of the ventricular septum anteriorly, membranous septum and right fibrous trigone (central fibrous body) medially, and aortic-to-mitral continuity posteriorly. The infero-septal commissure of the mitral valve is located at the inferior apex of this infero-septal recess. The postero-lateral free wall of the right ventricular outflow tract, corresponding to the supraventricular crest, lies anterior to the right coronary aortic sinus. The primary septum at the floor of the fossa ovalis is transilluminated. The paired section of this image is Figure 76.

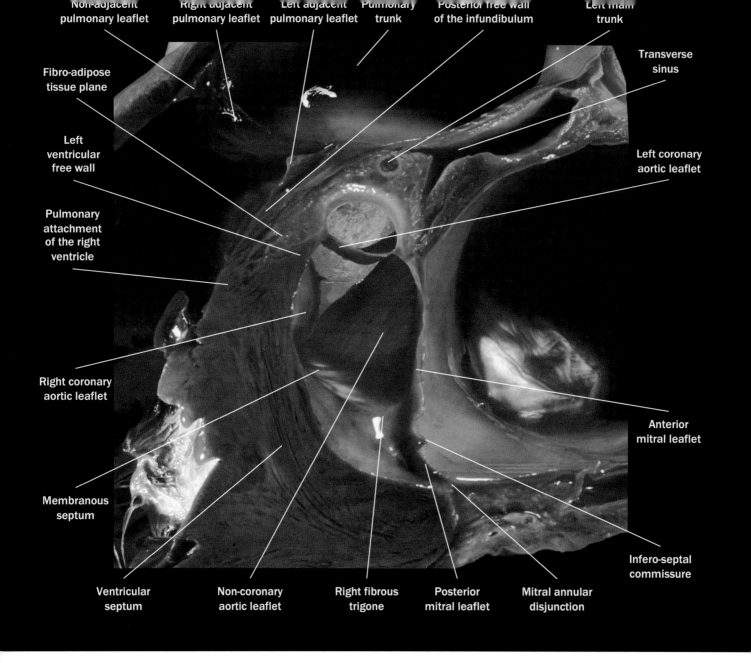

Non-adjacent pulmonary leaflet | Right adjacent pulmonary leaflet | Left adjacent pulmonary leaflet | Pulmonary trunk | Posterior free wall of the infundibulum | Left main trunk

Transverse sinus

Fibro-adipose tissue plane

Left coronary aortic leaflet

Left ventricular free wall

Pulmonary attachment of the right ventricle

Right coronary aortic leaflet

Anterior mitral leaflet

Membranous septum

Infero-septal commissure

Ventricular septum | Non-coronary aortic leaflet | Right fibrous trigone | Posterior mitral leaflet | Mitral annular disjunction

Figure 129   Sagittal sections of the left ventricular outflow tract.[1]

The bisected heart is viewed from the right (left) and left (right) directions. In this section, the left ventricular outflow tract is not a circular-shaped space, demarcated by the left coronary aortic leaflet superior, the left ventricular free wall supporting the left coronary aortic sinus antero-superior, ventricular septum anterior, membranous septum, right fibrous trigone (central fibrous body) medial (right), and aortic-to-mitral (aortomitral) continuity/anterior mitral leaflet posterior. Note the beak-shaped, thin myocardium of the basal superior left ventricular free wall supporting the left coronary aortic sinus.[3] During systole, due to the consequence of the systolic bulging of the aortic-to-mitral continuity, the shape of the left ventricular outflow tract becomes more circular than during diastole.[4] In the left image, the aortic root, the membranous septum, and

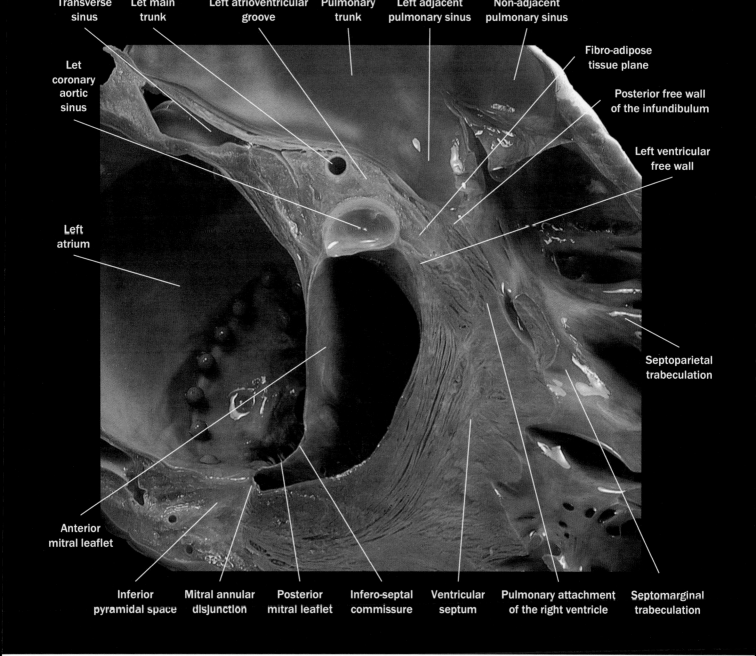

Transverse sinus | Let main trunk | Left atrioventricular groove | Pulmonary trunk | Left adjacent pulmonary sinus | Non-adjacent pulmonary sinus

Fibro-adipose tissue plane

Posterior free wall of the infundibulum

Left ventricular free wall

Let coronary aortic sinus

Left atrium

Septoparietal trabeculation

Anterior mitral leaflet

Inferior pyramidal space | Mitral annular disjunction | Posterior mitral leaflet | Infero-septal commissure | Ventricular septum | Pulmonary attachment of the right ventricle | Septomarginal trabeculation

the primary septum at the floor of the fossa ovalis are transilluminated. The membranous septum is the medial partition of the distal left ventricular outflow tract. The mitral annular disjunction is observed at the attachment of medial (P3) scallop.[5] The posterior free wall of the right ventricular outflow tract starts to separate from the left ventricle anterior to the left coronary aortic sinus. Therefore, the fibro-adipose tissue plane on the left ventricular summit separates the left ventricular free wall from the posterior free wall of the right ventricular outflow tract. The pulmonary root, specifically the left adjacent pulmonary sinus, overrides the left coronary aortic sinus. The pulmonary trunk then lies superior to the left main trunk of the left coronary artery. Refer to Figures 87 and 100.

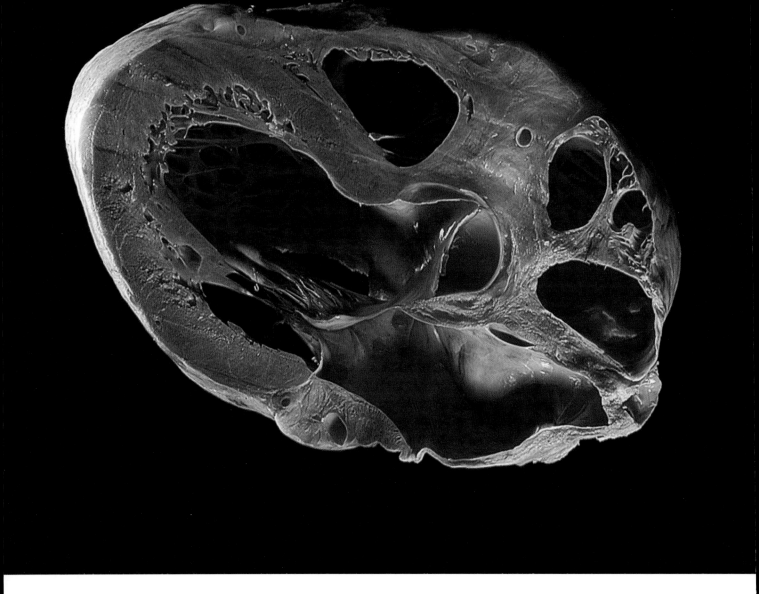

Figure 130 The horizontal plane at the level of the left ventricular outflow tract viewed from the superior direction.[1]

The posterior (lateral) and anterior (septal) wall of the left ventricular outflow tract is demarcated by the anterior mitral leaflet and crest of the ventricular septum, respectively. The left ventricular outflow tract is located posterior to the right ventricular outflow tract. No discrete structure can be defined at the bottom of the left ventricular outflow tract. It is wide open toward the basal infero-septum—in other words, the infero-septal process of the left ventricle. The interleaflet triangle between the right and non-coronary aortic sinuses is a part of the aortic root, but it is hemodynamically part of the left

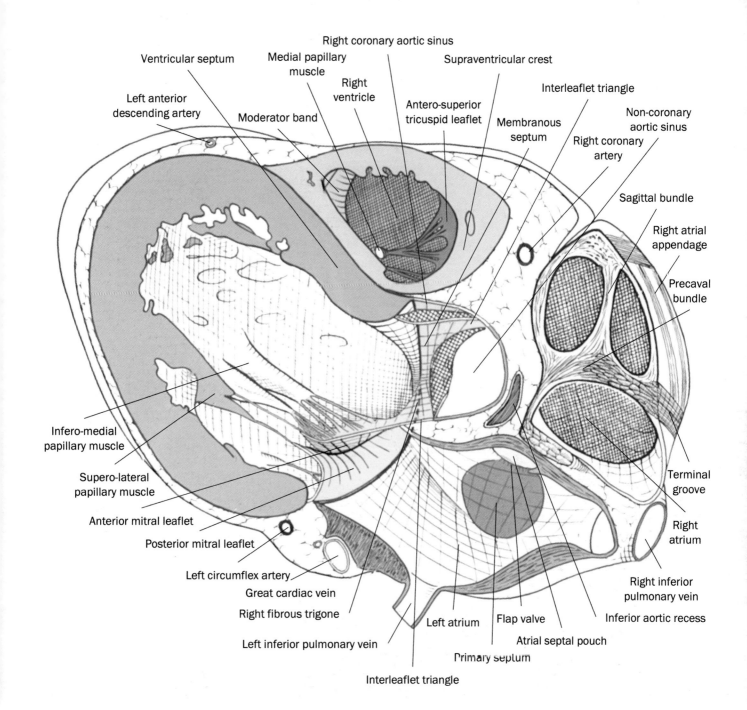

Right coronary aortic sinus

Ventricular septum

Medial papillary muscle

Supraventricular crest

Left anterior descending artery

Right ventricle

Interleaflet triangle

Moderator band

Antero-superior tricuspid leaflet

Non-coronary aortic sinus

Membranous septum

Right coronary artery

Sagittal bundle

Right atrial appendage

Precaval bundle

Infero-medial papillary muscle

Supero-lateral papillary muscle

Terminal groove

Anterior mitral leaflet

Right atrium

Posterior mitral leaflet

Left circumflex artery

Right inferior pulmonary vein

Great cardiac vein

Right fibrous trigone

Left atrium

Flap valve

Inferior aortic recess

Left inferior pulmonary vein

Atrial septal pouch

Primary septum

Interleaflet triangle

ventricular outflow tract.[6] The left ventricular outflow tract is angled relative to the left ventricular longitudinal axis. The difference in the distance from the left inferior pulmonary vein to the lateral mitral annulus and the distance from the right inferior pulmonary vein to the medial mitral annulus is remarkable. The flap valve of the primary septum and atrial septal pouch is observed at the atrial septum. Note the superior part of the right atrial appendage is divided into basal and apical rooms by the sagittal bundle.[7] The paired section of this image is Figure 131.

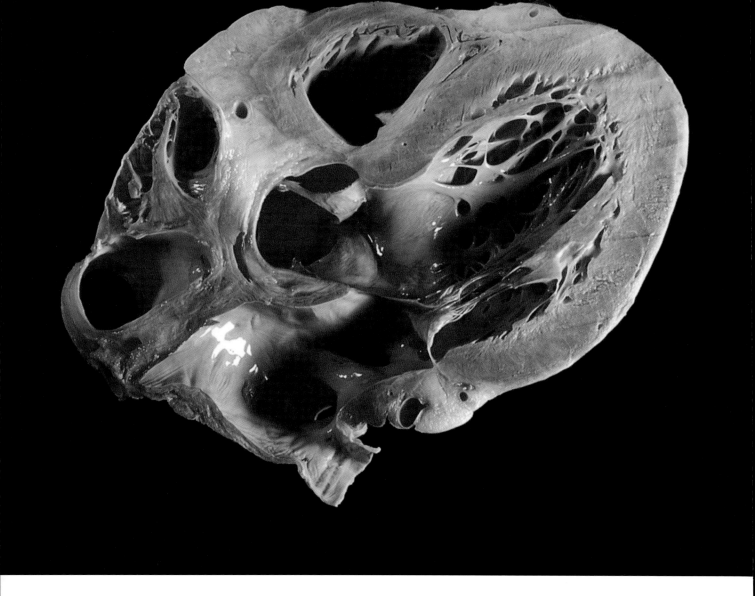

Figure 131 The horizontal plane at the level of the left ventricular outflow tract viewed from the inferior direction.[1]

The posterior (lateral) and anterior (septal) wall of the left ventricular outflow tract is demarcated by the anterior mitral leaflet and the crest of the ventricular septum, respectively. The left ventricular outflow tract is located posterior to the right ventricular outflow tract. The medial and superior roof of the left ventricular outflow tract is the crest of the ventricular

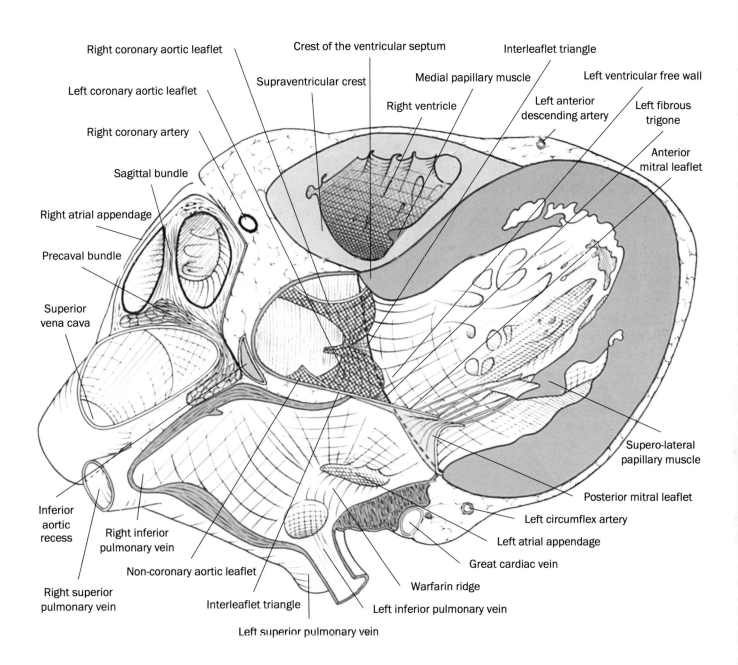

Right coronary aortic leaflet

Left coronary aortic leaflet

Right coronary artery

Sagittal bundle

Right atrial appendage

Precaval bundle

Superior vena cava

Inferior aortic recess

Right superior pulmonary vein

Right inferior pulmonary vein

Non-coronary aortic leaflet

Interleaflet triangle

Left superior pulmonary vein

Crest of the ventricular septum

Supraventricular crest

Right ventricle

Medial papillary muscle

Interleaflet triangle

Left ventricular free wall

Left anterior descending artery

Left fibrous trigone

Anterior mitral leaflet

Supero-lateral papillary muscle

Posterior mitral leaflet

Left circumflex artery

Left atrial appendage

Great cardiac vein

Warfarin ridge

Left inferior pulmonary vein

septum supporting the right coronary aortic sinus and left ventricular free wall supporting the left coronary aortic sinus, respectively. The interleaflet triangle between the left and right coronary aortic sinuses is a part of the aortic root, but it is hemodynamically part of the left ventricular outflow tract.[2] The paired section of this image is Figure 130.

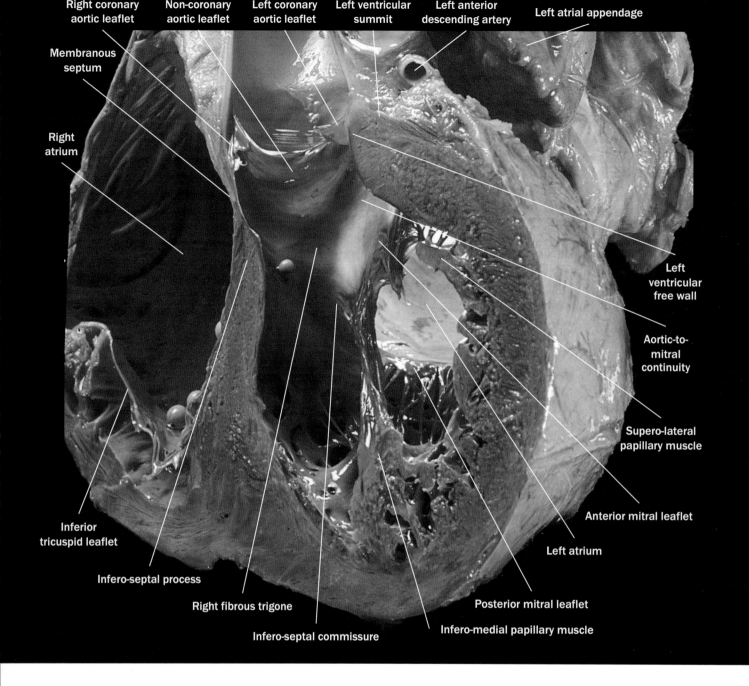

Right coronary aortic leaflet

Non-coronary aortic leaflet

Left coronary aortic leaflet

Left ventricular summit

Left anterior descending artery

Left atrial appendage

Membranous septum

Right atrium

Left ventricular free wall

Aortic-to-mitral continuity

Supero-lateral papillary muscle

Anterior mitral leaflet

Left atrium

Inferior tricuspid leaflet

Infero-septal process

Right fibrous trigone

Infero-septal commissure

Posterior mitral leaflet

Infero-medial papillary muscle

Figure 132 The anterior mitral leaflet and its relationship to the left ventricular outflow tract viewed from the left anterior oblique direction.[1]

In this section, the left ventricular outflow is the surrounded by the left ventricular free wall (supero-lateral side), aortic-to-mitral (aortomitral) continuity/anterior mitral leaflet (lateral side), right fibrous trigone (basal side), atrioventricular portion of the membranous septum and infero-septal process of the basal medial left ventricle[8] facing to the right atrium (medial side). The bottom of the left ventricular outflow tract is wide open to the base of the infero-septal process. The right fibrous trigone is the fibrous tissue supporting the medial part of the anterior mitral leaflet, between the nadir of the non-coronary aortic sinus and the infero-septal commissure. As seen in this image, three-dimensional shape of the left ventricular outflow tract is not a simple tube and not consistent throughout the cardiac cycle. The rest of the free wall (superior side) and crest of the ventricular septum and interventricular portion of the membranous septum (medial to supero-medial side) are necessary to close this left ventricular outflow tract.

References

1. McAlpine WA. Digitized collection of all the images created by Dr. McAlpine at UCLA. Copyright UCLA Cardiac Arrhythmia Center. Part of this collection appeared in *Heart and Coronary Arteries: An Anatomical Atlas for Clinical Diagnosis, Radiological Investigation, and Surgical Treatment*. New York: Springer-Verlag; 1975.

2. Mori S, Fukuzawa K, Takaya T, et al. Clinical cardiac structural anatomy reconstructed within the cardiac contour using multi-detector-row computed tomography: Left ventricular outflow tract. *Clin Anat*. 2016;29:353–363.

3. Toh H, Mori S, Tretter JT, et al. Living anatomy of the ventricular myocardial crescents supporting the coronary aortic sinuses. *Semin Thorac Cardiovasc Surg*. 2020;32:230–241.

4. Suchá D, Tuncay V, Prakken NH, et al. Does the aortic annulus undergo conformational change throughout the cardiac cycle? A systematic review. *Eur Heart J Cardiovasc Imaging*. 2015;16:1307–1317.

5. Toh H, Mori S, Izawa Y, et al. Prevalence and extent of mitral annular disjunction in structurally normal hearts: Comprehensive 3D analysis using cardiac computed tomography. *Eur Heart J Cardiovasc Imaging*. 2021;22:614–622.

6. Mori S, Fukuzawa K, Takaya T, et al. Optimal angulations for obtaining an *en face* view of each coronary aortic sinus and the interventricular septum: Correlative anatomy around the left ventricular outflow tract. *Clin Anat*. 2015;28:494–505.

7. Igawa O. Focus on the atrial structure: Useful anatomical information for catheter ablation. *J Arrhythm*. 2011;27:268–288.

8. Li A, Zuberi Z, Bradfield JS, et al. Endocardial ablation of ventricular ectopic beats arising from the basal inferoseptal process of the left ventricle. *Heart Rhythm*. 2018;15:1356–1362.

20

Aortic Valve

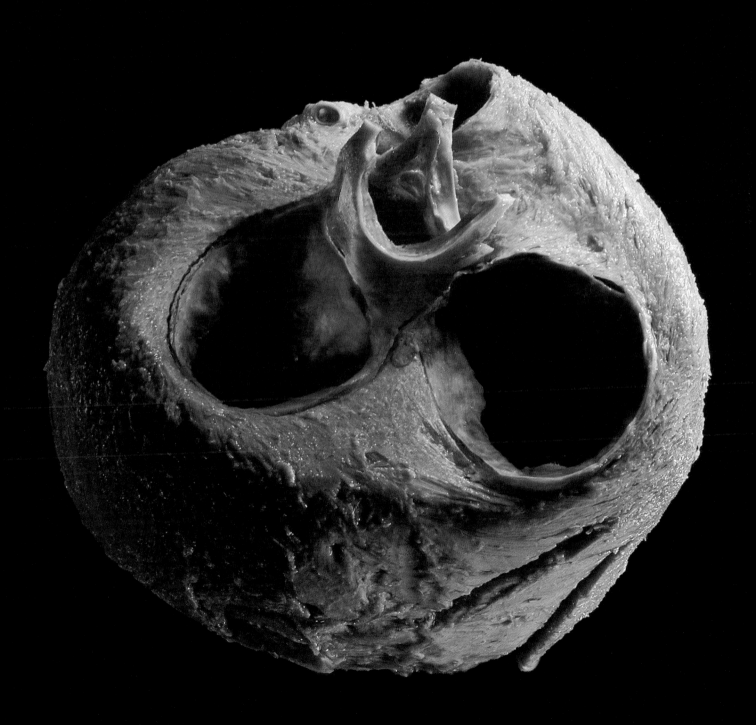

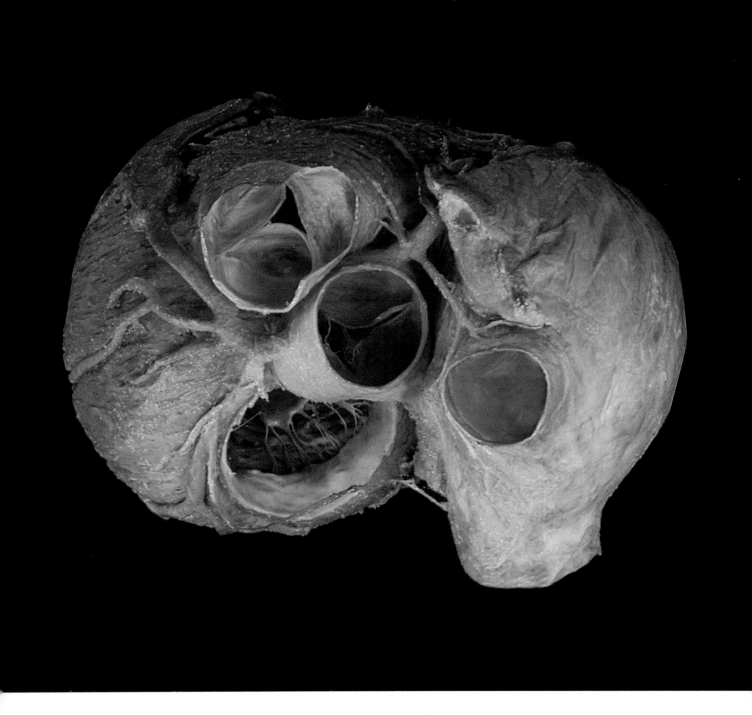

Figure 133 The structural relationship surrounding the aortic root.[1]

The heart is viewed from the superior direction. The aortic root wedges into the superior crux of the heart between the bilateral atrioventricular junctions. The aortic root directs toward the right antero-superior direction, whereas the pulmonary root directs toward the postero-superior direction. The pulmonary root is located left antero-superior to the aortic root. The right atrial appendage is located right anterior to the aortic root, covering the right atrioventricular groove involving the right coronary artery. The superior vena cava is located right posterior to the aortic root.[2] The left atrium is located posterior to the aortic root. The right coronary aortic leaflet is located anterior, whereas the left and non-coronary aortic leaflets are located left posterior and right posterior, respectively. The postero-lateral free wall of the right ventricular outflow tract (infundibulum) is located anterior to the right coronary aortic sinus. The apex of the interleaflet triangle between the right and left coronary aortic sinuses is adjacent to the apex of the interleaflet triangle between the right and left adjacent pulmonary sinuses. The myocardium supporting the anterior half of the left coronary

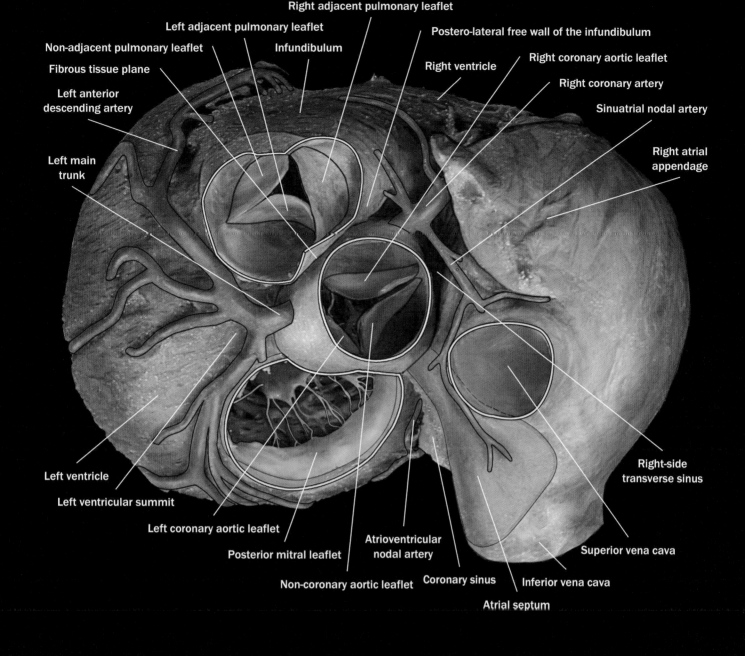

Right adjacent pulmonary leaflet

Left adjacent pulmonary leaflet

Non-adjacent pulmonary leaflet

Fibrous tissue plane

Left anterior descending artery

Left main trunk

Infundibulum

Postero-lateral free wall of the infundibulum

Right ventricle

Right coronary aortic leaflet

Right coronary artery

Sinuatrial nodal artery

Right atrial appendage

Left ventricle

Left ventricular summit

Left coronary aortic leaflet

Posterior mitral leaflet

Atrioventricular nodal artery

Non-coronary aortic leaflet

Coronary sinus

Inferior vena cava

Atrial septum

Superior vena cava

Right-side transverse sinus

aortic sinus is the basal superior left ventricular free wall, the epicardial side of which is referred to as the left ventricular summit,[1,3] carrying the proximal left coronary artery on it. The posterior half of the non-coronary aortic sinus and posterior half of the left coronary aortic sinus are adjacent to the left atrium, and the anterior half of the non-coronary aortic sinus is adjacent to the right atrium. The interleaflet triangles between the right coronary and non-coronary aortic sinuses, non-coronary and left coronary aortic sinuses, and left and right coronary aortic sinuses face to the right-side transverse sinus medial to the right atrial appendage, the transverse sinus, and the fibrous tissue plane between the aortic and pulmonary root, respectively. Thus, all of the interleaflet triangle is facing toward the extracardiac plane.[4] Against the central axis of the aortic root, the orifices of the both coronary arteries are not located opposite each other, but they are located approximately 150 degrees apart on average.[5]

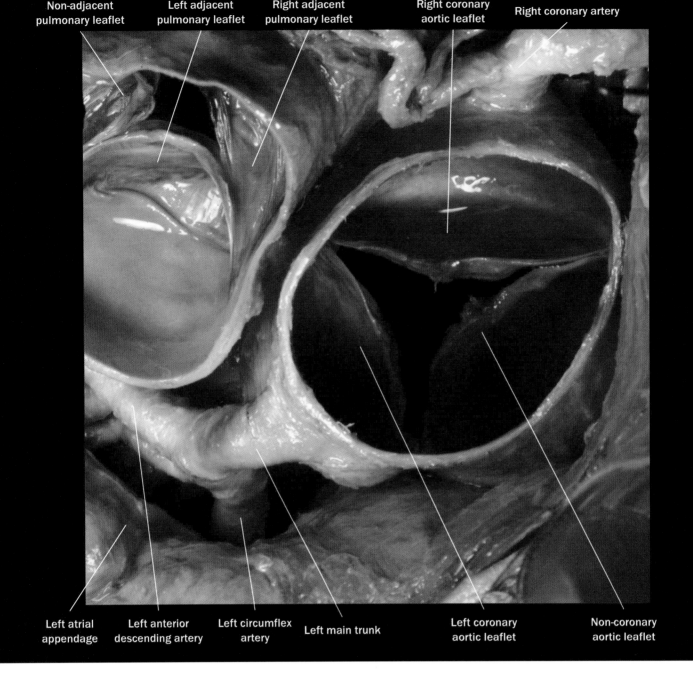

Non-adjacent pulmonary leaflet

Left adjacent pulmonary leaflet

Right adjacent pulmonary leaflet

Right coronary aortic leaflet

Right coronary artery

Left atrial appendage

Left anterior descending artery

Left circumflex artery

Left main trunk

Left coronary aortic leaflet

Non-coronary aortic leaflet

Figure 134   The *en face* view of the aortic valvular orifice and non-coronary aortic sinus/leaflet.[1]

The heart is viewed from the right antero-superior direction (left). The pulmonary valve is not on the same plane with the aortic valve. Its orifice tilts posterior relative to the orifice of the aortic valve. The right image is the *en face* endocardial view of the non-coronary aortic leaflet. The commissures are located at the level of the sinutubular junction plane. On the

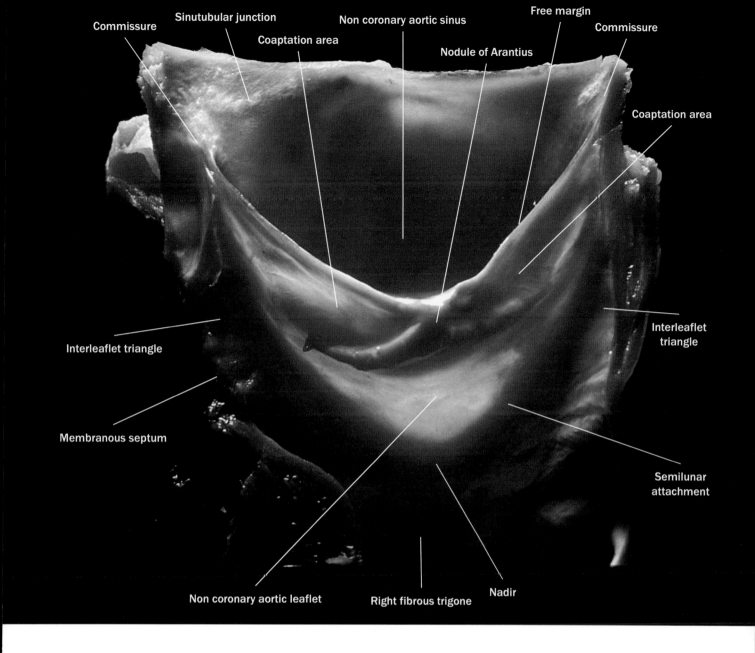

Commissure · Sinutubular junction · Coaptation area · Non coronary aortic sinus · Free margin · Commissure

Nodule of Arantius · Coaptation area

Interleaflet triangle · Interleaflet triangle

Membranous septum · Semilunar attachment

Non coronary aortic leaflet · Right fibrous trigone · Nadir

contrary, the central zone of coaptation is lower than the plane of the sinutubular junction,[6] approximately at half of its height.[7] Each leaflet has semilunar attachment to the aortic root, creating the interleaflet triangle between each sinus.[8] The nodule of Arantius is found at the central zone of coaptation.

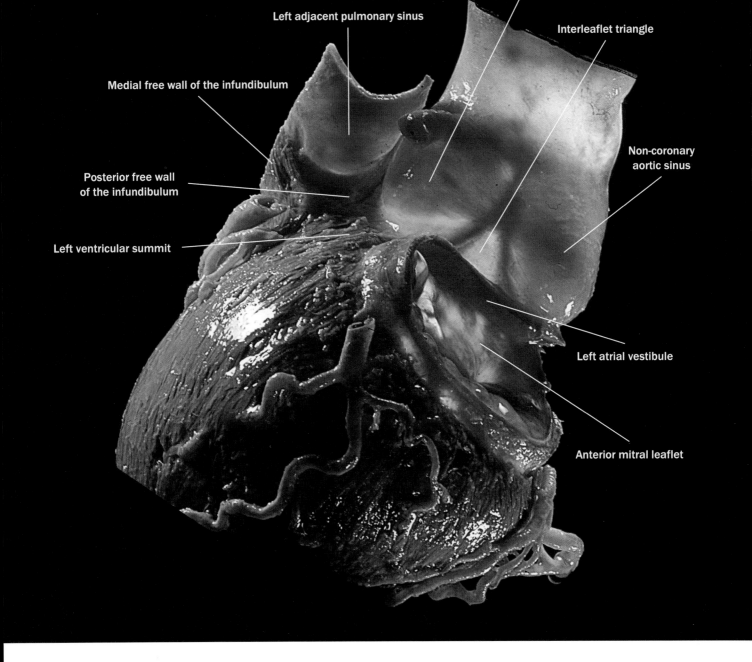

Left adjacent pulmonary sinus

Interleaflet triangle

Medial free wall of the infundibulum

Non-coronary aortic sinus

Posterior free wall of the infundibulum

Left ventricular summit

Left atrial vestibule

Anterior mitral leaflet

Figure 135   The posterior view of the aortic root.[1]

The interleaflet triangle between the non-coronary and left coronary aortic sinuses is in continuity with the anterior mitral leaflet, divided by the attachment of the left atrial anterior wall. This triangle faces to the transverse sinus. The posterior free wall of the right ventricular outflow tract (infundibulum) starts to separate from the left ventricle anterior to the left coronary aortic sinus (left). Then, the pulmonary root/trunk overrides the left coronary aortic sinus and the proximal left

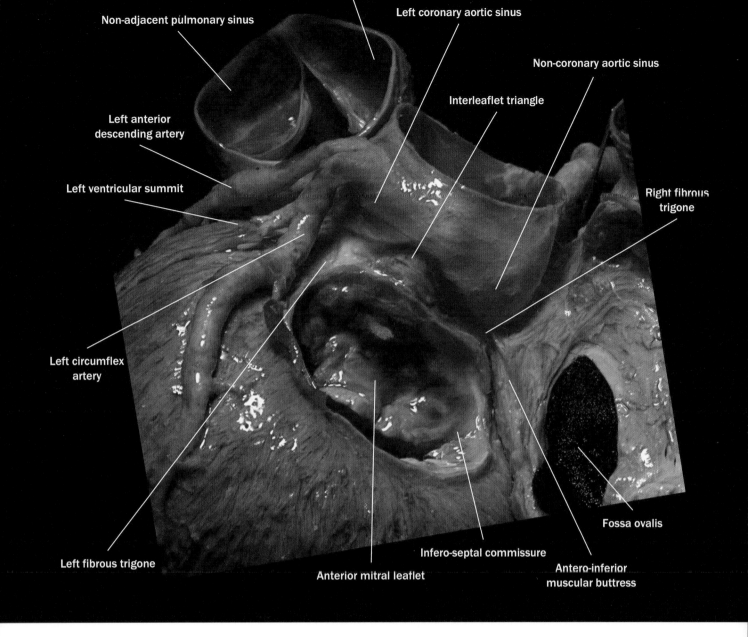

Non-adjacent pulmonary sinus

Left coronary aortic sinus

Non-coronary aortic sinus

Left anterior
descending artery

Interleaflet triangle

Left ventricular summit

Right fibrous
trigone

Left circumflex
artery

Left fibrous trigone

Fossa ovalis

Infero-septal commissure

Anterior mitral leaflet

Antero-inferior
muscular buttress

coronary artery. The left ventricular free wall myocardium supports the anterior half of the left coronary aortic sinus.[4] The epicardial side of this region corresponds to the left ventricular summit.[1,9] The pulmonary valve is not on the same plane with the aortic valve (right). The pulmonary root is located left antero-superior to the aortic root and tilts posterior relative to the aortic root.

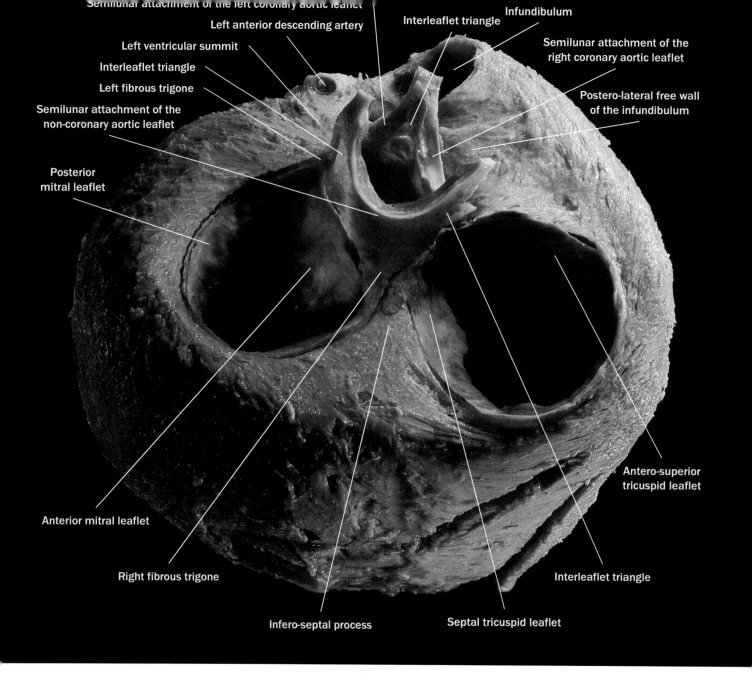

Semilunar attachment of the left coronary aortic leaflet
Left anterior descending artery
Left ventricular summit
Interleaflet triangle
Left fibrous trigone
Semilunar attachment of the non-coronary aortic leaflet
Posterior mitral leaflet
Anterior mitral leaflet
Right fibrous trigone
Infero-septal process

Infundibulum
Interleaflet triangle
Semilunar attachment of the right coronary aortic leaflet
Postero-lateral free wall of the infundibulum
Antero-superior tricuspid leaflet
Interleaflet triangle
Septal tricuspid leaflet

Figure 136 Progressive dissection of the ventricular mass.[1]

The dissection shows the ventricular mass with the semilunar hingelines and interleaflet triangles (left). The aortic root is located central to the ventricular mass. In the right image, the aortic root, the mitral valve, and the membranous septum in the left image are removed to show the left ventricular ostium.[1,10] The left ventricular ostium is the anatomical concept involving the basal left ventricular myocardium[1] that surrounds inflow and outflow of the left ventricular cone. This dissection is feasible as there is no ventricular myocardium intervening between the mitral orifice and the left ventricular outflow tract. In contrast, in the right ventricle, the inflow and outflow tracts are separated by the infundibulum. The

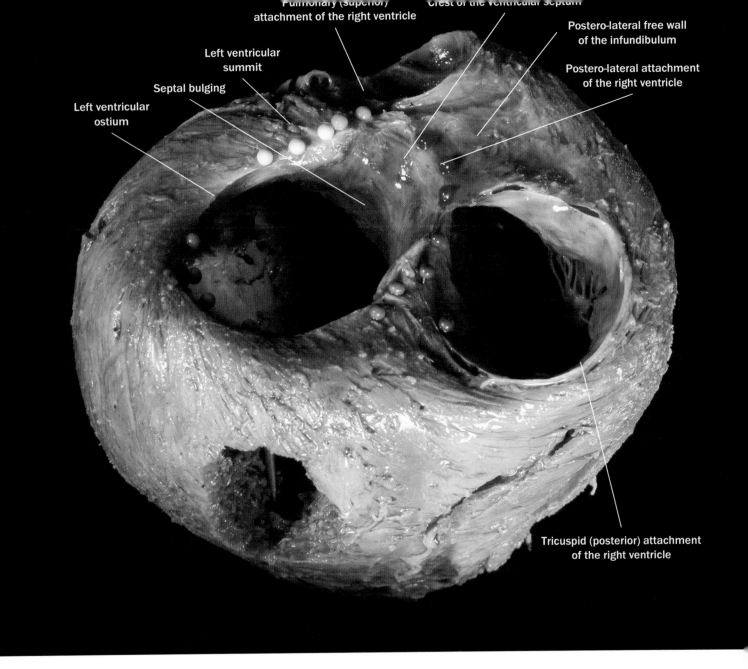

Pulmonary (superior)
attachment of the right ventricle

Crest of the ventricular septum

Postero-lateral free wall
of the infundibulum

Left ventricular
summit

Postero-lateral attachment
of the right ventricle

Septal bulging

Left ventricular
ostium

Tricuspid (posterior) attachment
of the right ventricle

yellow beads denote the left ventricular free wall supporting the left coronary aortic sinus. The red beads show the crest of the ventricular septum supporting the right coronary aortic sinus, which is extensive (14 mm) than the yellow beads (4 mm). The crest of the ventricular septum also supports the base of the membranous septum. Refer to Figure 85. White beads indicated the left fibrous trigone. The green beads are the septal attachment of the septal tricuspid leaflet. The blue beads are the location of the atrioventricular node. The membranous septum is located between the blue and red beads.[1]

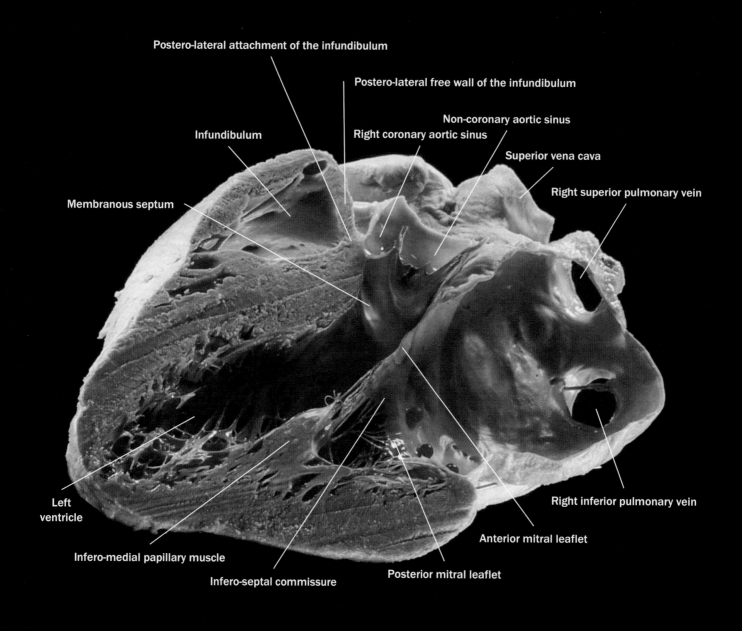

Postero-lateral attachment of the infundibulum

Postero-lateral free wall of the infundibulum

Non-coronary aortic sinus

Infundibulum

Right coronary aortic sinus

Superior vena cava

Right superior pulmonary vein

Membranous septum

Left
ventricle

Right inferior pulmonary vein

Infero-medial papillary muscle

Anterior mitral leaflet

Infero-septal commissure

Posterior mitral leaflet

Figure 137   The pair of the parasternal left ventricular long-axis sections.[1]

The left image corresponds to the parasternal long-axis section, and the right image is the paired section. The membranous septum and fossa ovalis in the left image, and the left atrial appendage in the right image are transilluminated. The aortic valve is bisected between the center of the right coronary aortic sinus and interleaflet triangle between the non-coronary and left coronary aortic sinuses.[11] This is the section that can bisect the anterior and posterior mitral leaflets. The crest of the ventricular septum supports the anterior base of the right coronary aortic sinus. This part corresponds to the

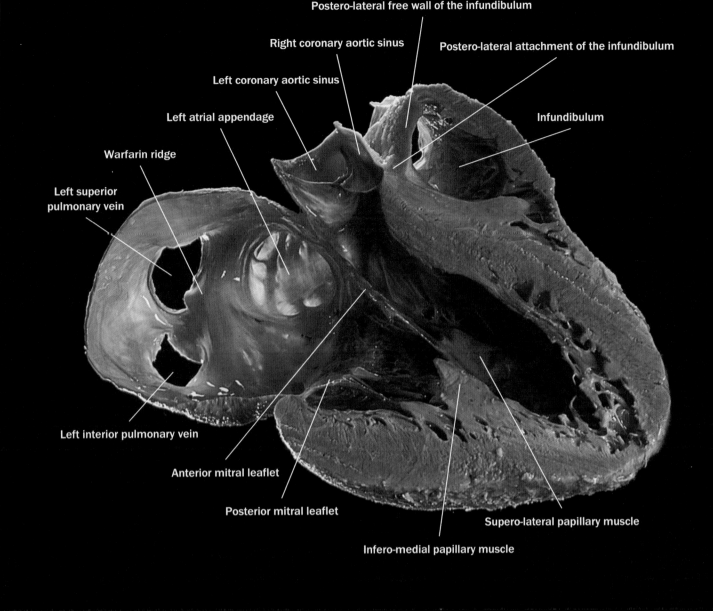

Postero-lateral free wall of the infundibulum

Right coronary aortic sinus

Postero-lateral attachment of the infundibulum

Left coronary aortic sinus

Left atrial appendage

Infundibulum

Warfarin ridge

Left superior
pulmonary vein

Left interior pulmonary vein

Anterior mitral leaflet

Posterior mitral leaflet

Supero-lateral papillary muscle

Infero-medial papillary muscle

postero-lateral attachment of the right ventricle, identical to the ventriculo-arterial junction at the right coronary aortic sinus. The ventriculo-arterial junction is the inferior limit of the postero-lateral free wall of the right ventricular outflow tract (infundibulum) located anterior to the right coronary aortic sinus. The membranous septum extends at the base of the right and non-coronary aortic sinuses. The relationship with the virtual basal ring and the membranous septum shows the individual variation.[12] Refer to Figures 101 and 102.

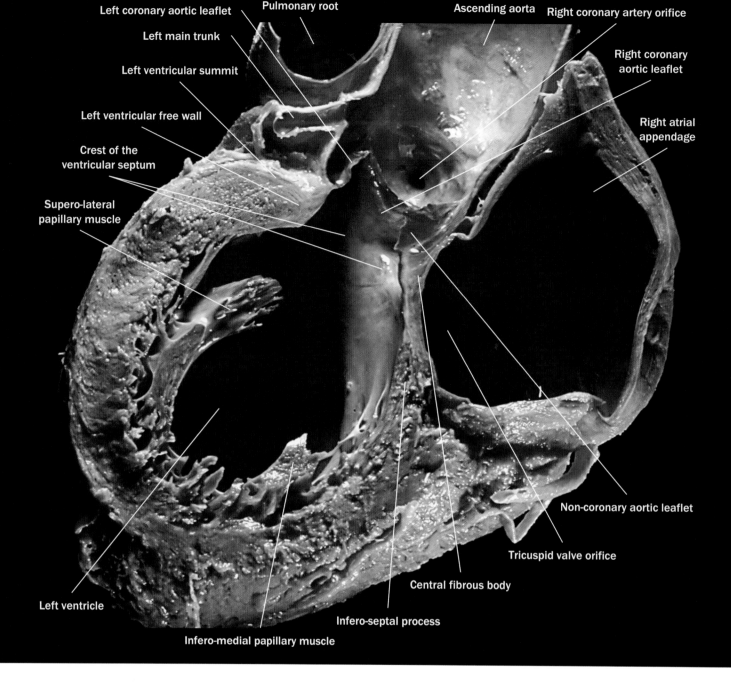

Left coronary aortic leaflet
Pulmonary root
Ascending aorta
Right coronary artery orifice
Left main trunk
Right coronary aortic leaflet
Left ventricular summit
Left ventricular free wall
Right atrial appendage
Crest of the ventricular septum
Supero-lateral papillary muscle
Non-coronary aortic leaflet
Tricuspid valve orifice
Central fibrous body
Left ventricle
Infero-septal process
Infero-medial papillary muscle

Figure 138 The pair of the frontal section cut at the level of the left coronary artery orifice.[1]

The left and right images are viewed from the posterior and anterior directions, respectively. The right coronary aortic sinus is supported by the crest of the ventricular septum. Refer to Figure 136. The left ventricular free wall supports the anterior half of the left coronary aortic sinus. The left ventricular summit is the epicardial region of this left ventricular free wall. The myocardial thickness supporting the left coronary aortic sinus is thin,[5] indicating the distance between the virtual basal ring and the ventriculo-arterial junction at this region is short. This distance corresponds to the thickness of the myocardial crescent incorporated at the base of the left coronary aortic sinus.[5] The average value of the thickness of the myocardial crescent is 6.4 mm at the right coronary aortic sinus supported by the crest of the ventricular septum,

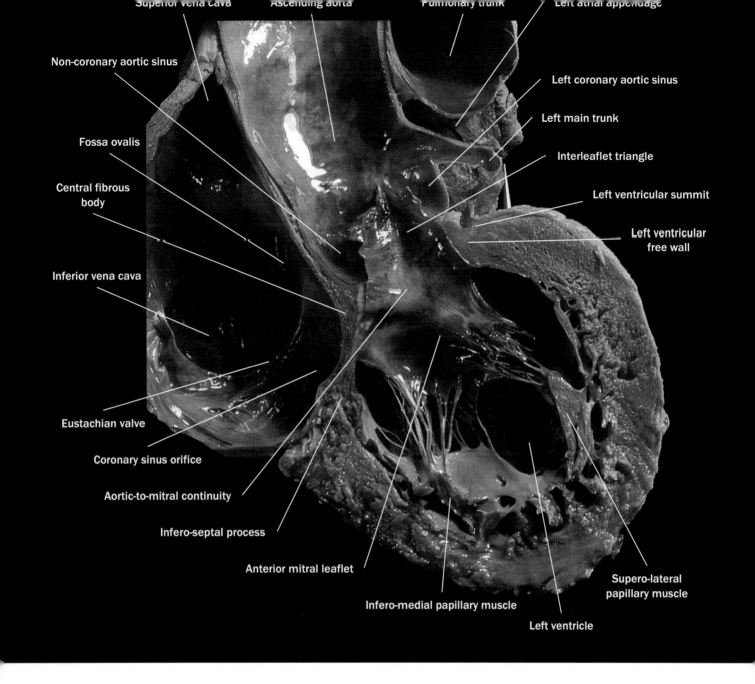

Superior vena cava Ascending aorta Pulmonary trunk Left atrial appendage

Non-coronary aortic sinus

Left coronary aortic sinus

Left main trunk

Fossa ovalis

Interleaflet triangle

Central fibrous body

Left ventricular summit

Left ventricular free wall

Inferior vena cava

Eustachian valve

Coronary sinus orifice

Aortic-to-mitral continuity

Infero-septal process

Anterior mitral leaflet

Supero-lateral papillary muscle

Infero-medial papillary muscle

Left ventricle

whereas it is 2.9 mm at the left coronary aortic sinus supported by the free wall.[5] The left main trunk of the left coronary artery is located within the epicardial adipose tissue on the left ventricular summit. The pulmonary root/trunk overrides the left coronary aortic sinus and the left main trunk. The interleaflet triangle between the left and non-coronary aortic sinuses are in continuity with the anterior mitral leaflet. The thick fibrous tissue supporting the nadir of the non-coronary aortic sinus, between the right atrium and the left ventricular outflow tract is the part of the central fibrous body, also referred to as the right fibrous trigone.[1,13] The compact atrioventricular node is located on the right atrial side of this fibrous tissue.

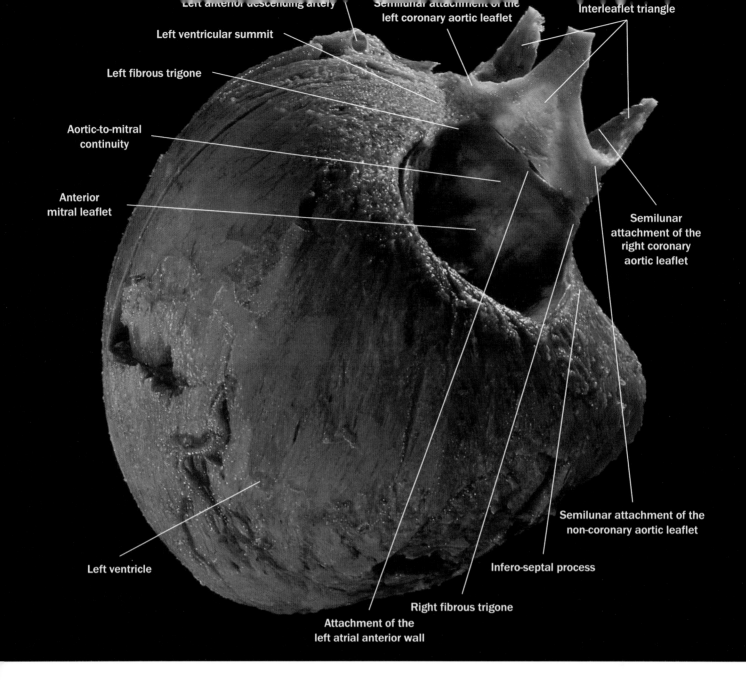

Left anterior descending artery

Left ventricular summit

Left fibrous trigone

Aortic-to-mitral continuity

Anterior mitral leaflet

Left ventricle

Semilunar attachment of the left coronary aortic leaflet

Interleaflet triangle

Semilunar attachment of the right coronary aortic leaflet

Semilunar attachment of the non-coronary aortic leaflet

Infero-septal process

Right fibrous trigone

Attachment of the left atrial anterior wall

Figure 139   The left ventricular cone and three-pointed coronet of the aortic root.[1]

As the interleaflet fibrous triangle within the aortic root is a part of the left ventricular outflow tract hemodynamically, this is the shape of the hemodynamic left ventricle. The infero-septal process directs to the right fibrous trigone (central fibrous body) at the nadir of the non-coronary aortic sinus. The left ventricular free wall located at the left ventricular summit supports the nadir of the left coronary aortic sinus.[4] McAlpine terms this part of the free wall as the left ostial process[1] in relation with the extent of the left fibrous trigone at the nadir of the left coronary aortic sinus. The interleaflet triangle between the non-coronary and left coronary aortic sinuses is in continuity with the anterior mitral leaflet. The aortic-to-mitral (aortomitral) continuity extends approximately between the level of the virtual basal ring to the hingeline of the anterior mitral leaflet between the supero-lateral and infero-septal commissures. The aortic-to-mitral continuity is hardly distinguishable from the anterior mitral leaflet,[14] as there is no specific boundary. The attachment of the left atrial anterior wall divides the interleaflet triangle from the aortic-to-mitral continuity.

References

1. McAlpine WA. Digitized collection of all the images created by Dr. McAlpine at UCLA. Copyright UCLA Cardiac Arrhythmia Center. Part of this collection appeared in *Heart and Coronary Arteries: An Anatomical Atlas for Clinical Diagnosis, Radiological Investigation, and Surgical Treatment*. New York: Springer-Verlag; 1975.
2. Mori S, Tretter JT, Spicer DE, et al. What is the real cardiac anatomy? *Clin Anat*. 2019;32:288–309.
3. Bradfield JS. Redefining optimal targets for intramural ventricular arrhythmias: Planning for combat! *JACC Clin Electrophysiol*. 2020;6:1349–1352.
4. Mori S, Fukuzawa K, Takaya T, et al. Clinical cardiac structural anatomy reconstructed within the cardiac contour using multi-detector-row computed tomography: Left ventricular outflow tract. *Clin Anat*. 2016;29:353–363.
5. Toh H, Mori S, Tretter JT, et al. Living anatomy of the ventricular myocardial crescents supporting the coronary aortic sinuses. *Semin Thorac Cardiovasc Surg*. 2020;32:230–241.
6. Mori S, Izawa Y, Shimoyama S, et al. Three-dimensional understanding of complexity of the aortic root anatomy as the basis of routine Two-dimensional echocardiographic measurements. *Circ J*. 2019;83:2320–2323.
7. Izawa Y, Mori S, Tretter JT, et al. Normative aortic valvar measurements in adults using cardiac computed tomography: A potential guide to further sophisticate aortic valve-sparing surgery. *Circ J*. 2021;85:1059–1067.
8. Tretter JT, Spicer DE, Mori S, et al. The significance of the interleaflet triangles in determining the morphology of congenitally abnormal aortic valves: Implications for noninvasive imaging and surgical management. *J Am Soc Echocardiogr*. 2016;29:1131–1143.
9. Yamada T, McElderry HT, Doppalapudi H, et al. Idiopathic ventricular arrhythmias originating from the left ventricular summit: Anatomic concepts relevant to ablation. *Circ Arrhythm Electrophysiol*. 2010;3:616–623.
10. Yamada T, Litovsky SH, Kay GN. The left ventricular ostium: An anatomic concept relevant to idiopathic ventricular arrhythmias. *Circ Arrhythm Electrophysiol*. 2008;1:396–404.
11. Mori S, Anderson RH, Tahara N, et al. The differences between bisecting and off-center cuts of the aortic root: The three-dimensional anatomy of the aortic root reconstructed from the living heart. *Echocardiography*. 2017;34:453–461.
12. Mori S, Tretter JT, Toba T, et al. Relationship between the membranous septum and the virtual basal ring of the aortic root in candidates for transcatheter implantation of the aortic valve. *Clin Anat*. 2018;31:525–534.
13. Zimmerman J, Bailey CP. The surgical significance of the fibrous skeleton of the heart. *J Thorac Cardiovasc Surg*. 1962;44:701–712.
14. David TE, Kuo J, Armstrong S. Aortic and mitral valve replacement with reconstruction of the intervalvular fibrous body. *J Thorac Cardiovasc Surg*. 1997;114:766–771.

21

Coronary Arteries

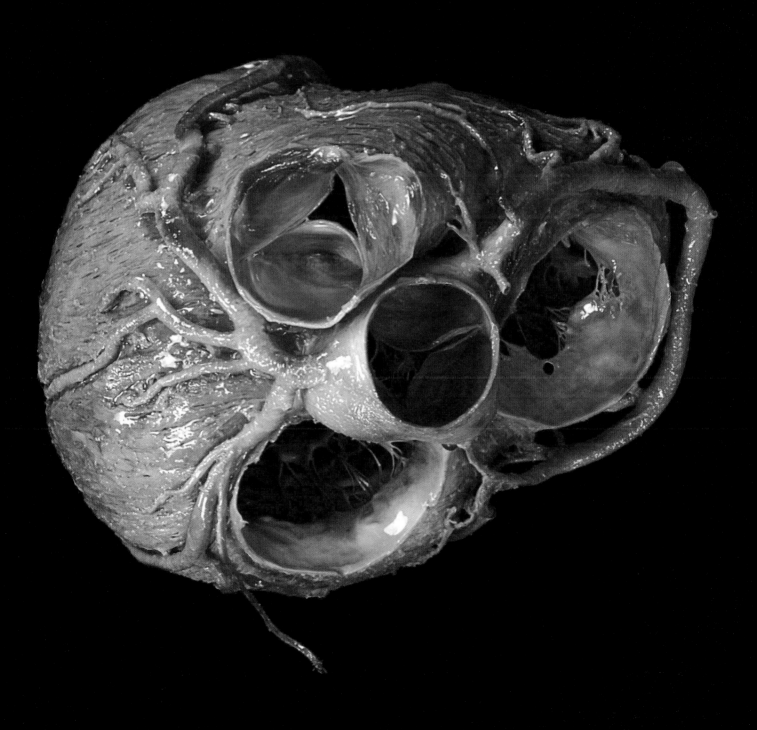

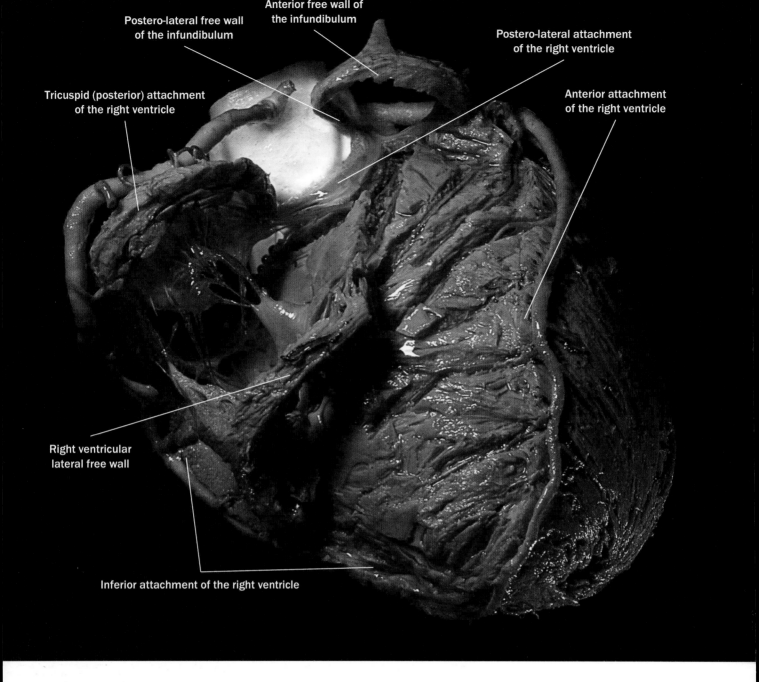

Figure 140 The septal branches.[1]

The heart is viewed from the anterior direction. The septal branches are dissected from the right ventricular septal surface. The first septal branch runs close to the medial papillary muscle, that is located close to the proximal right bundle branch. The first septal branch enters into the basal superior ventricular septum from the pulmonary (superior) attachment of the right ventricle, where the posterior free wall of the right ventricular outflow tract (infundibulum) starts to separate from the left ventricle to override the left coronary aortic sinus and proximal left coronary artery. Refer to Figure 80. After

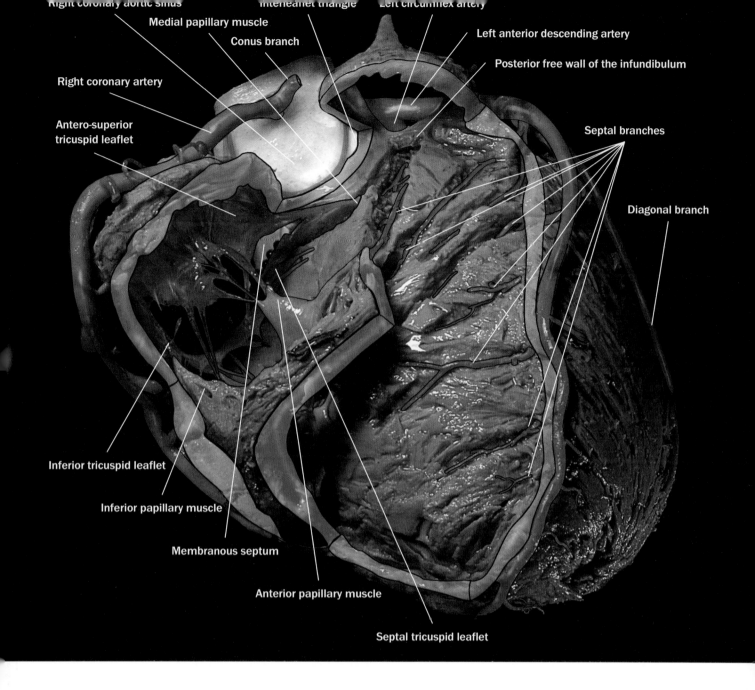

Right coronary aortic sinus

Medial papillary muscle

Conus branch

Interleaflet triangle

Left circumflex artery

Left anterior descending artery

Posterior free wall of the infundibulum

Right coronary artery

Antero-superior tricuspid leaflet

Septal branches

Diagonal branch

Inferior tricuspid leaflet

Inferior papillary muscle

Membranous septum

Anterior papillary muscle

Septal tricuspid leaflet

running nearly horizontally behind the left adjacent pulmonary sinus to skirt the pulmonary root, the left anterior descending artery changes its course toward the antero-inferior direction along the anterior interventricular groove. Thus, the base of the pulmonary root is located between the aortic root and this bending point of the left anterior descending artery. Multiple septal branches are seen in the superior half of the ventricular septum that is related to the region of the superior fascicle,[2] also conventionally referred to as the anterior fascicle of the left bundle branch.

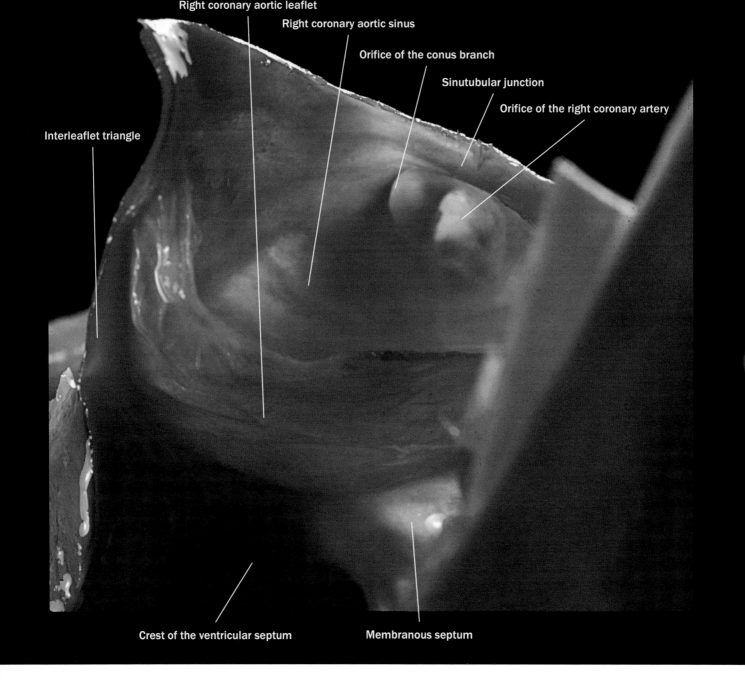

Right coronary aortic leaflet

Right coronary aortic sinus

Orifice of the conus branch

Sinutubular junction

Orifice of the right coronary artery

Interleaflet triangle

Crest of the ventricular septum

Membranous septum

Figure 141   The coronary orifices.[1]

The coronary orifice of the right coronary artery is located at the right side of the right coronary aortic sinus near the sinutubular junction with the separated orifice of the conus branch (left). The orifice of the left coronary artery is located at the center of the sinus near the sinutubular junction (right).[3] The aortic valvular leaflets in the right case show

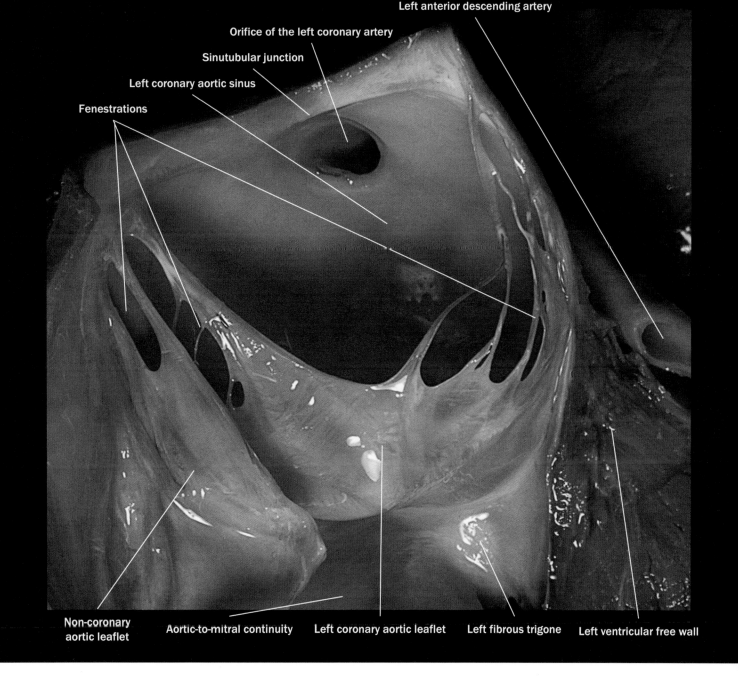

Left anterior descending artery

Orifice of the left coronary artery

Sinutubular junction

Left coronary aortic sinus

Fenestrations

Non-coronary aortic leaflet

Aortic-to-mitral continuity

Left coronary aortic leaflet

Left fibrous trigone

Left ventricular free wall

fenestration.[4] Fenestration matters clinically only if it extends beyond the zone of coaptation, or the fibrous cords tear.[5] Average height of the orifices of the right and left coronary arteries from the virtual basal ring plane are 17.7 mm and 14.8 mm, respectively.[3]

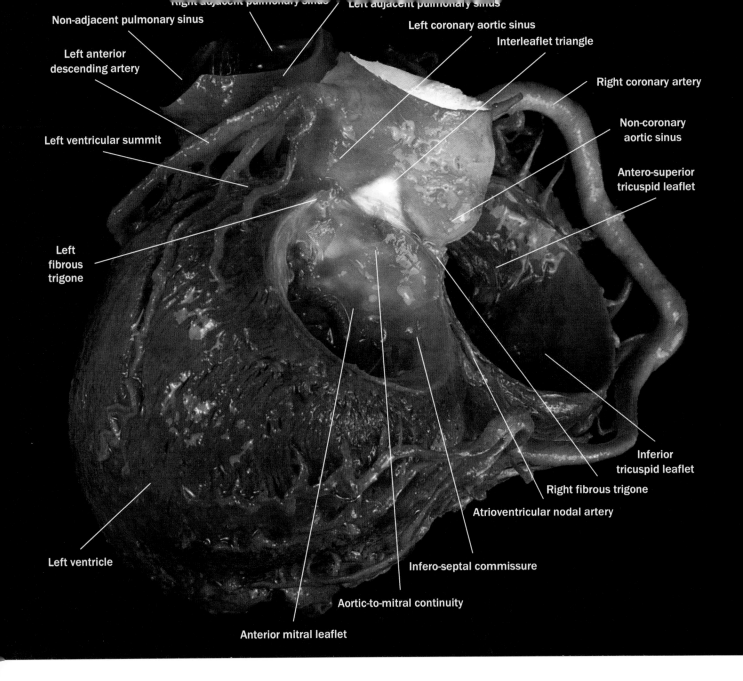

Non-adjacent pulmonary sinus

Left anterior
descending artery

Left ventricular summit

Left
fibrous
trigone

Left ventricle

Left coronary aortic sinus

Interleaflet triangle

Right coronary artery

Non-coronary
aortic sinus

Antero-superior
tricuspid leaflet

Inferior
tricuspid leaflet

Right fibrous trigone

Atrioventricular nodal artery

Infero-septal commissure

Aortic-to-mitral continuity

Anterior mitral leaflet

Figure 142 The right and left coronary arteries.[1] Anaglyph 17.

In the left image, the heart is viewed from the posterior direction. The left and non-coronary aortic sinuses are located posterior, in contrast to the anteriorly located right coronary aortic sinus. The right coronary artery is dominant in this heart, which runs along the right atrioventricular groove, gives rise to the atrioventricular nodal artery at the inferior crux of the heart, and distributes to the inferior and infero-lateral region of the left ventricle. Refer to Figure 114. In the right image, the heart is viewed from the left anterior oblique and cranial direction, which shows the heart in the Valentine

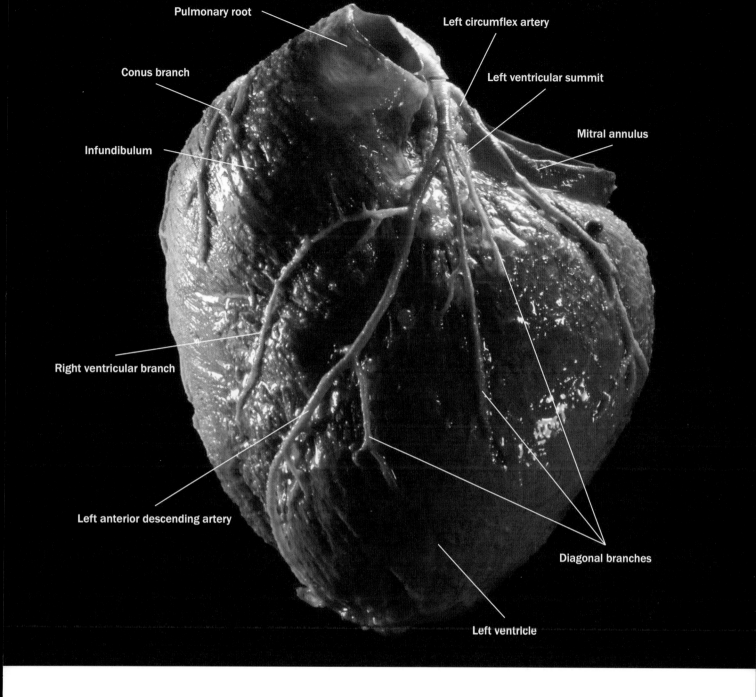

Pulmonary root

Left circumflex artery

Conus branch

Left ventricular summit

Infundibulum

Mitral annulus

Right ventricular branch

Left anterior descending artery

Diagonal branches

Left ventricle

position;[2] the heart standing on its apex. This left anterior oblique and cranial view, and the left anterior oblique and caudal view are the best angulation to separate the proximal part of the left coronary artery in each dorsal/vertical and ventral/horizontal hearts, respectively. The *en face* view of the left ventricular summit can be also obtained from this direction, with deep cranial angulation.

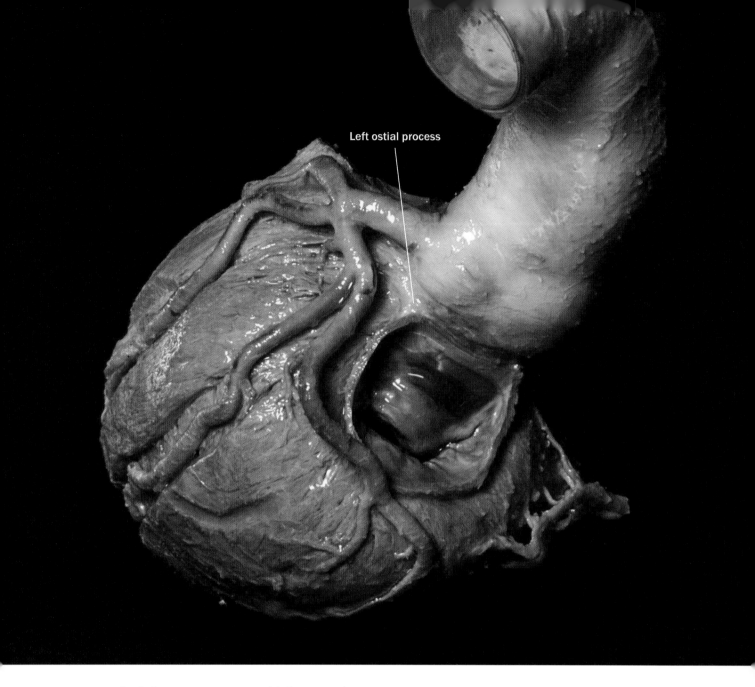

Left ostial process

Figure 143 The left coronary artery and left ventricular summit.[1]

The proximal left coronary artery covers the basal superior free wall of the left ventricle. The epicardial side of this basal superior free wall supporting the left coronary aortic sinus is referred to as the left ventricular summit.[1,6] Refer to Figure 135. McAlpine refers to the angled myocardium found at the left fibrous trigone as the left ostial process.[1] It is this left ostial process, at the postero-inferior part of the left ventricular summit, that is mistakenly termed as aortic-to-mitral

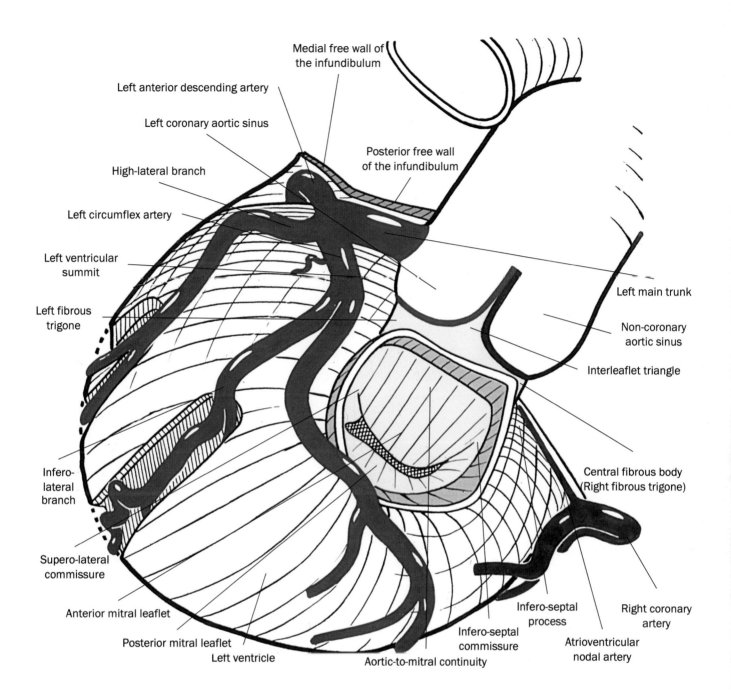

Medial free wall of
the infundibulum

Left anterior descending artery

Left coronary aortic sinus

High-lateral branch

Left circumflex artery

Left ventricular
summit

Left fibrous
trigone

Infero-
lateral
branch

Supero-lateral
commissure

Anterior mitral leaflet

Posterior mitral leaflet

Left ventricle

Posterior free wall
of the infundibulum

Left main trunk

Non-coronary
aortic sinus

Interleaflet triangle

Central fibrous body
(Right fibrous trigone)

Infero-septal
process

Right coronary
artery

Infero-septal
commissure

Atrioventricular
nodal artery

Aortic-to-mitral continuity

(aortomitral) continuity in the field of electrophysiology.[7,8] Actually, the aortic-to-mitral continuity is the region between the interleaflet triangle and anterior mitral leaflet. After running horizontally behind the pulmonary root, the left anterior descending artery turns its course toward the anterior interventricular groove. The small, high-lateral branch enters into the left ventricular summit.

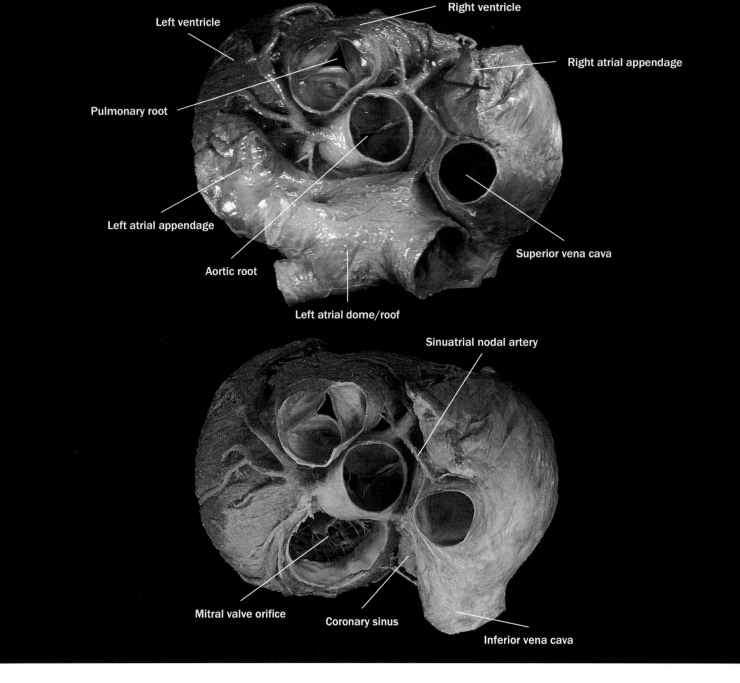

Figure 144 The progressive dissection showing the course of the coronary arteries.[1]

The hearts are viewed from the superior direction. From the heart with intact cardiac chambers (upper image on the left page), the left atrium and the right atrium are progressively removed in the lower image on the left page and image on the right page, respectively. The left atrial appendage covers the diagonal branch, high-lateral branch, and circumflex artery.

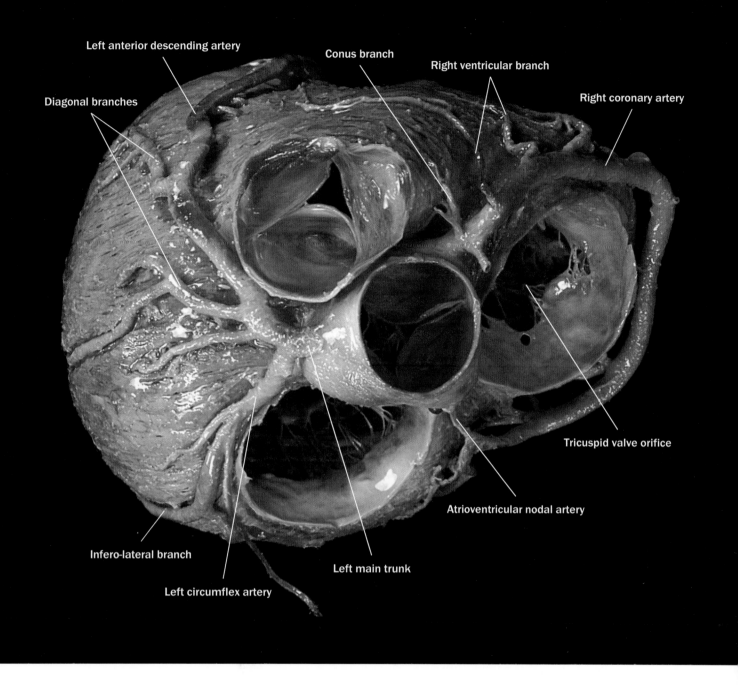

Left anterior descending artery

Diagonal branches

Conus branch

Right ventricular branch

Right coronary artery

Tricuspid valve orifice

Atrioventricular nodal artery

Infero-lateral branch

Left circumflex artery

Left main trunk

The right atrial appendage covers the right coronary artery and sinuatrial nodal artery. The right coronary artery directs toward the right anterior oblique direction. The orifices of the right and left coronary arteries are separated by 150-degree angulation on average.[3]

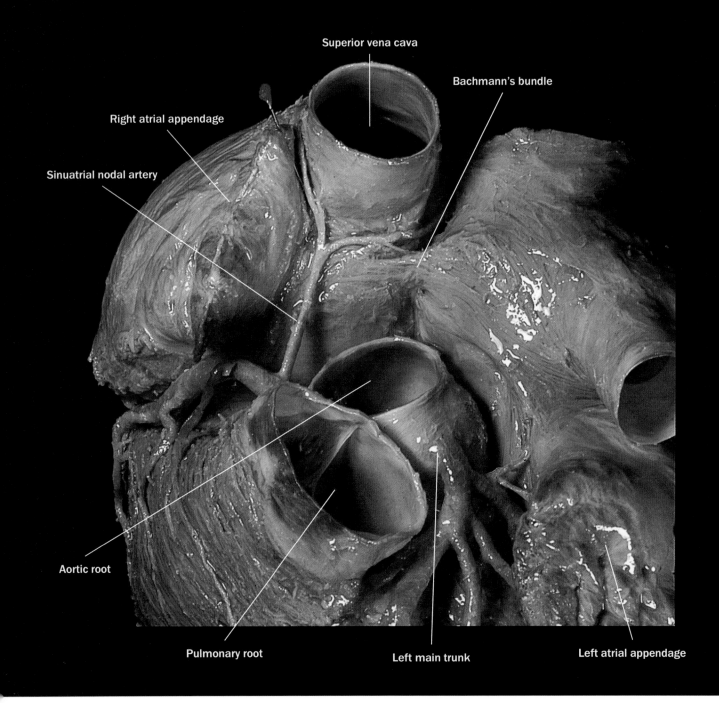

Superior vena cava

Bachmann's bundle

Right atrial appendage

Sinuatrial nodal artery

Aortic root

Pulmonary root

Left main trunk

Left atrial appendage

Figure 145 The variation in the course of the sinuatrial nodal artery.[1]

The sinuatrial nodal artery commonly originates from either right coronary artery or the left circumflex artery. The course of the artery as well as its final relationship between the superior vena cava are variable.[9] Dual supply is not infrequent.[10] The sinuatrial nodal artery is also common arterial supply for the Bachmann's bundle.[11] The left image shows the Y-shaped terminal of the right sinuatrial nodal artery originating from the proximal right coronary artery, running medial to the right atrial appendage. The red bead indicates the location of the sinuatrial node. The upper image on the right page shows the left sinuatrial nodal artery emerging from the just proximal circumflex artery, running anterior to the orifice of the left

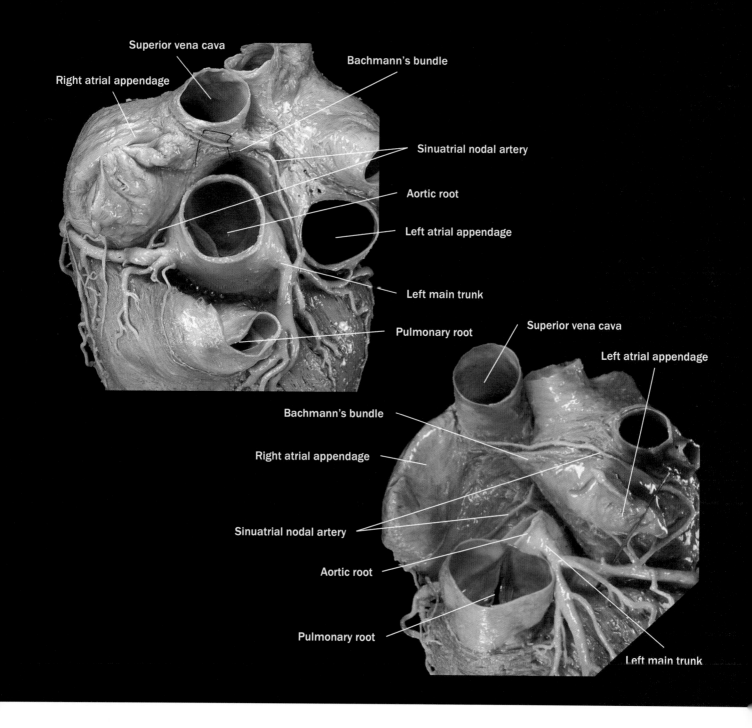

Superior vena cava

Right atrial appendage

Bachmann's bundle

Sinuatrial nodal artery

Aortic root

Left atrial appendage

Left main trunk

Pulmonary root

Superior vena cava

Left atrial appendage

Bachmann's bundle

Right atrial appendage

Sinuatrial nodal artery

Aortic root

Pulmonary root

Left main trunk

atrial appendage, left atrial anterior wall within the Bachmann's bundle, and anterior to the superior vena cava to reach the sinuatrial node. The lower image on the right page shows the left sinuatrial nodal artery originating from the proximal circumflex artery, running posterior to the orifice of the left atrial appendage within the fold between the left pulmonary veins, which is the location of the vein of Marshall. Then, it runs anterior to the left atrial anterior wall on the Bachmann's bundle and the superior vena cava to reach the sinuatrial node on the terminal groove. When the right or left sinuatrial nodal artery has anastomosis with the atrioventricular nodal artery,[12] that anastomosis is referred to as the Kugel's artery.[13]

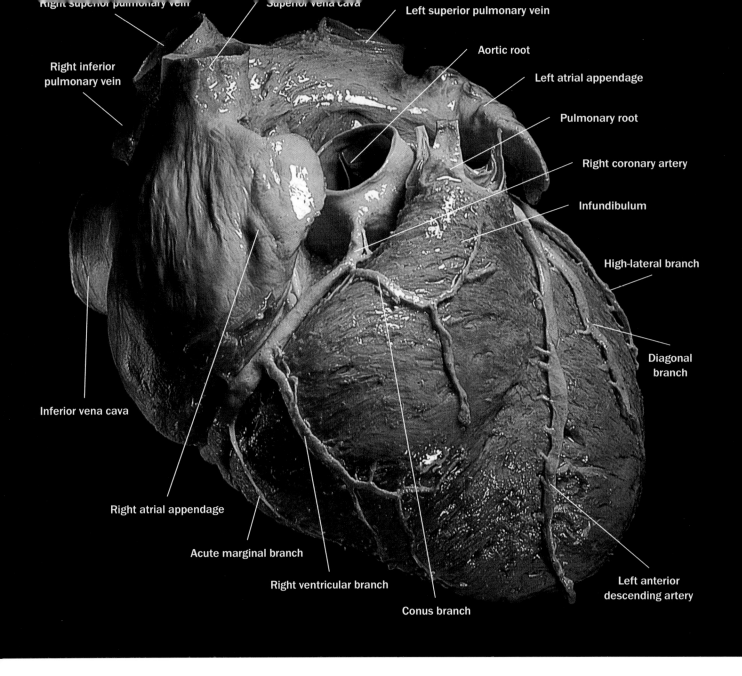

Right superior pulmonary vein

Superior vena cava

Left superior pulmonary vein

Aortic root

Right inferior pulmonary vein

Left atrial appendage

Pulmonary root

Right coronary artery

Infundibulum

High-lateral branch

Diagonal branch

Inferior vena cava

Right atrial appendage

Acute marginal branch

Right ventricular branch

Conus branch

Left anterior descending artery

Figure 146   The conus branch.[1]

The heart is viewed from the anterior direction. The conus branch, also referred to as the conal artery,[14] perfuses anterior right ventricular outflow tract corresponding to the area right beneath the third to fourth intercostal space along the left sternal border.[15] The isolated acute occlusion of this artery induces isolated right ventricular infarction, which is known to show ST-segment elevation prominent in the V2 lead,[15] similar to the characteristic coved-type ST-segment elevation in Brugada syndrome. When the right conus branch forms anastomosis with the left conus branch originating from the proximal left anterior descending artery, it is referred to as the Vieussens' ring.[16] The Vieussens' ring can work as the critical collateral source in the setting of occlusion of the proximal left anterior descending artery or the left main trunk.[17]

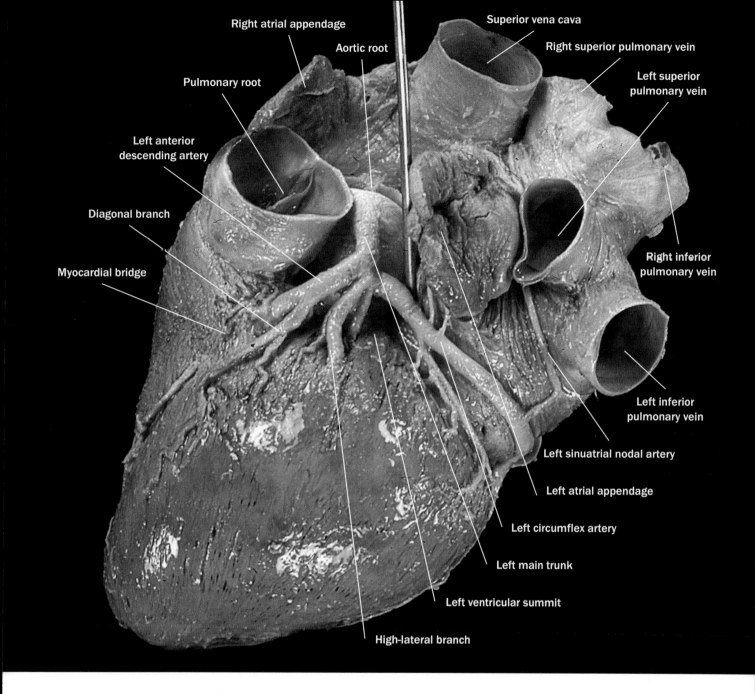

Right atrial appendage

Aortic root

Pulmonary root

Left anterior
descending artery

Diagonal branch

Myocardial bridge

Superior vena cava

Right superior pulmonary vein

Left superior
pulmonary vein

Right inferior
pulmonary vein

Left inferior
pulmonary vein

Left sinuatrial nodal artery

Left atrial appendage

Left circumflex artery

Left main trunk

Left ventricular summit

High-lateral branch

Figure 147   The myocardial bridges.[1]

The mid-left anterior descending artery shows the myocardial bridge. The diagonal and high-lateral branches also show the intra-mural course, rendering the lateral epicardial wall to look avascular. The myocardial bridge is likely to be usually benign anatomical variation found in normal individuals and not necessarily lead to coronary artery ischemia.[18] With improved imaging modalities, it is increasingly and readily recognized.[19,20] The left sinuatrial nodal artery takes a posterior course relative to the left atrial appendage. Small atrial branches are found anterior to the orifice of the left atrial appendage.

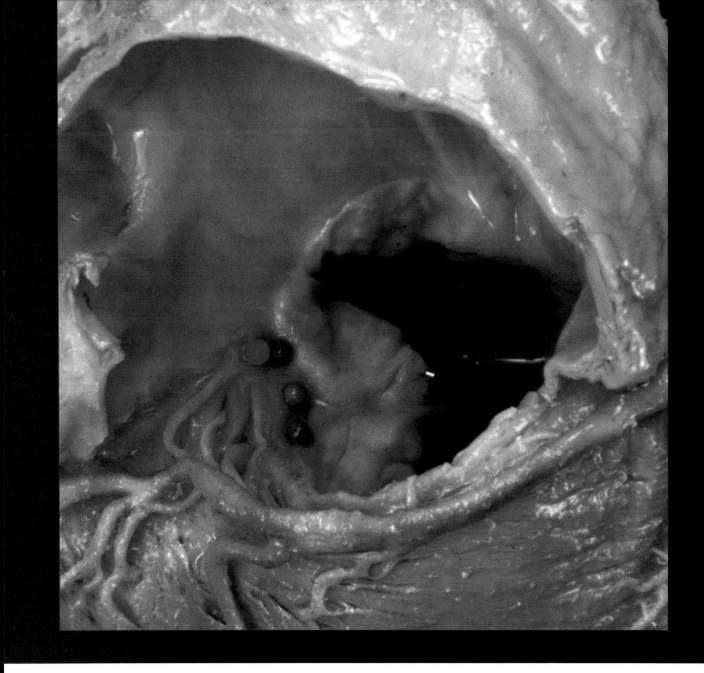

Figure 148 The atrioventricular nodal artery.[1]

The right atrial wall at the floor of the triangle of Koch is removed to show the inferior pyramidal space involving the atrioventricular nodal arteries.[21] The inferior pyramidal space is the epicardial adipose tissue wedging deeply from the inferior crux of the heart.[21] The inferior pyramidal space (removed in this specimen) lies on the epicardial surface of the basal infero-medial left ventricular mass, referred to as the infero-septal process.[22] The red bead at the apex of the triangle

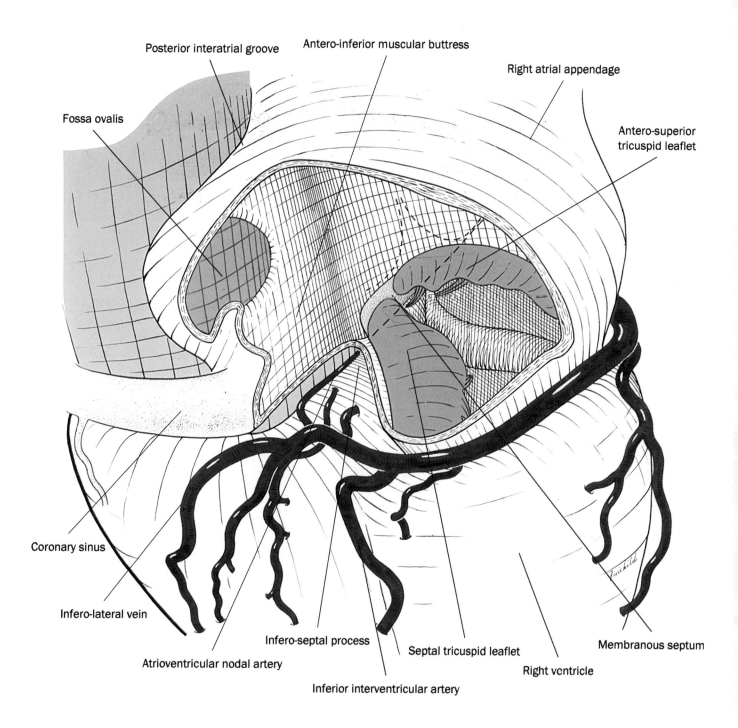

Posterior interatrial groove

Antero-inferior muscular buttress

Right atrial appendage

Fossa ovalis

Antero-superior tricuspid leaflet

Coronary sinus

Infero-lateral vein

Infero-septal process

Septal tricuspid leaflet

Membranous septum

Atrioventricular nodal artery

Right ventricle

Inferior interventricular artery

of Koch marks the location of the atrioventricular node. The blue beads denote the septal attachment of the septal tricuspid leaflet. These atrioventricular nodal arteries as well as the atrioventricular node are thus epicardial structures, sandwiched between the right atrium and the left ventricle.[23] Multiple atrioventricular nodal arteries are common.[24]

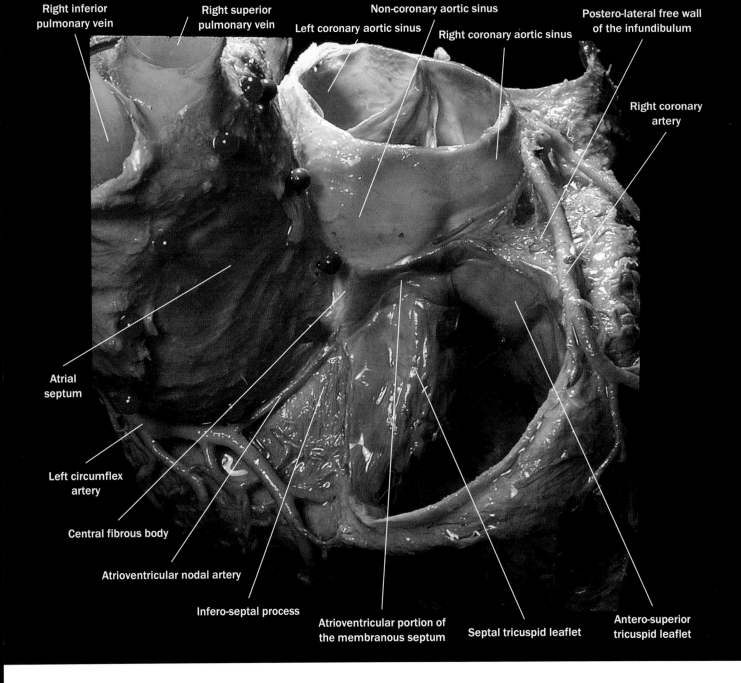

Right inferior pulmonary vein

Right superior pulmonary vein

Non-coronary aortic sinus

Left coronary aortic sinus

Right coronary aortic sinus

Postero-lateral free wall of the infundibulum

Right coronary artery

Atrial septum

Left circumflex artery

Central fibrous body

Atrioventricular nodal artery

Infero-septal process

Atrioventricular portion of the membranous septum

Septal tricuspid leaflet

Antero-superior tricuspid leaflet

Figure 149   The left and right atrioventricular nodal arteries.[1]

The left and right images show the left and right atrioventricular nodal arteries. The atrioventricular nodal artery originates from the right coronary artery in nine-tenths of the patients.[9] Regardless of its origin from the distal left circumflex artery or distal right coronary artery, the atrioventricular nodal artery is located within the inferior pyramidal space at

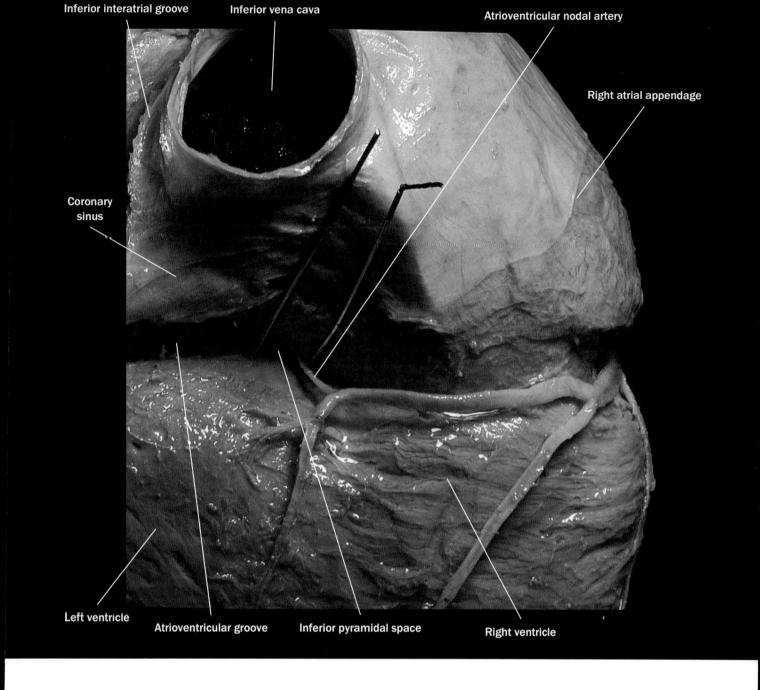

Inferior interatrial groove · Inferior vena cava · Atrioventricular nodal artery · Right atrial appendage · Coronary sinus · Left ventricle · Atrioventricular groove · Inferior pyramidal space · Right ventricle

the epicardial side of the infero-septal process, and ascends toward the central fibrous body located at the bottom of the non-coronary aortic sinus.[25]

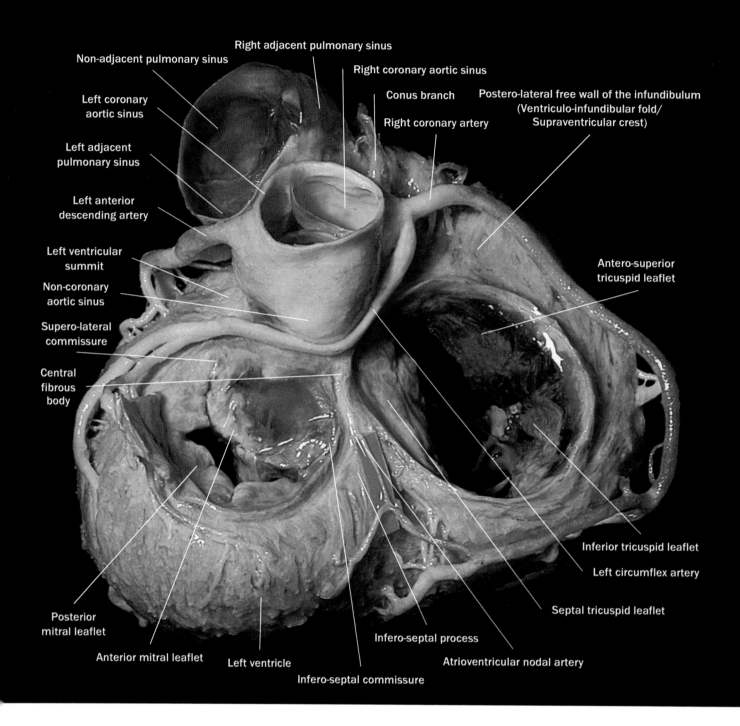

Figure 150 Anomalous origin of the left circumflex artery from the right coronary aortic sinus.[1]

The heart is viewed from the right posterior direction. The abnormal left circumflex artery originates from the right coronary aortic sinus with a common orifice with the right coronary artery. It runs right postero-inferior to the aortic root, crossing the bottom of the non-coronary aortic sinus and interleaflet triangle above the aortic-to-mitral (aortomitral) continuity. In this particular anomaly, the medial anterior wall of the right and left atria, corresponding to the right and left aortic mounds,[26] are in close contact with this anomalous artery. The right atrioventricular nodal artery ascends toward the central fibrous body on the epicardial side of the infero-septal process.

References

1. McAlpine WA. Digitized collection of all the images created by Dr. McAlpine at UCLA. Copyright UCLA Cardiac Arrhythmia Center. Part of this collection appeared in *Heart and Coronary Arteries: An Anatomical Atlas for Clinical Diagnosis, Radiological Investigation, and Surgical Treatment*. New York: Springer-Verlag; 1975.
2. Mori S, Spicer DE, Anderson RH. Revisiting the anatomy of the living heart. *Circ J*. 2016;80:24–33.
3. Toh H, Mori S, Tretter JT, et al. Living anatomy of the ventricular myocardial crescents supporting the coronary aortic sinuses. *Semin Thorac Cardiovasc Surg*. 2020;32:230–241.
4. Akiyama K, Hirota J, Taniyasu N, et al. Pathogenetic significance of myxomatous degeneration in fenestration-related massive aortic regurgitation. *Circ J*. 2004;68:439–443.
5. Akasaka K, Saito E, Higuchi T, et al. Aortic regurgitation caused by fibrous strand rupture in a fenestrated aortic valve. *J Echocardiogr*. 2012;10:151–153.
6. Yamada T, McElderry HT, Doppalapudi H, et al. Idiopathic ventricular arrhythmias originating from the left ventricular summit: Anatomic concepts relevant to ablation. *Circ Arrhythm Electrophysiol*. 2010;3:616–623.
7. Kumagai K, Fukuda K, Wakayama Y, et al. Electrocardiographic characteristics of the variants of idiopathic left ventricular outflow tract ventricular tachyarrhythmias. *J Cardiovasc Electrophysiol*. 2008;19:495–501.
8. Steven D, Roberts-Thomson KC, Seiler J, et al. Ventricular tachycardia arising from the aortomitral continuity in structural heart disease: Characteristics and therapeutic considerations for an anatomically challenging area of origin. *Circ Arrhythm Electrophysiol*. 2009;2:660–666.
9. Saremi F, Abolhoda A, Ashikyan O, et al. Arterial supply to sinuatrial and atrioventricular nodes: imaging with multidetector CT. *Radiology*. 2008;246:99–107.
10. Kawashima T, Sasaki H. The morphological significance of the human sinuatrial nodal branch (artery). *Heart Vessels*. 2003;18:213–219.
11. Saremi F, Channual S, Krishnan S, et al. Bachmann Bundle and its arterial supply: Imaging with multidetector CT—implications for interatrial conduction abnormalities and arrhythmias. *Radiology*. 2008;248:447–457.
12. Nerantzis CE, Marianou SK, Koulouris SN, et al. Kugel's artery: An anatomical and angiographic study using a new technique. *Tex Heart Inst J*. 2004;31:267–270.
13. Kugel MA. Anatomical studies on the coronary arteries and their branches. I. Arteria anastomotica auricularis magna. *Am Heart J*. 1927;3:260–270.
14. Loukas M, Patel S, Cesmebasi A, et al. The clinical anatomy of the conal artery. *Clin Anat*. 2016;29:371–379.
15. Mori S, Takamiya M, Suzuki K, et al. Three-dimensional relationship between the conus branch and the precordial leads confirmed by 64-multidetector-row computed tomography. *J Electrocardiol*. 2009;42:118.e1–5.
16. Loukas M, Clarke P, Tubbs RS, et al. Raymond de Vieussens. *Anat Sci Int*. 2007;82:233–236.
17. Malik SA, Goldsweig AM. The circle of life: Vieussens' arterial ring. *JACC Cardiovasc Interv*. 2019;12:e73–e74.
18. Möhlenkamp S, Hort W, Ge J, Erbel R. Update on myocardial bridging. *Circulation*. 2002;106:2616–2622.
19. Nakaura T, Awai K, Yamashita Y. Incidence of myocardial bridging observed on MDCT. *AJR Am J Roentgenol*. 2006;187:W662.
20. Loukas M, Von Kriegenbergh K, Gilkes M, et al. Myocardial bridges: A review. *Clin Anat*. 2011;24:675–683.
21. Mori S, Fukuzawa K, Takaya T, et al. Clinical structural anatomy of the Inferior pyramidal space reconstructed within the cardiac contour using multidetector-row computed tomography. *J Cardiovasc Electrophysiol*. 2015;26:705–712.
22. Li A, Zuberi Z, Bradfield JS, et al. Endocardial ablation of ventricular ectopic beats arising from the basal inferoseptal process of the left ventricle. *Heart Rhythm*. 2018;15:1356–1362.
23. Shimizu S. [Topographical anatomy of the atrioventricular node of Tawara—findings by macro-microscopic dissection under dissecting microscope] (in Japanese). *Nihon Kyobu Geka Gakkai Zasshi*. 1989;37:227–233.
24. Kawashima T, Sato F. Clarifying the anatomy of the atrioventricular node artery. *Int J Cardiol*. 2018;269:158–164.
25. Mori S, Nishii T, Takaya T, et al. Clinical structural anatomy of the inferior pyramidal space reconstructed from the living heart: Three-dimensional visualization using multidetector-row computed tomography. *Clin Anat*. 2015;28:878–887.
26. Mori S, Nishii T, Tretter JT, et al. Demonstration of living anatomy clarifies the morphology of interatrial communications. *Heart*. 2018;104:2003–2009.

22

Coronary Veins

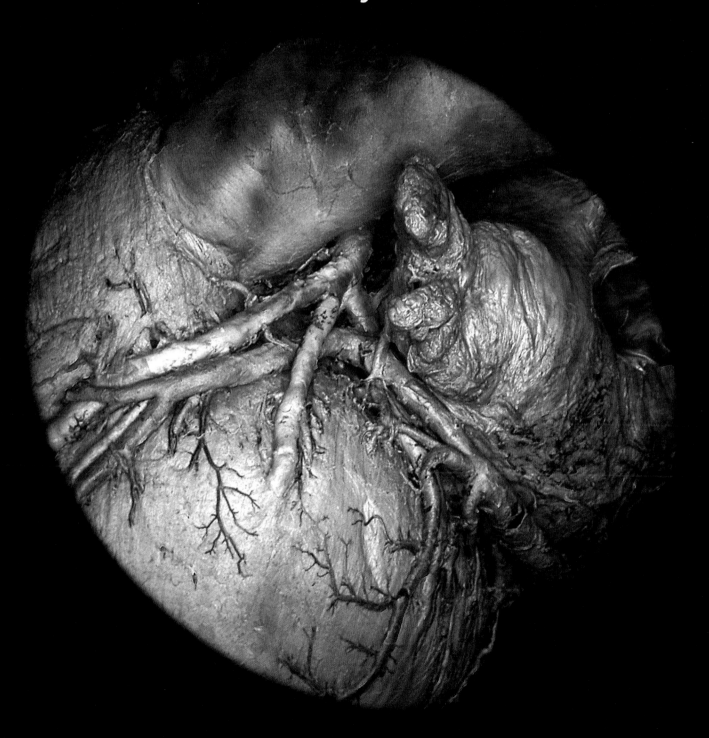

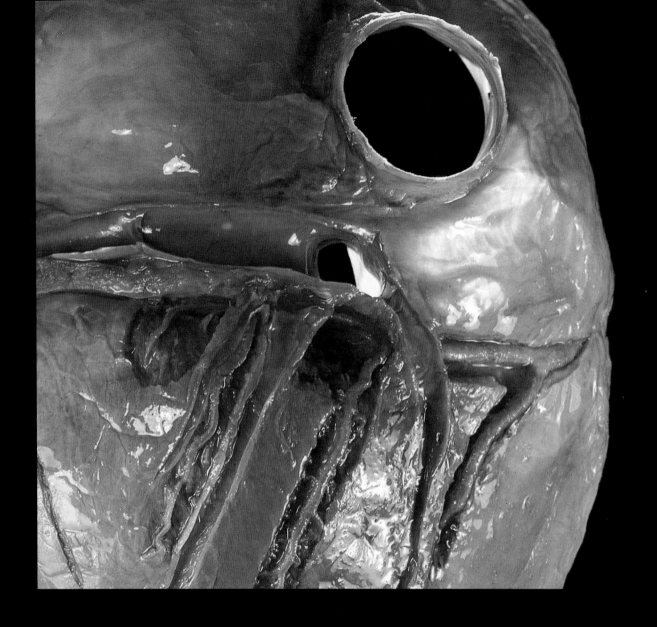

Figure 151   The coronary sinus.[1]

The heart is viewed from the inferior direction. The coronary sinus and its tributaries are opened. The coronary sinus runs to the atrial side relative to the distal right coronary artery running along the right and left atrioventricular junction. The

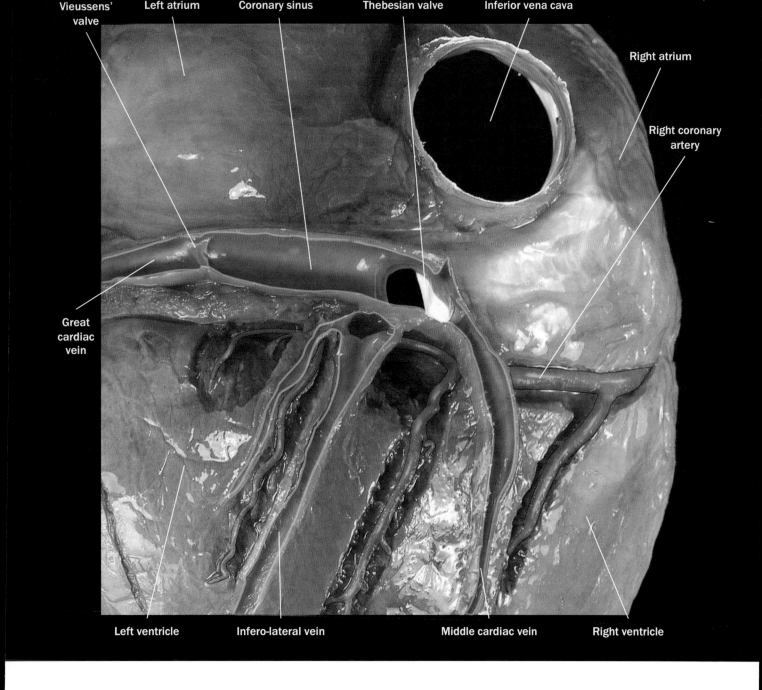

Vieussens' valve | Left atrium | Coronary sinus | Thebesian valve | Inferior vena cava

Right atrium

Right coronary artery

Great cardiac vein

Left ventricle | Infero-lateral vein | Middle cardiac vein | Right ventricle

Vieussens' valve is located at infero-lateral portion,[2] which is used to define the anatomical border between the coronary sinus and the great cardiac vein.

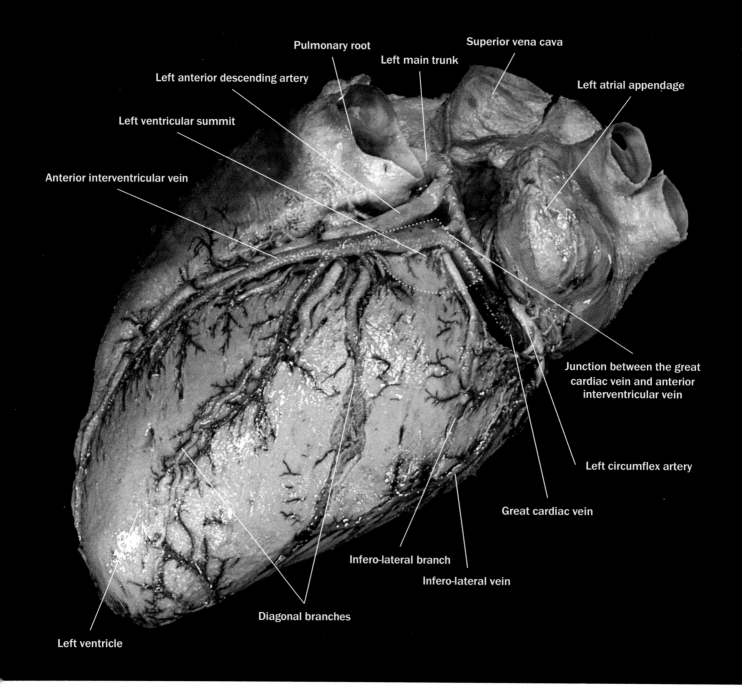

Pulmonary root

Left main trunk

Superior vena cava

Left anterior descending artery

Left atrial appendage

Left ventricular summit

Anterior interventricular vein

Junction between the great
cardiac vein and anterior
interventricular vein

Left circumflex artery

Great cardiac vein

Infero-lateral branch

Infero-lateral vein

Diagonal branches

Left ventricle

Figure 152   The great cardiac vein and anterior interventricular vein.[1]

The great cardiac vein runs along the left circumflex artery covered by the left atrial appendage. The relationship between the coronary veins and coronary arteries,[3] coronary veins and mitral annulus,[4] coronary veins and the phrenic nerve on the pericardium,[5] and branching pattern of the coronary veinous tributaries,[6,7] are highly variable. In the left image, the anterior interventricular vein runs along the left anterior descending artery on its lateral side. The great cardiac vein is located apical

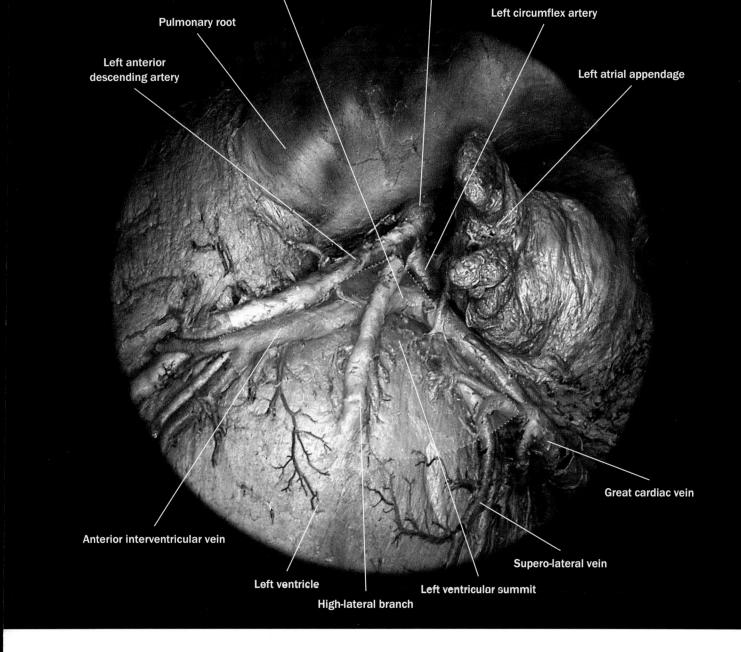

Pulmonary root

Left anterior descending artery

Left circumflex artery

Left atrial appendage

Great cardiac vein

Anterior interventricular vein

Supero-lateral vein

Left ventricle

High-lateral branch

Left ventricular summit

to the left circumflex artery. The anterior interventricular vein-great cardiac vein junction crosses over the proximal obtuse marginal artery. In the right image, the thick septal branch of the anterior interventricular vein overrides the left anterior descending artery. The anterior interventricular vein-great cardiac vein junction is located beneath the high-lateral branch. In both hearts, multiple small veins are detected on the left ventricular summit (yellow, fan-shape areas).

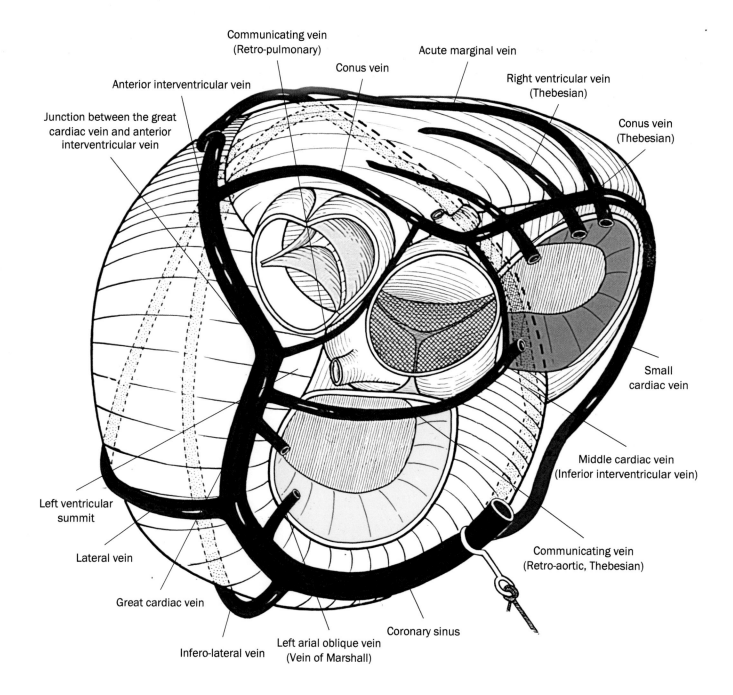

Figure 153 The illustration showing the variable course of the coronary veins.[1]

Distal anastomosis is common among coronary venous tributaries. The communicating vein is illustrated as the vein running between the pulmonary and aortic roots (image on the left page).[8] Several other veins on the left ventricular summit and septal veins[9,10] are also illustrated (images on the right page), which can be the potential route for ethanol ablation for the ventricular arrhythmias originating from the left ventricular summit[11] or intraventricular septum.[12,13] Several Thebesian

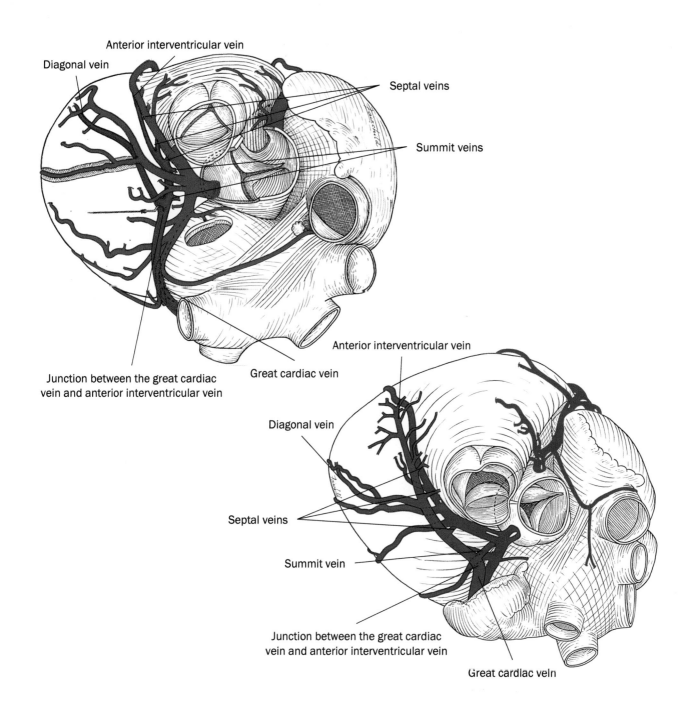

Anterior interventricular vein

Diagonal vein

Septal veins

Summit veins

Junction between the great cardiac
vein and anterior interventricular vein

Great cardiac vein

Anterior interventricular vein

Diagonal vein

Septal veins

Summit vein

Junction between the great cardiac
vein and anterior interventricular vein

Great cardiac vein

veins[14] are also common that directly drain back to the right atrium from the medial or lateral free wall of the right atrial appendage, as illustrated as the retro-aortic communicating vein, conus vein, right ventricular vein, and acute marginal vein (image on the left page). The topographic relationship between the coronary veins and the coronary artery is also variable (images on the right page). The angulation of the junction of the anterior interventricular vein-great cardiac vein and its distance from the aortic root are also variable.[11]

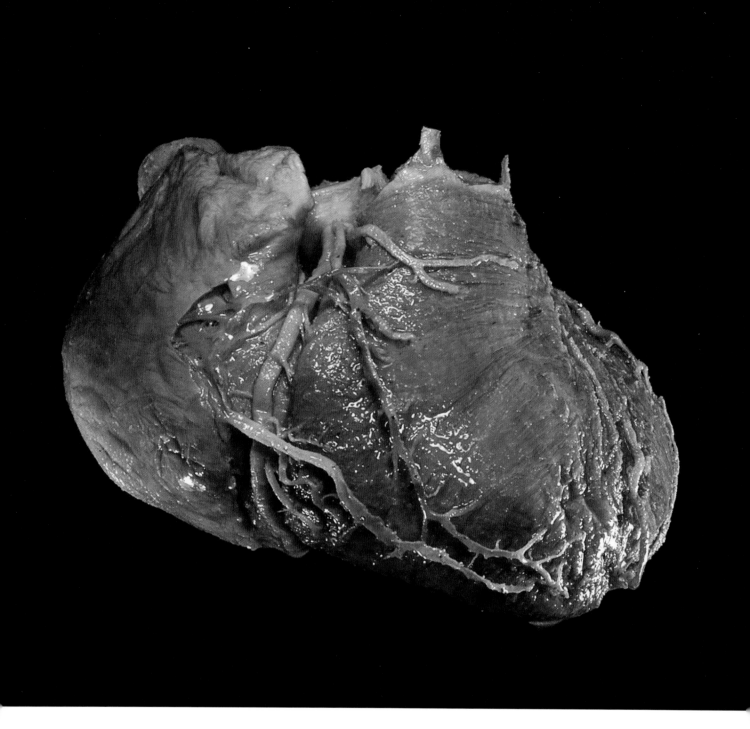

Figure 154   The Thebesian veins draining into the lateral right appendage.[1]

The heart is viewed from the right anterior oblique direction. The coronary venous tributaries draining the region of the infundibulum (conus vein) and acute margin (acute marginal vein) return directly to the lateral right atrial appendage after crossing over the right coronary artery. These Thebesian veins, the coronary veins directly returning to the right atrium

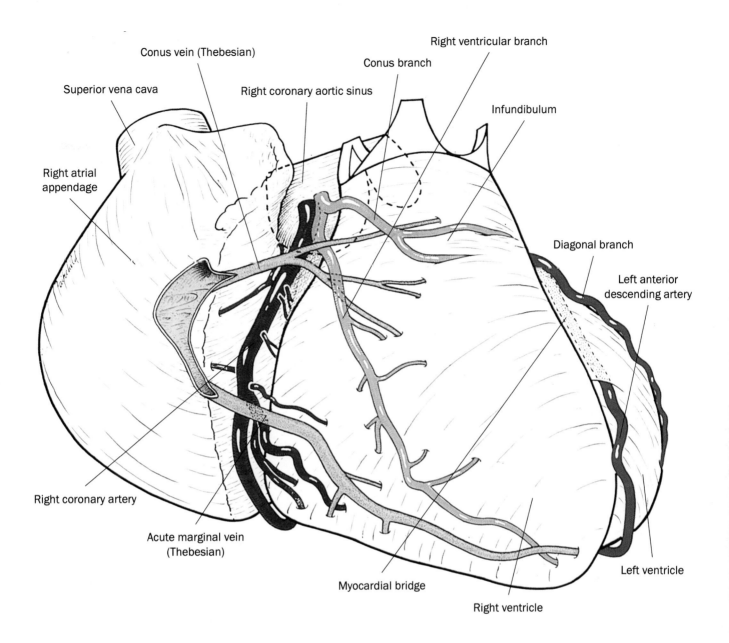

Conus vein (Thebesian)

Superior vena cava

Right coronary aortic sinus

Right atrial appendage

Right ventricular branch

Conus branch

Infundibulum

Diagonal branch

Left anterior descending artery

Right coronary artery

Acute marginal vein (Thebesian)

Myocardial bridge

Left ventricle

Right ventricle

without joining into the coronary sinus, are normal anatomical findings. However, in the setting of coronary sinus stenosis/atresia, prominent Thebesian veins can be found as the alternative route for venous drainage.[15] Conversely, incidental observation of a prominent or unusual Thebesian vein suggests the coronary sinus stenosis/atresia.

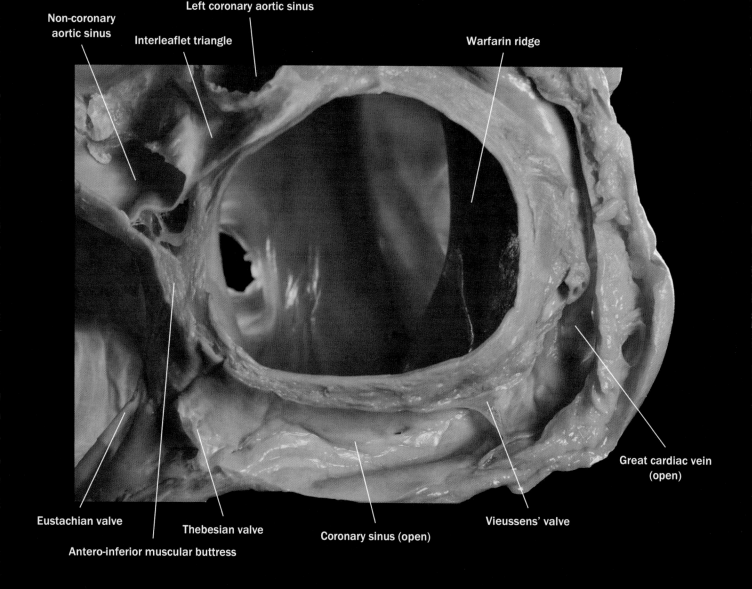

Non-coronary aortic sinus

Left coronary aortic sinus

Interleaflet triangle

Warfarin ridge

Great cardiac vein (open)

Eustachian valve

Thebesian valve

Coronary sinus (open)

Vieussens' valve

Antero-inferior muscular buttress

Figure 155 The Vieussens' valve.

The heart is sectioned along the left atrioventricular groove. The coronary sinus and the great cardiac vein are opened and viewed from the left anterior oblique direction. At the infero-lateral segment, the Vieussens' valve is observed (left), demarcating the margin between the coronary sinus and the great cardiac vein.[2] At the inferior orifice of the coronary sinus, the Thebesian valve is also observed.[16] When the Vieussens' valve is removed (right), the orifice of the oblique vein of the left

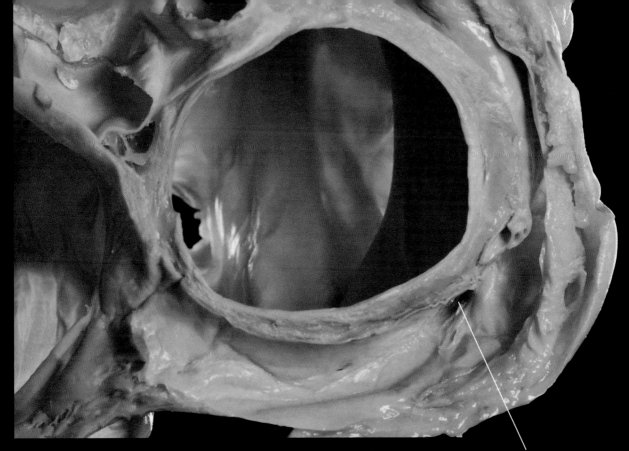

**Orifice of the oblique vein of the left atrium
(Vein of Marshall)**

atrium, also referred to as the vein of Marshall,[17] appears at the nadir of the attachment of the Vieussens' valve. The warfarin (Coumadin) ridge is observed between the left pulmonary veins and the orifice of the left arial appendage.[18] Epicardial side of the warfarin ridge, the fold between the left pulmonary veins and left atrial appendage, is the route for the vein of Marshall or persistent left superior vena cava draining into the coronary sinus.

References

1. McAlpine WA. Digitized collection of all the images created by Dr. McAlpine at UCLA. Copyright UCLA Cardiac Arrhythmia Center. Part of this collection appeared in *Heart and Coronary Arteries: An Anatomical Atlas for Clinical Diagnosis, Radiological Investigation, and Surgical Treatment.* New York: Springer-Verlag; 1975.

2. Zawadzki M, Pietrasik A, Pietrasik K, et al. Endoscopic study of the morphology of Vieussens' valve. *Clin Anat.* 2004;17:318–321.

3. Spencer JH, Sundaram CC, Iaizzo PA. The relative anatomy of the coronary arterial and venous systems: implications for coronary interventions. *Clin Anat.* 2014;27:1023–1029.

4. Choure AJ, Garcia MJ, Hesse B, et al. In vivo analysis of the anatomical relationship of coronary sinus to mitral annulus and left circumflex coronary artery using cardiac multidetector computed tomography: Implications for percutaneous coronary sinus mitral annuloplasty. *J Am Coll Cardiol.* 2006;48:1938–1945.

5. Noheria A, DeSimone CV, Lachman N, et al. Anatomy of the coronary sinus and epicardial coronary venous system in 620 hearts: An electrophysiology perspective. *J Cardiovasc Electrophysiol.* 2013;24:1–6.

6. Jongbloed MR, Lamb HJ, Bax JJ, et al. Noninvasive visualization of the cardiac venous system using multislice computed tomography. *J Am Coll Cardiol.* 2005;45:749–753.

7. Saremi F, Muresian H, Sánchez-Quintana D. Coronary veins: Comprehensive CT-anatomic classification and review of variants and clinical implications. *Radiographics.* 2012;32:E1–32.

8. Komatsu Y, Nogami A, Shinoda Y, et al. Idiopathic ventricular arrhythmias originating from the vicinity of the communicating vein of cardiac venous systems at the left ventricular summit. *Circ Arrhythm Electrophysiol.* 2018;11:e005386.

9. Bradfield JS. Redefining optimal targets for intramural ventricular arrhythmias: Planning for combat! *JACC Clin Electrophysiol.* 2020;6:1349–1352.

10. Briceño DF, Enriquez A, Liang JJ, et al. Septal coronary venous mapping to guide substrate characterization and ablation of intramural septal ventricular arrhythmia. *JACC Clin Electrophysiol.* 2019;5:789–800.

11. Tavares L, Fuentes S, Lador A, et al. Venous anatomy of the left ventricular summit: Therapeutic implications for ethanol infusion. *Heart Rhythm.* 2021;18:1557–1565.

12. Yokokawa M, Good E, Chugh A, et al. Intramural idiopathic ventricular arrhythmias originating in the intraventricular septum: Mapping and ablation. *Circ Arrhythm Electrophysiol.* 2012;5:258–263.

13. Kreidieh B, Rodríguez-Mañero M, Schurmann P, et al. Retrograde coronary venous ethanol infusion for ablation of refractory ventricular tachycardia. *Circ Arrhythm Electrophysiol.* 2016;9:e004352.

14. Ansari A. Anatomy and clinical significance of ventricular Thebesian veins. *Clin Anat.* 2001;14:102–110.

15. Weng S, Tang M, Zhou B, et al. Supraventricular tachycardia in patients with coronary sinus stenosis/atresia: Prevalence, anatomical features, and ablation outcomes. *J Cardiovasc Electrophysiol.* 2020;31:3223–3231.

16. Hołda MK, Klimek-Piotrowska W, Koziej M, et al. Anatomical variations of the coronary sinus valve (Thebesian valve): Implications for electrocardiological procedures. *Europace.* 2015;17:921–927.

17. Marshall J. On the development of the great anterior veins in man and mammalia: Including an account of certain remnants of foetal structure found in the adult, a comparative view of these great veins in the different mammalia, and an analysis of their occasional peculiarities in the human subject. *Phil Trans R Soc Lond.* 1850;140:133–169.

18. Piątek-Koziej K, Hołda J, Tyrak K, et al. Anatomy of the left atrial ridge (coumadin ridge) and possible clinical implications for cardiovascular imaging and invasive procedures. *J Cardiovasc Electrophysiol.* 2020;31:220–226.

23

Pericardial Space

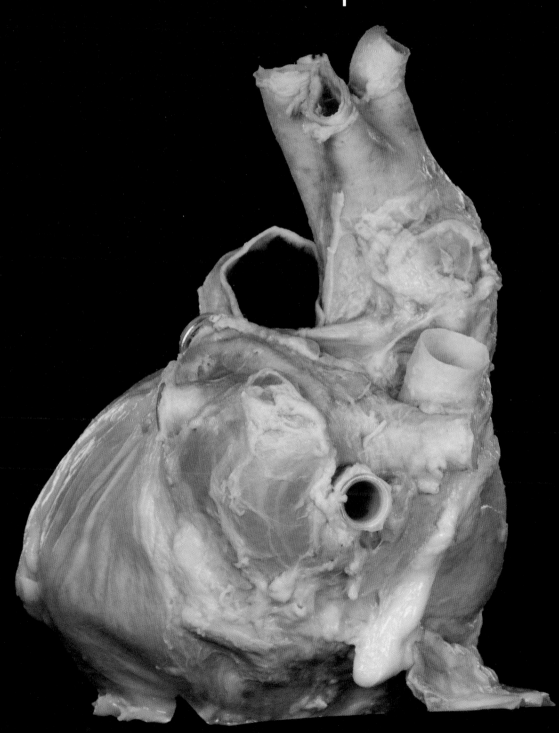

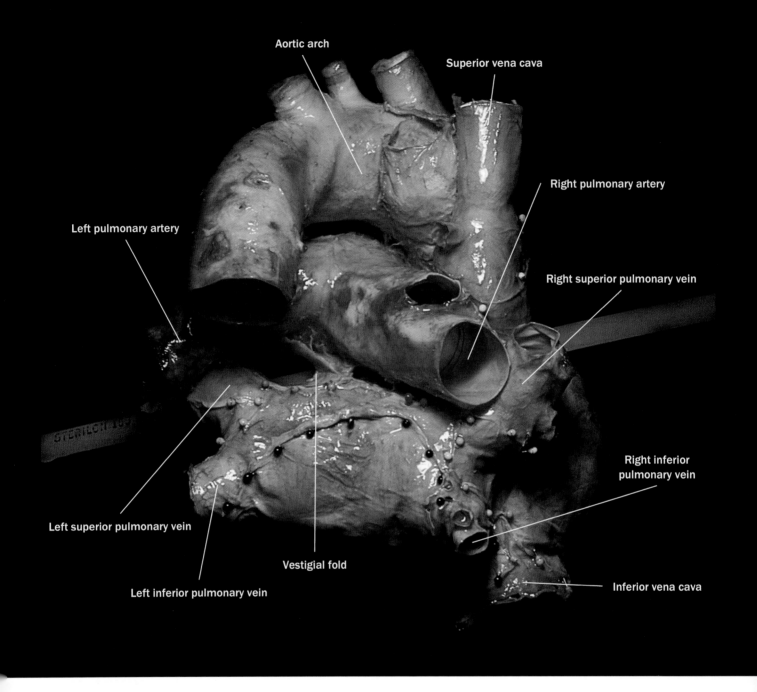

Figure 156   The posterior hilum of the heart.[1]

The heart is viewed from the postero-superior direction. The bar passes through the transverse sinus. The posterior hilum of the heart, mainly located at the pulmonary venous component of the left atrium (left atrial dome/roof), is the venous pole of the heart. It is surrounded by the pericardial reflection around the pulmonary veins and both superior and inferior vena cavae. Compared to the superior hilum, which is the arterial pole of the heart around the arterial trunks, the posterior

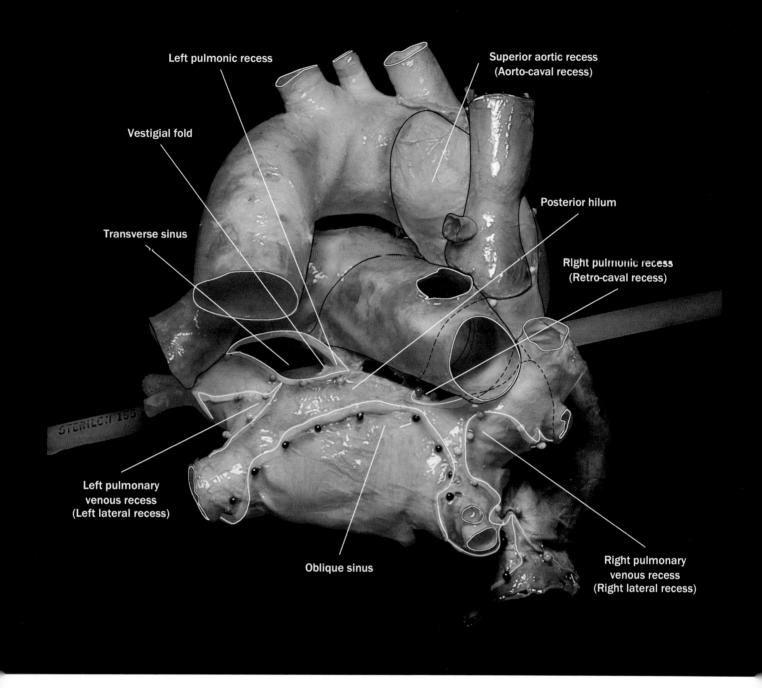

Left pulmonic recess

Vestigial fold

Transverse sinus

Superior aortic recess
(Aorto-caval recess)

Posterior hilum

Right pulmonic recess
(Retro-caval recess)

Left pulmonary
venous recess
(Left lateral recess)

Oblique sinus

Right pulmonary
venous recess
(Right lateral recess)

hilum has more complicated shape due to the multiple recesses and oblique sinus.[2] The posterior hilum is directly adjacent to the mediastinal space. Both hila of the heart work as the entrances/exits for the extracardiac nerves and vessels. Refer to Figure 163.

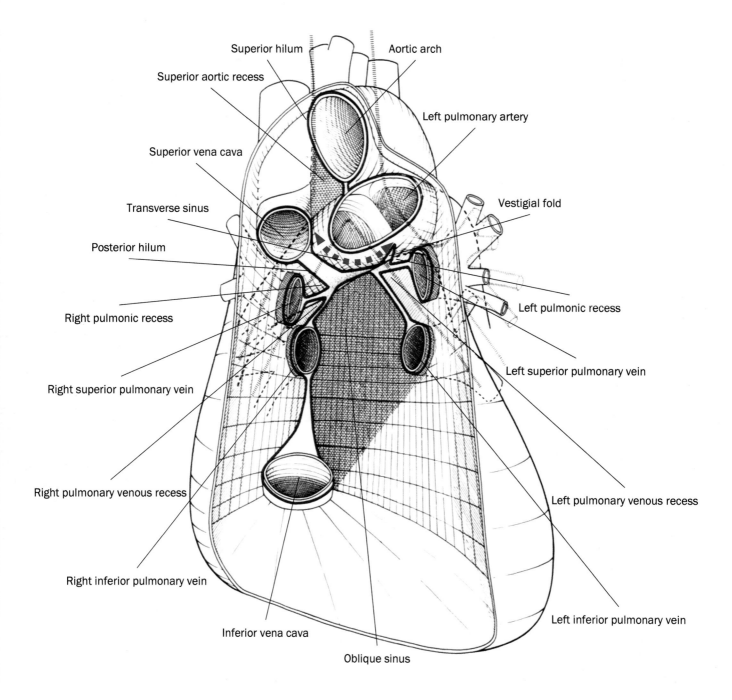

Figure 157 The illustration showing the pericardial reflections and hilum of the heart.[1]

The heart is viewed from the anterior (left) and posterior (right) directions. The superior and posterior hila (areas surrounded by thick lines in the left image) involve arterial and venous poles, respectively. The shape of the posterior hilum is complicated and variable due to the recesses, deep oblique sinus, and vestigial fold.[3] The posterior hilum is close to the

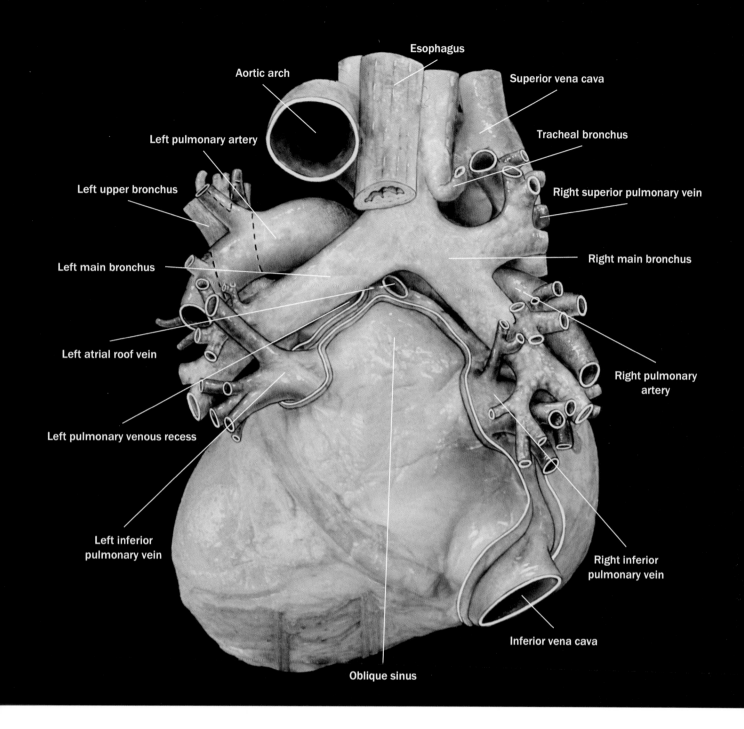

Esophagus

Aortic arch

Superior vena cava

Left pulmonary artery

Tracheal bronchus

Left upper bronchus

Right superior pulmonary vein

Left main bronchus

Right main bronchus

Left atrial roof vein

Right pulmonary artery

Left pulmonary venous recess

Left inferior pulmonary vein

Right inferior pulmonary vein

Inferior vena cava

Oblique sinus

pulmonary bifurcation, right pulmonary artery, tracheal carina, and bronchus. The entrance of the oblique sinus opens in oblique fashion between the inferior vena cava and the left inferior pulmonary vein. The transverse sinus is located between the superior hilum and posterior hilum of the heart.

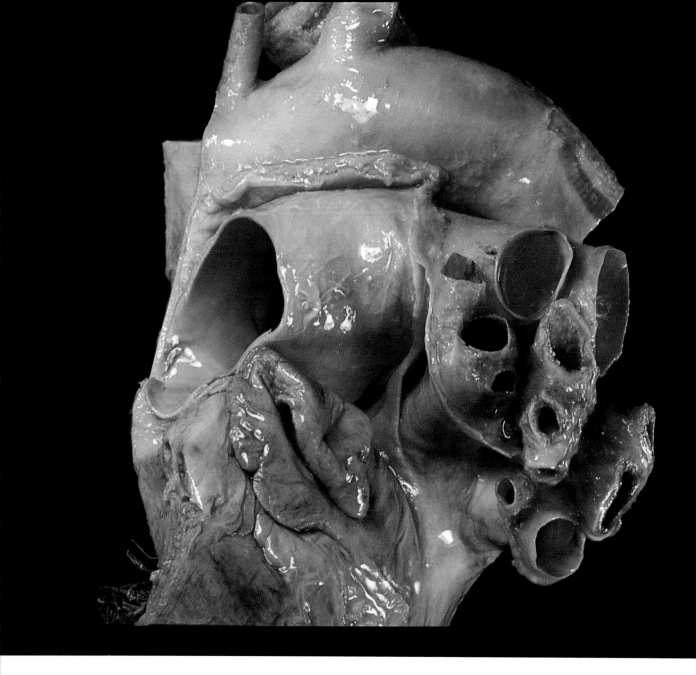

Figure 158 The left lateral view showing the transverse sinus and vestigial fold.[1] ▭▬ Anaglyph 18.

The heart is viewed from the left lateral direction. The vestigial fold is sandwiched by the anteriorly located transverse sinus and the posteriorly located left pulmonic recess. In contrast to the transverse sinus, the left pulmonic recess and the left pulmonary venous recess are the blind-end.

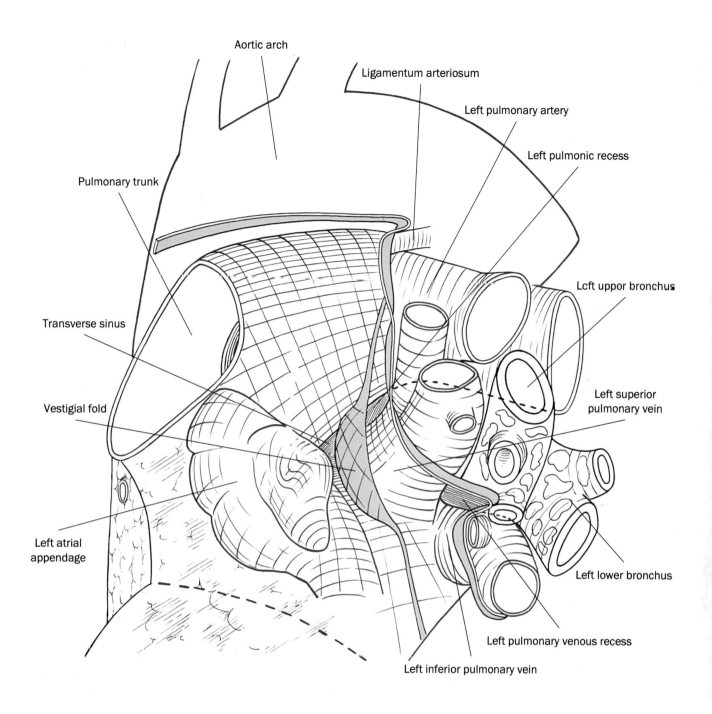

Aortic arch

Ligamentum arteriosum

Left pulmonary artery

Left pulmonic recess

Pulmonary trunk

Left upper bronchus

Transverse sinus

Left superior
pulmonary vein

Vestigial fold

Left atrial
appendage

Left lower bronchus

Left pulmonary venous recess

Left inferior pulmonary vein

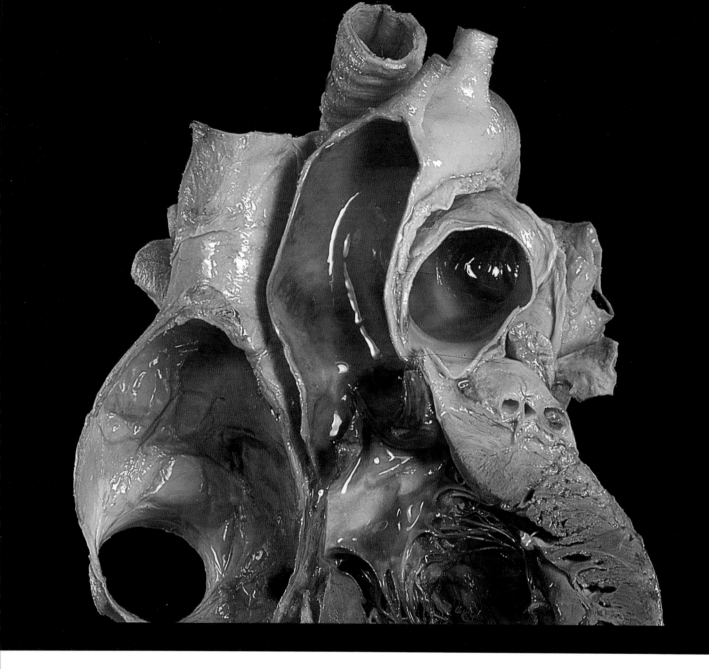

Figure 159   The frontal section showing the structural anatomy anterior to the transverse sinus.[1]

The heart is viewed from the anterior direction. The arrow in the right image indicates the transverse sinus. The transverse sinus is located posterior to the arterial trunks. The lateral entrances are guarded by bilateral atrial appendages. The transverse sinus has deep superior and inferior extension right posterior to the aortic root. They are referred to as the superior and

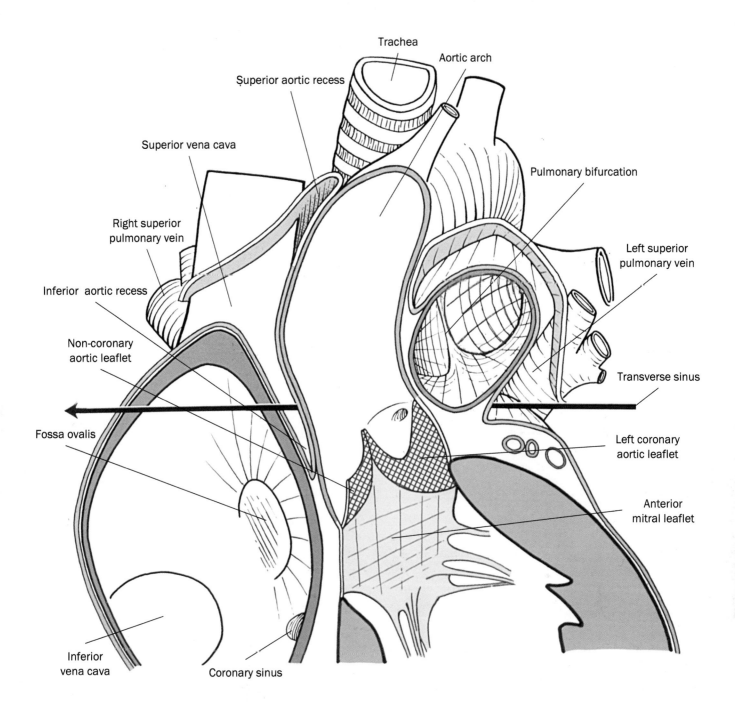

Trachea

Aortic arch

Superior aortic recess

Superior vena cava

Pulmonary bifurcation

Right superior
pulmonary vein

Left superior
pulmonary vein

Inferior aortic recess

Non-coronary
aortic leaflet

Transverse sinus

Fossa ovalis

Left coronary
aortic leaflet

Anterior
mitral leaflet

Inferior
vena cava

Coronary sinus

inferior aortic recesses, respectively. The inferior aortic recess extends close to the nadir of the non-coronary aortic sinus. The superior aortic recess extends to the aortic arch. The superior aortic recess is also referred to as the aorto-caval recess.

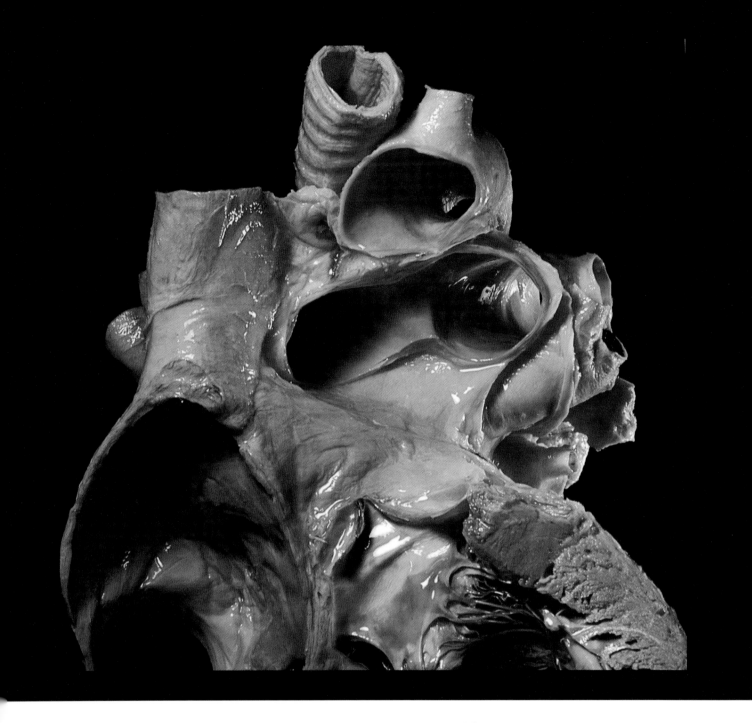

Figure 160 The frontal section showing the transverse sinus and vestigial fold.[1]

The heart in Figure 159 is further dissected by removing arterial trunks and viewed from the anterior direction. The vestigial fold is sandwiched between the anteriorly located transverse sinus and the posteriorly located left pulmonic recess.

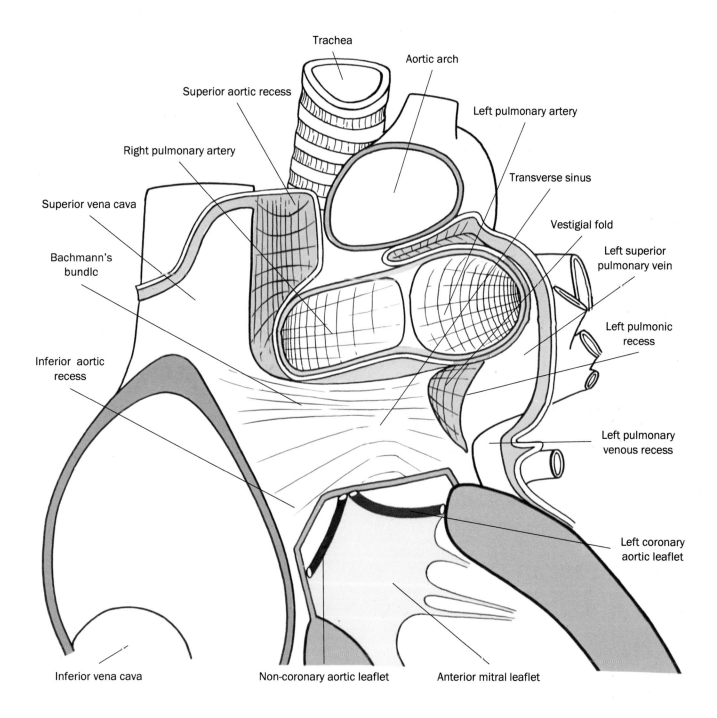

Trachea

Aortic arch

Superior aortic recess

Left pulmonary artery

Right pulmonary artery

Transverse sinus

Superior vena cava

Vestigial fold

Bachmann's bundlc

Left superior pulmonary vein

Inferior aortic recess

Left pulmonic recess

Left pulmonary venous recess

Left coronary aortic leaflet

Inferior vena cava

Non-coronary aortic leaflet

Anterior mitral leaflet

The transverse sinus is located inferior to the pulmonic bifurcation, anterior to the left atrial anterior wall, posterior to the arterial trunks.

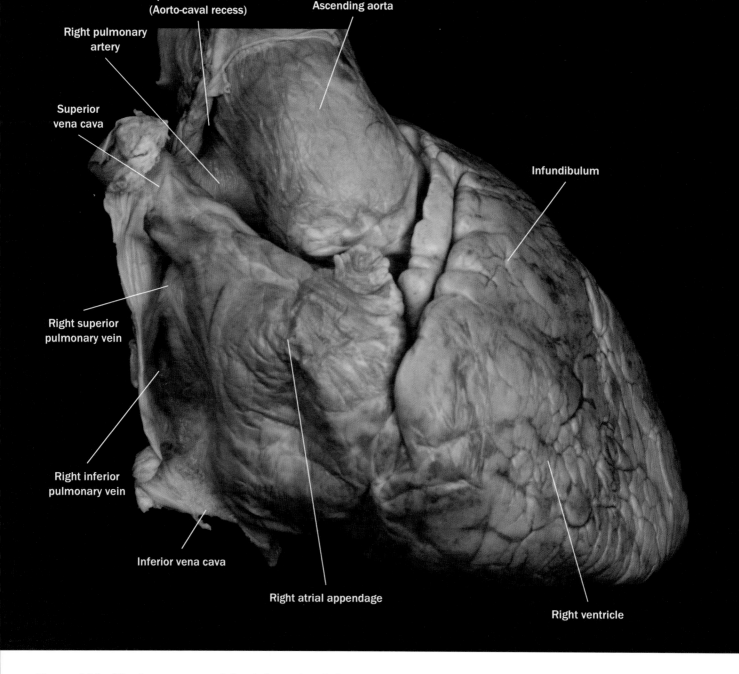

(Aorto-caval recess)
Ascending aorta
Right pulmonary
artery
Superior
vena cava
Infundibulum
Right superior
pulmonary vein
Right inferior
pulmonary vein
Inferior vena cava
Right atrial appendage
Right ventricle

Figure 161   The inner aspect of the right pericardial recesses.

Perfused fixed heart with the remained posterior pericardium shows the right lateral aspects of the entrance/exit of the pericardial recesses and sinuses. In contrast to the transverse sinus, the right pulmonic recess and right pulmonary venous recess are generally blind-ended without communication with the transverse or oblique sinuses.

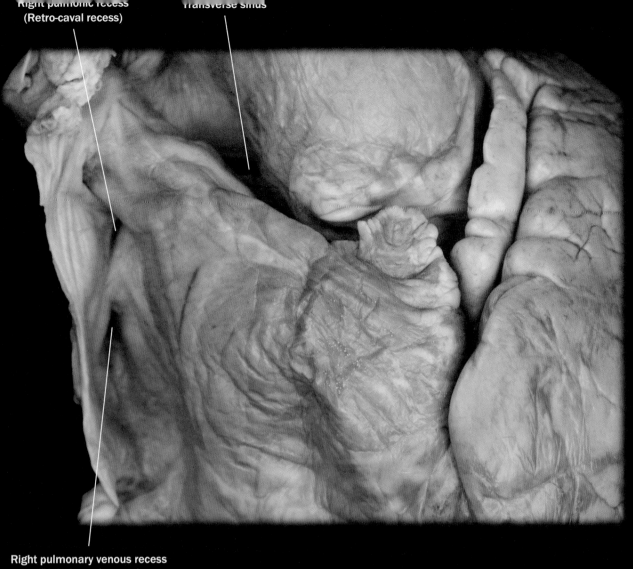

Right pulmonic recess
(Retro-caval recess)

Transverse sinus

Right pulmonary venous recess
(Right lateral recess)

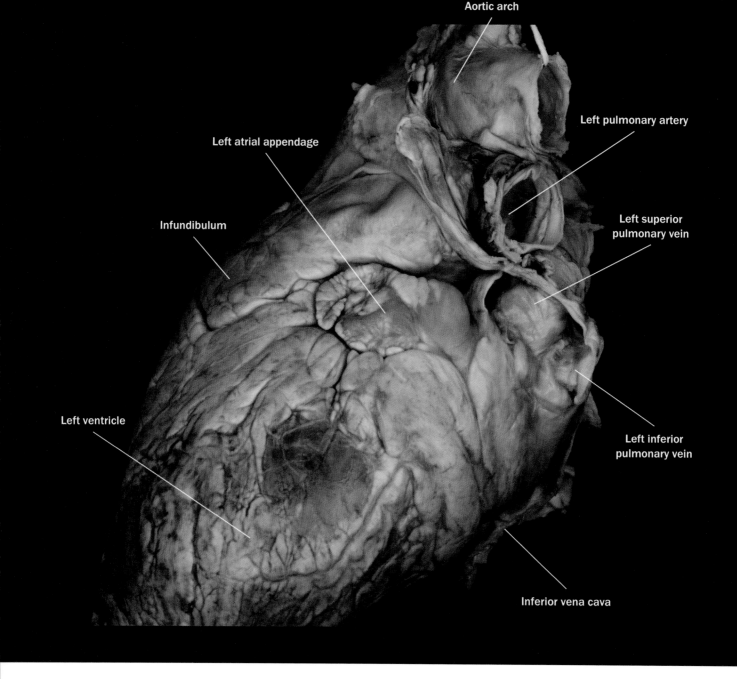

Figure 162 The inner aspect of the left pericardial recesses.

Perfused fixed heart with the remained posterior pericardium shows the left lateral aspects of the entrance/exit of the pericardial recesses and sinuses. In contrast to the transverse sinus, the left pulmonic recess and left pulmonary venous recess

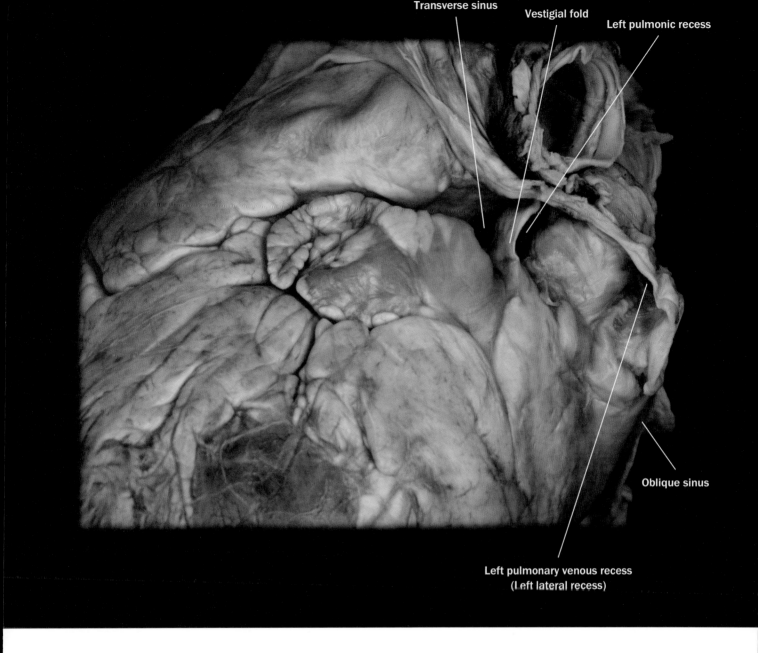

Transverse sinus

Vestigial fold

Left pulmonic recess

Oblique sinus

Left pulmonary venous recess
(Left lateral recess)

are generally blind-ended. The left pulmonic recess is located posterior to the vestigial fold, separated from the anteriorly located transverse sinus.

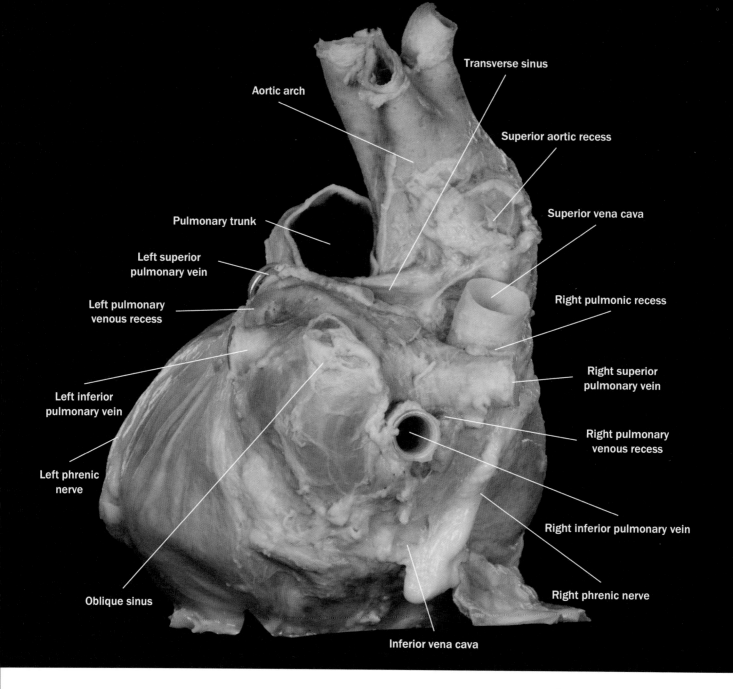

Figure 163 The outer aspect of the pericardial recesses, sinuses, and hila of the heart. [icon] Anaglyphs 19 and 20.

The heart is dissected with the pericardium remaining intact. The pericardial space is replaced with blue-colored agar. The heart is viewed from the posterior (left) and right postero-superior (right) directions, respectively. The red and blue strings mark the pericardial reflections of the superior (arterial) hilum and posterior (venous) hilum, respectively. The superior hilum encircles the ascending aorta and pulmonary trunk. The posterior hilum encircles pulmonary and both superior and inferior vena cavae. Both of the hila are separated by the transverse sinus.[2] Both of the hila serve as the exclusive entrances/

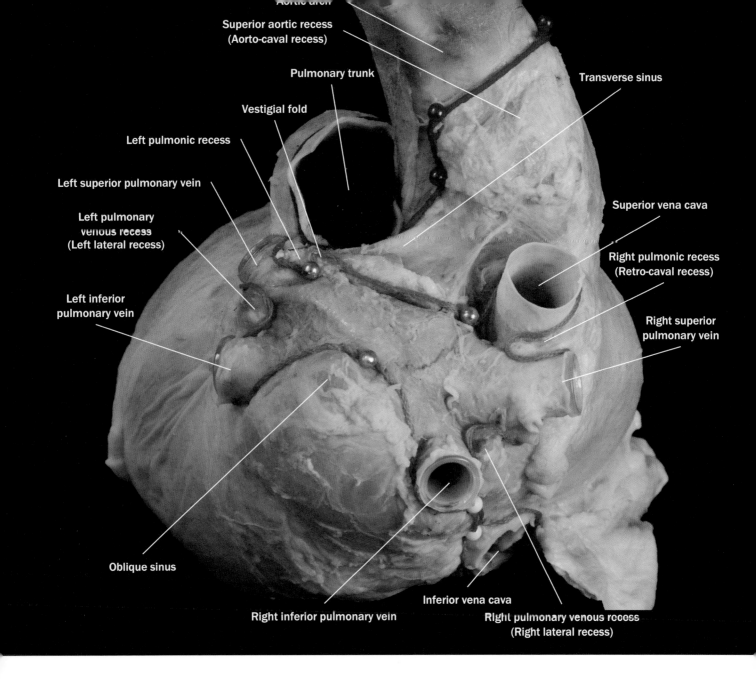

Aortic arch

Superior aortic recess
(Aorto-caval recess)

Pulmonary trunk

Transverse sinus

Vestigial fold

Left pulmonic recess

Left superior pulmonary vein

Superior vena cava

Left pulmonary
venous recess
(Left lateral recess)

Right pulmonic recess
(Retro-caval recess)

Left inferior
pulmonary vein

Right superior
pulmonary vein

Oblique sinus

Inferior vena cava

Right inferior pulmonary vein

Right pulmonary venous recess
(Right lateral recess)

exits for the extracardiac nerves and vessels. The pulmonary venous component of the left atrium, corresponding to the left atrial dome/roof is the exact location of the posterior hilum directly facing to the mediastinum. The distance between the transverse and oblique sinuses, corresponding to the width of the posterior hilum is 18.5 mm in this particular heart, which is variable.[3]

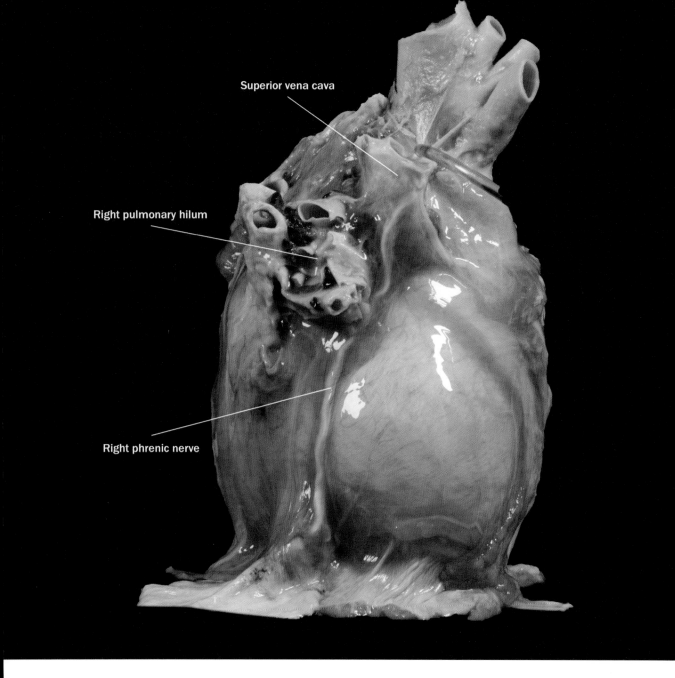

Superior vena cava

Right pulmonary hilum

Right phrenic nerve

Figure 164   The phrenic nerve.

The heart with intact pericardium is viewed from the right lateral (left), and left lateral (right) directions. Fluid fills the pericardial space. Both phrenic nerves typically arise from the C4 cervical root, then descend on the anterior scalenus muscle, which is located anterior to the subclavian artery. Then, it descends behind the clavicula to enter the thoracic cavity, and continues descending between the pericardium and parietal pleura to reach the diaphragm. Both phrenic nerves are identically located anterior to both pulmonary hila.[4] In contrast, both vagus nerves are identically located posterior to the

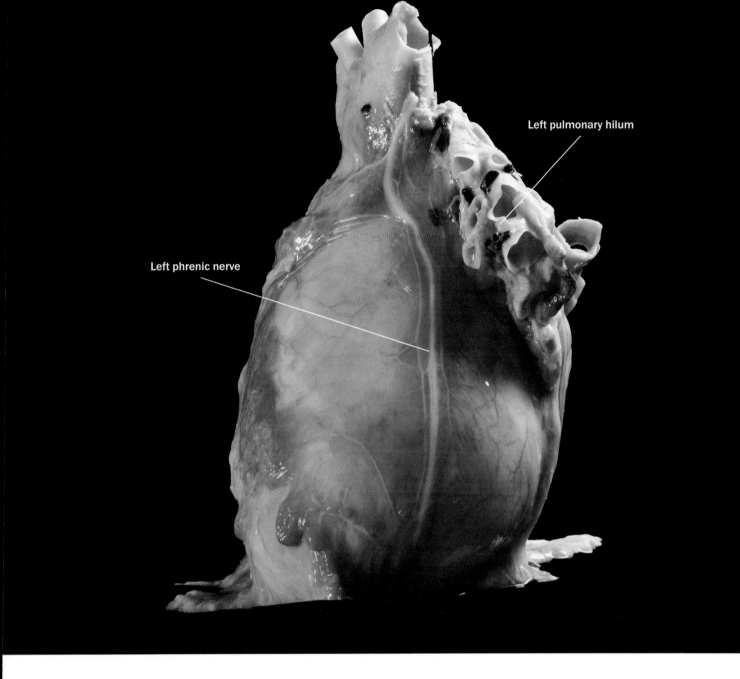

Left pulmonary hilum

Left phrenic nerve

both pulmonary hila. The right phrenic nerve is commonly related to the postero-lateral portion of sinus venarum and anterior portion of right pulmonary veins. The left phrenic nerve is commonly related to the left atrial appendage and basal-mid left ventricular lateral wall.[5] However, this spatial relationship is affected by the variation in the size and rotation of individual hearts within the pericardium. Note the closer relationship the right pulmonary hilum and right phrenic nerve have in this heart compared to the left side.

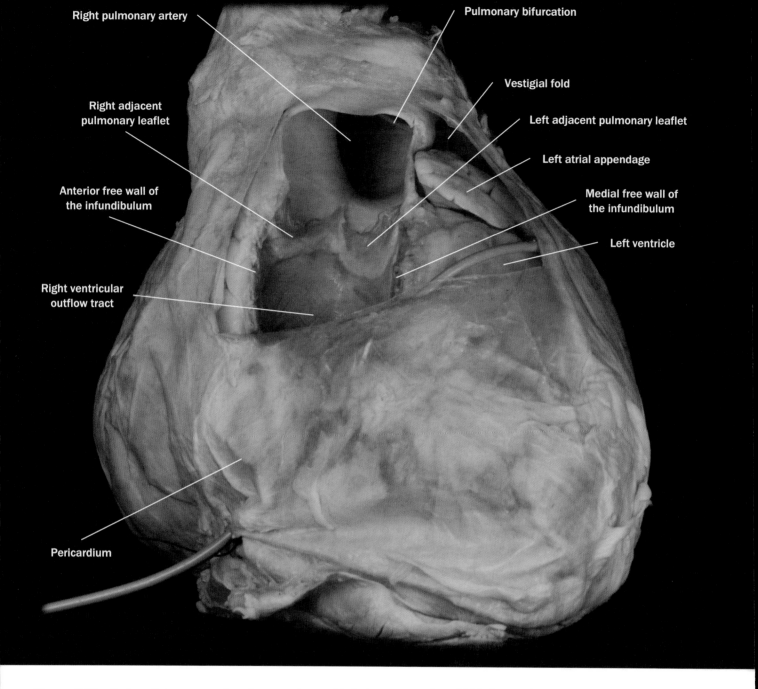

Right pulmonary artery

Pulmonary bifurcation

Vestigial fold

Right adjacent
pulmonary leaflet

Left adjacent pulmonary leaflet

Left atrial appendage

Anterior free wall of
the infundibulum

Medial free wall of
the infundibulum

Left ventricle

Right ventricular
outflow tract

Pericardium

Figure 165   Epicardial access using the anterior and inferior approaches. ⬜🔴 Anaglyph 21.

The hearts are viewed from the left anterior oblique direction. Epicardial access using the anterior (left) and inferior (right) approaches are replicated.[6,7] The pericardial window is created to show the infundibulum, pulmonary root, and left atrial appendage. Anterior and medial free wall of the infundibulum is partially removed in part, as well as the corresponding

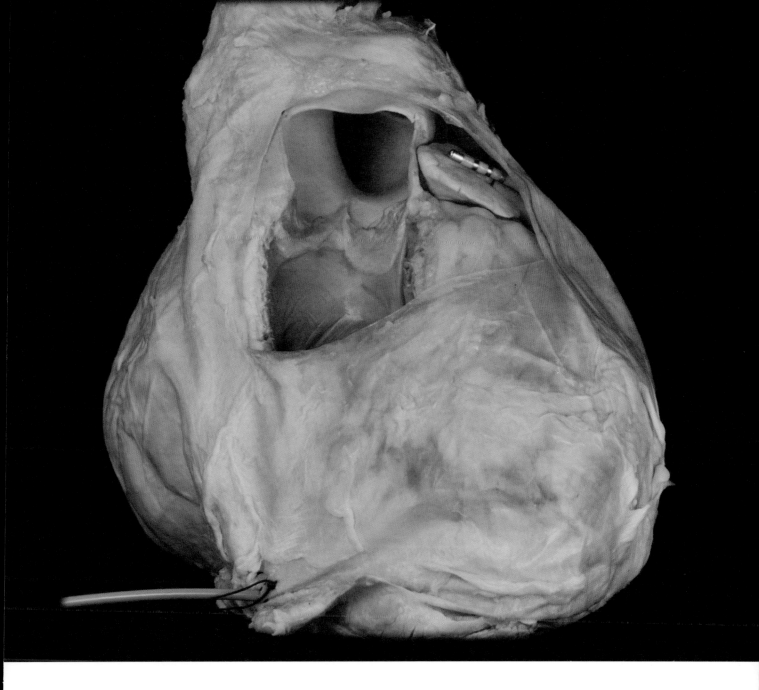

left anterior part of the pulmonary root involving the non-adjacent pulmonary sinus. In the anterior approach (left), note the catheter takes a sigmoid shape. In the inferior approach (right), the tip of the catheter is placed on the left atrial appendage after passing around the inferior and infero-lateral region of the left ventricle.

References

1. McAlpine WA. Digitized collection of all the images created by Dr. McAlpine at UCLA. Copyright UCLA Cardiac Arrhythmia Center. Part of this collection appeared in *Heart and Coronary Arteries: An Anatomical Atlas for Clinical Diagnosis, Radiological Investigation, and Surgical Treatment.* New York: Springer-Verlag; 1975.

2. Mori S, Hanna P, Dacey MJ, et al. Comprehensive anatomy of the pericardial space and the cardiac hilum: Anatomical dissections with Intact pericardium. *JACC Cardiovasc Imaging.* 2021. DOI: 10.1016/j.jcmg.2021.04.016. Online ahead of print.

3. Chaffanjon P, Brichon PY, Faure C, et al. Pericardial reflection around the venous aspect of the heart. *Surg Radiol Anat.* 1997;19:17–21.

4. Rodriguez ER, Tan CD. Structure and anatomy of the human pericardium. *Prog Cardiovasc Dis.* 2017;59:327–340.

5. Wang YJ, Liu L, Zhang MC, et al. Imaging of pericardiophrenic bundles using multislice spiral computed tomography for phrenic nerve anatomy. *J Cardiovasc Electrophysiol.* 2016;27:961–971.

6. Fukuzawa K, Nagamatsu Y, Mori S, et al. Percutaneous Pericardiocentesis With the Anterior Approach: Demonstration of the Precise Course With Computed Tomography. JACC Clin Electrophysiol. 2019;5:730-741.

7. Mori S, Bradfield JS, Peacock WJ, et al. Living Anatomy of the Pericardial Space: A Guide for Imaging and Interventions. *JACC Clin Electrophysiol.* 2021;7:1628-1644.

24

Cardiac Innervation

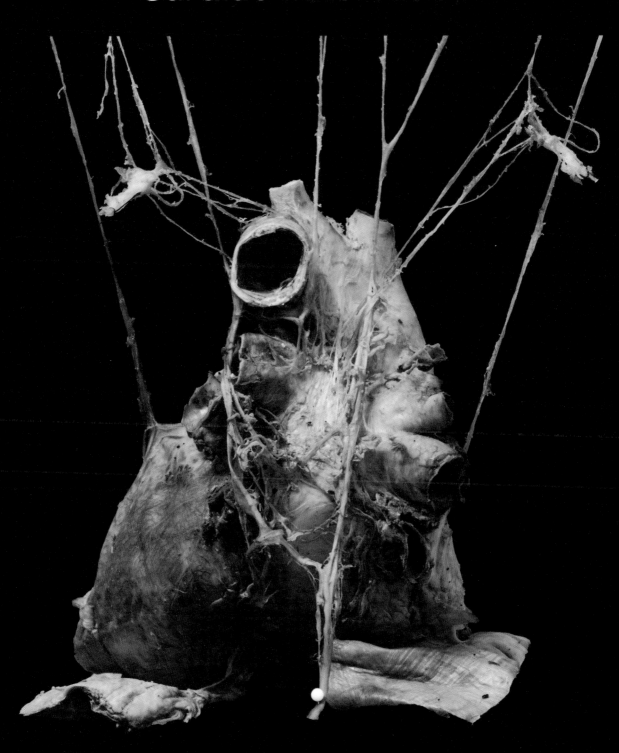

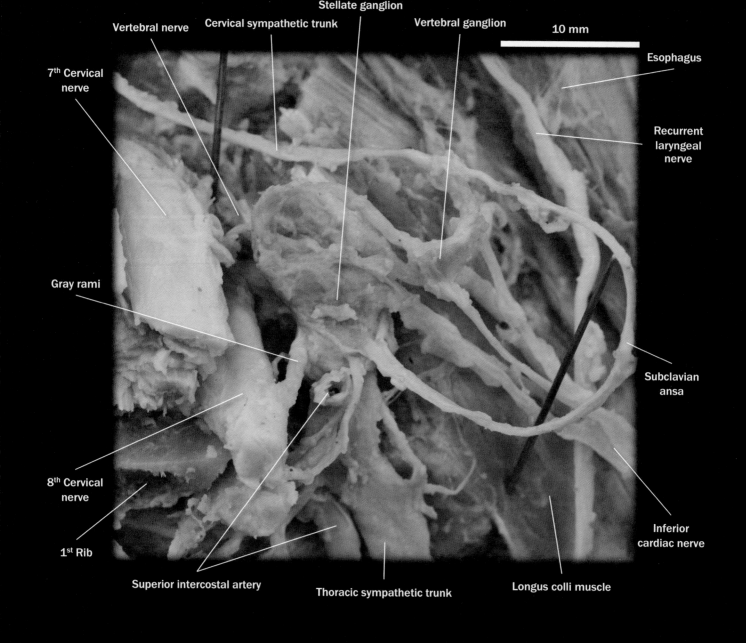

Stellate ganglion

Vertebral nerve   Cervical sympathetic trunk   Vertebral ganglion   10 mm

Esophagus

7th Cervical nerve

Recurrent laryngeal nerve

Gray rami

Subclavian ansa

8th Cervical nerve

Inferior cardiac nerve

1st Rib

Superior intercostal artery

Thoracic sympathetic trunk   Longus colli muscle

Figure 166   The stellate ganglia. Anaglyphs 22 and 23.

The right (left) and left (right) stellate ganglia are dissected focusing on their superior halves, referred to as the inferior cervical ganglion. In the left image, the pleura and subclavian artery are removed to show the inferior half of the stellate ganglion, corresponding to the Th1 ganglion, and the continuing thoracic sympathetic trunk. The subclavian ansa, also referred to as the Vieussens' ansa/loop,[1] as well as vertebral ganglion can be observed. In the right image, the pleura and subclavian artery is preserved. The pleura is transilluminated by the light source placed within the pleural cavity. The

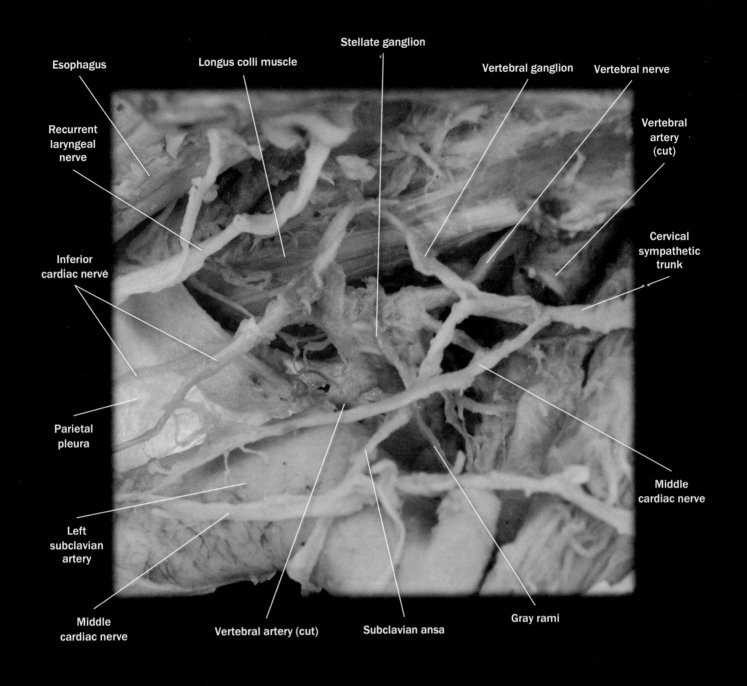

Esophagus

Recurrent
laryngeal
nerve

Inferior
cardiac nerve

Parietal
pleura

Left
subclavian
artery

Middle
cardiac nerve

Longus colli muscle

Stellate ganglion

Vertebral ganglion   Vertebral nerve

Vertebral
artery
(cut)

Cervical
sympathetic
trunk

Middle
cardiac nerve

Vertebral artery (cut)   Subclavian ansa   Gray rami

stellate ganglion is located on the apex of the pleura outside the pleural cavity. The superior half of the stellate ganglion, the inferior cervical ganglion, is located in front of the first rib close to its costotransverse joint. The inferior cervical ganglion gives rise to many branches like a star,[2] combined with the middle cervical and vertebral ganglia. Those branches include the subclavian ansa,[1] multiple middle and inferior cardiac nerves,[3] gray rami to the brachial plexus,[4] and vertebral nerves.[5] The size and shape of the stellate ganglion are variable.[6]

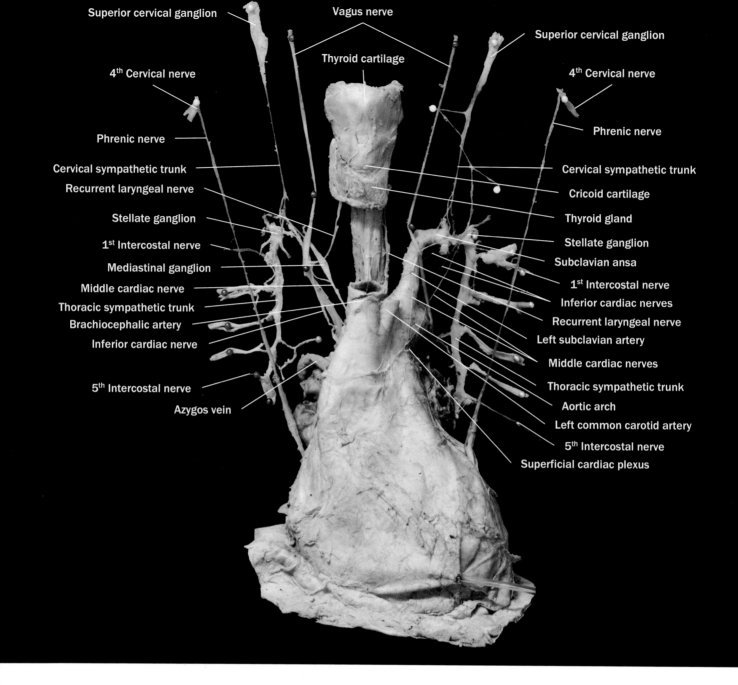

Superior cervical ganglion

Vagus nerve

Superior cervical ganglion

Thyroid cartilage

4th Cervical nerve

4th Cervical nerve

Phrenic nerve

Phrenic nerve

Cervical sympathetic trunk

Cervical sympathetic trunk

Recurrent laryngeal nerve

Cricoid cartilage

Stellate ganglion

Thyroid gland

1st Intercostal nerve

Stellate ganglion

Mediastinal ganglion

Subclavian ansa

Middle cardiac nerve

1st Intercostal nerve

Thoracic sympathetic trunk

Inferior cardiac nerves

Brachiocephalic artery

Recurrent laryngeal nerve

Inferior cardiac nerve

Left subclavian artery

Middle cardiac nerves

5th Intercostal nerve

Thoracic sympathetic trunk

Azygos vein

Aortic arch

Left common carotid artery

5th Intercostal nerve

Superficial cardiac plexus

Figure 167 The anterior view of cardiac innervation. [glasses icon] Anaglyph 24.

Bilateral vagus nerves, sympathetic trunks, and phrenic nerves are isolated with the heart, esophagus, trachea, bronchi, thyroid/cricoid cartilages, and thyroid gland. The part of the trachea is removed to show the esophagus behind. The pericardium is kept intact.[7]

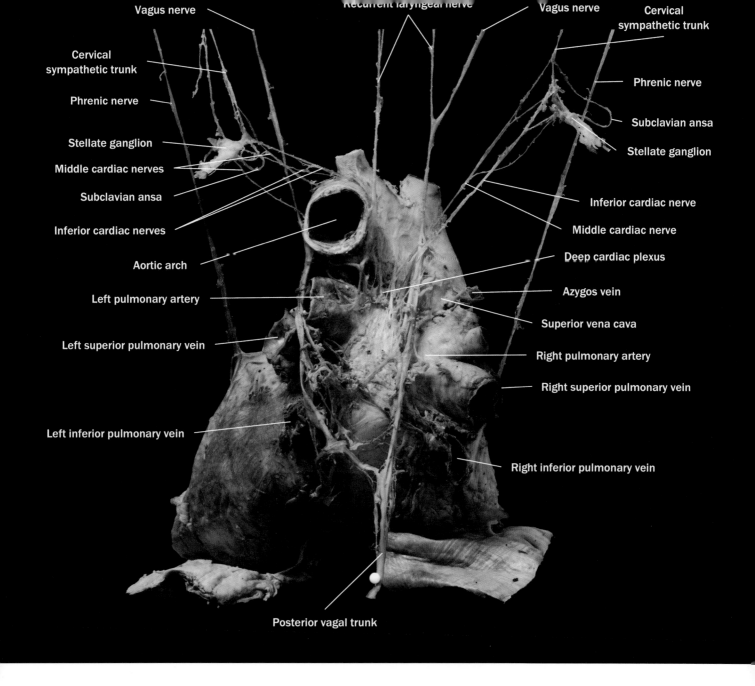

Vagus nerve

Recurrent laryngeal nerve

Vagus nerve

Cervical sympathetic trunk

Cervical sympathetic trunk

Phrenic nerve

Phrenic nerve

Subclavian ansa

Stellate ganglion

Stellate ganglion

Middle cardiac nerves

Subclavian ansa

Inferior cardiac nerve

Inferior cardiac nerves

Middle cardiac nerve

Aortic arch

Deep cardiac plexus

Left pulmonary artery

Azygos vein

Superior vena cava

Left superior pulmonary vein

Right pulmonary artery

Right superior pulmonary vein

Left inferior pulmonary vein

Right inferior pulmonary vein

Posterior vagal trunk

Figure 168 The posterior view of cardiac sympathetic innervation. Anaglyph 25.

Bilateral vagus nerves, stellate ganglia, and phrenic nerves are isolated with the heart. The esophagus, trachea, bronchi, thyroid/cricoid cartilages, and thyroid gland in the Figure 167 are removed. The deep cardiac plexus behind the aortic arch and pulmonary bifurcation is shown. The pericardium is kept intact.[7]

References

1. Loukas M, Zhan XL, Tubbs RS, et al. The ansa subclavia: A review of the literature. *Folia Morphol (Warsz).* 2008;67:166–170.

2. Janes RD, Brandys JC, Hopkins DA, et al. Anatomy of human extrinsic cardiac nerves and ganglia. *Am J Cardiol.* 1986;57:299–309.

3. Kawashima T. The autonomic nervous system of the human heart with special reference to its origin, course, and peripheral distribution. *Anat Embryol (Berl).* 2005;209:425–438.

4. Kuntz A. Distribution of the sympathetic rami to the brachial plexus: Its relation to sympathectomy affecting the upper extremity. *Arch Surg.* 1927;15:871–877.

5. Tubbs RS, Loukas M, Remy AC, et al. The vertebral nerve revisited. *Clin Anat.* 2007;20:644–647.

6. Marcer N, Bergmann M, Klie A, et al. An anatomical investigation of the cervicothoracic ganglion. *Clin Anat.* 2012;25:444–451.

7. Mori S, Hanna P, Dacey MJ, et al. Comprehensive anatomy of the pericardial space and the cardiac hilum: Anatomical dissections with Intact pericardium. *JACC Cardiovasc Imaging.* 2021. DOI: 10.1016/j.jcmg.2021.04.016. Online ahead of print.

APPENDIX OF REPRESENTATIVE FIGURES

Figures for terms may appear more than once in this book. In this appendix, the figures noted are the most representative of the term listed.